10 50

RESPIRATION

IN HEALTH AND DISEASE

By

R. M. CHERNIACK, M.D., M.Sc., F.R.C.P.(C.)

*Assistant Professor of Medicine, University of Manitoba School of Medicine;
Director, Respiratory Division, Clinical Investigation Unit, and Assistant Physician, Winnipeg General Hospital; Consultant in Respiratory Diseases to Children's Hospital and Municipal Hospitals, Winnipeg, Canada*

L. CHERNIACK, M.D., B.Sc., M.R.C.P.(Lond.), F.R.C.P.(C.), F.A.C.P.

*Assistant Professor of Medicine, University of Manitoba School of Medicine;
Associate Physician, Winnipeg General Hospital; Physician, Division of Medicine, Winnipeg Clinic, Winnipeg, Canada*

Illustrated by

NANCY JOY, A.O.C.A.

*Assistant Professor of Medical Illustration, University of Manitoba School of Medicine,
Winnipeg, Canada*

W. B. SAUNDERS COMPANY

Philadelphia   *London*

TO

PROFESSOR JOSEPH DOUPE

OUR SEVEREST CRITIC

FOREWORD

THE TITLE of this book, *Respiration in Health and Disease,* suggests at once that the authors have a fresh and unconventional approach to the understanding of respiratory disorders. This impression is confirmed by a glance at the Table of Contents. The book is divided into four sections. The first section is entitled "Basic Considerations" and offers a concise presentation of the newest concepts of respiratory physiology and anatomy, together with those biochemical principles which are applicable to respiration and its disorders. This section lays a firm foundation of basic knowledge upon which the authors later develop their ideas about the mechanisms of respiratory disease. The second section deals with "The Manifestations of Respiratory Disease," and here we find an excellent account of the signs and symptoms of pulmonary disorders interpreted in terms of applied physiology and structural change. In the third section the authors have extended their concepts to more particular areas, such as bronchial disease, pulmonary parenchymal disease, etc., emphasizing the mechanisms rather than the morbid anatomy of specific respiratory diseases. The final section of the book outlines in some detail the clinical, radiological, functional, bacteriological and pathological assessment of respiratory disease. This section is an excellent summing-up of the many facets of any respiratory disease which must be studied in order to make a comprehensive appraisal of pulmonary dysfunction.

Throughout the text, the various steps which lead to a clear understanding of respiration in health and disease are illustrated by a series of diagrams and line drawings by Miss Nancy Joy. These illustrations serve to interpret the authors' ideas with remarkable clarity and simplicity.

The authors of this book are brothers, and both are admirably equipped for their joint authorship. Dr. Louis Cherniack has had a long and varied experience in the clinical aspects of chest disease; Dr. Reuben Cherniack, in addition to clinical experience, has had intensive training in respiratory investigation and has made many significant contributions in that field. Together, they have combined their special skills and knowledge to produce a stimulating and readable book which follows the important modern trend toward analyzing the actual mechanisms of diseases, rather than merely describing them. Because of this fresh and logical approach, *Respiration in Health and Disease* should help to fill the gap between the technical treatises on pulmonary physiology, on the one hand, and the purely descriptive text books on respiratory diseases on the other.

LENNOX G. BELL
M.B.E., M.D., F.R.C.P. (LOND.), F.R.C.P.(C.)

Dean, Faculty of Medicine, University of Manitoba; Professor and Head of the Department of Medicine, University of Manitoba; Physician-in-Chief, Winnipeg General Hospital, Winnipeg, Canada

PREFACE

SINCE the days of Laennec, physicians have appreciated the necessity for a correlation between the clinical findings and the underlying pathological respiratory process. The classic approach of the clinician towards a patient who is suffering from respiratory disease has therefore been based on the determination of the morphology of the disease process by means of a thorough and systematic clinical, radiological and clinical-pathological assessment. This approach is still important, but, in addition to being able to determine the type of pathological process which has developed, the clinician must have an appreciation of the mechanism by which the symptoms and the abnormal signs are produced. In the course of many lectures to and tutorials with undergraduate and post-graduate "students" of respiratory disease, it became obvious to the authors that although there were some excellent textbooks available, there was no single text which encompassed this broad approach, which was felt to be so necessary for a complete and proper understanding of respiratory disease. It is the authors' hope that this manuscript will round out this grossly deficient area.

Respiratory disease manifests itself by certain symptoms and abnormal signs which develop as a result of a particular pathological pattern. The patterns of disease, such as atelectasis or pleural effusion, may result from many causes, but it is usually the pattern and not the etiological agent which is responsible for the symptoms and signs elicited by the clinician. It is therefore not the authors' intention to discuss in any detail the individual diseases such as tuberculosis or bronchogenic carcinoma. Such discussions are available in any number of good texts of pulmonary disease. Instead, it is our intention to elucidate the mechanisms by which the symptoms and abnormal signs are produced in the various patterns of respiratory disease. Nevertheless, certain disease processes are included because they are responsible for particular pathological patterns.

In recent years, great strides have been made in the treatment of respiratory disease because of advances in the estimation of cardio-pulmonary function. This book does not deal with therapy, but it is apparent that it is only with knowledge of the fundamentals of respiratory disease that the "respiratory physician" is able to assess adequately and treat these diseases.

Although our approach may occasionally be criticized as being didactic, we have attempted to present evidence whenever it is available, and when it is not available to point out where hypotheses or differences of opinion exist. A detailed bibliography has been deliberately omitted because it was felt that it would serve little useful purpose; to be of benefit at all, it would be so extensive as to be unwieldly and frightening to the student. However, a listing of suggested additional reading has been included as a guide.

The authors wish to acknowledge the helpful criticism of Professor Joseph Doupe, Drs. John Gemmell, William Fyles, Peter Warner and Morley Lertzman, and the many students who have been subjected to the numerous difficulties associated with the development of this book. We feel that a large measure of its value is due to their constructive criticism and the excellent illustrations which have been provided by Miss Nancy Joy. The secretarial assistance of Mrs. Donna Aspinall, Miss Nan Bell, Miss Alison Wood and Mrs. Anita Forster and the financial support of the University of Manitoba and the Winnipeg Clinic Research Institute are also gratefully acknowledged.

REUBEN M. CHERNIACK
LOUIS CHERNIACK

Winnipeg, Manitoba

CONTENTS

Section 1

BASIC CONSIDERATIONS

I. THE MECHANICS OF BREATHING 3

Action of the Respiratory Muscles 4
Lung Volumes 8
Forces and Resistances Involved in Breathing 10
Work of Breathing 27
Efficiency of the Respiratory Muscles 32

II. THE DISTRIBUTION OF GAS AND BLOOD AND
GASEOUS EXCHANGE 33

The Distribution of Gas 33
Gaseous Exchange 37
Alveolar Ventilation 41
Ventilation-Perfusion Ratios 44
True Venous Admixture 47
Diffusion of Gas 48

III. THE RESPIRATORY FUNCTION OF THE BLOOD 55

The Transport of Oxygen 55
The Transport of Carbon Dioxide 59
The pH of Blood 63
The Laboratory Estimation of Acid-Base Balance.... 66

IV. THE REGULATION OF RESPIRATION 68

The Respiratory Centers 68
Factors Which Influence Respiration 70

ix

The Work of Breathing and the Control of Respiration   80
The Regulation of Ventilation in Respiratory Disease .   82
Periodic Breathing   83

Section 2

THE MANIFESTATIONS OF RESPIRATORY DISEASE

V.   THE SYMPTOMS OF RESPIRATORY DISEASE   89

The Upper Respiratory Tract   89
The Defenses of the Respiratory Tract   91
The Expectoration of Sputum   96
Hemoptysis   97
Dyspnea   98
Chest Pain   102
Constitutional Symptoms   109

VI.   THE SIGNS OF RESPIRATORY DISEASE   113

Deformities of the Chest   113
Clubbing of the Digits   117
Signs of Inadequate Gaseous Exchange   120
Signs of Altered Physical Properties of the Thorax ...   128

Section 3

THE PATTERNS OF RESPIRATORY DISEASE

VII.   BRONCHIAL DISEASE   147

Bronchopulmonary Anatomy   147
Bronchial Obstruction   151
Bronchitis   157
Chronic Obstructive Emphysema   163
Bronchiectasis   173
Bronchial Asthma   179

VIII.   PULMONARY PARENCHYMAL DISEASE   183

Atelectasis   183
Pulmonary Consolidation   188

Pulmonary Abscess and Cavitation 194
Cysts of the Lung 199
Pulmonary Fibrosis 203

IX.   PULMONARY VASCULAR DISEASE 209

The Circulation of the Lung 209
Pulmonary Hypertension 212
Pulmonary Embolism and Infarction 216
Pulmonary Arteriovenous Aneurysm 222
Pulmonary Edema 225

X.   PLEURAL DISEASE 231

Anatomy 231
Pleural Effusion 232
Pneumothorax 241

XI.   MEDIASTINAL DISEASE 248

Anatomy 248
Obstruction of the Superior Vena Cava 252
Tumors of the Mediastinum 257
Inflammation of the Mediastinum 259
Mediastinal Air 263
Herniation of the Mediastinum 265

XII. DIAPHRAGMATIC DISEASE 266

Anatomy 266
Herniation of Abdominal Viscera 268
Diseases Affecting the Position of the Diaphragm 272
Inflammatory Diseases of the Diaphragm 274
Spasmodic Conditions Affecting the Diaphragm 275
Manifestations of Diaphragmatic Disease 275

XIII. DISEASES OF THE CHEST WALL AND THORACIC
      CAGE 279

Diseases Affecting Skin and Subcutaneous Tissues ... 279
Diseases Affecting the Respiratory Muscles 282
Diseases Affecting the Bony Thorax 283

XIV.   CARDIO-RESPIRATORY INSUFFICIENCY 289

Respiratory Insufficiency 289
Cardiac Insufficiency Secondary to Respiratory Insufficiency 292
Respiratory Insufficiency Secondary to Cardiac Insufficiency 294

Section 4

THE ASSESSMENT OF REPIRATORY DISEASE

XV.   THE CLINICAL ASSESSMENT 297

The History 297
The Physical Examination 303

XVI.   THE RADIOLOGICAL ASSESSMENT 329

The Radiological Appearance of the Normal Chest .. 329
Examination of the X-ray Film of the Chest 333
Special Radiographic Techniques 334
Fluoroscopic Examination of the Chest 337

XVII.   THE CLINICAL-PATHOLOGICAL ASSESSMENT 340

Abnormal Secretions 340
Bacteriological Diagnosis 346
Histological Diagnosis 354
Skin Tests 357
Special Tests in Blood 359
Nonspecific Tests 359

XVIII. THE FUNCTIONAL ASSESSMENT 362

Ventilatory Function 362
Gaseous Exchange 370

SUGGESTED ADDITIONAL READING 377

INDEX   383

SECTION

1

BASIC CONSIDERATIONS

THE MECHANICS OF BREATHING

THE DISTRIBUTION OF GAS AND BLOOD
AND GASEOUS EXCHANGE

THE RESPIRATORY FUNCTION OF THE
BLOOD

THE REGULATION OF RESPIRATION

CHAPTER I

The Mechanics of Breathing

BREATHING is brought about by the action of the respiratory muscles, which produce rhythmic changes in the volume of the chest cage. Expansion of the chest occurs when the inspiratory muscles contract, and air enters the lungs and distends the tracheobronchial tree (Fig. 1). During inspiration, all portions of the tracheobronchial tree become enlarged, but the greatest relative expansion takes place in the distal portions of the bronchi. On fluoroscopic examination, both roots of the lungs are seen to descend during inspiration, owing to the elongation of the trachea. In addition, fluoroscopy with radiopaque media placed in the bronchi demonstrates that the bronchi lengthen and increase in diameter during inspiration, whereas, during expiration, they return to their original length and diameter. These variations in size are due to

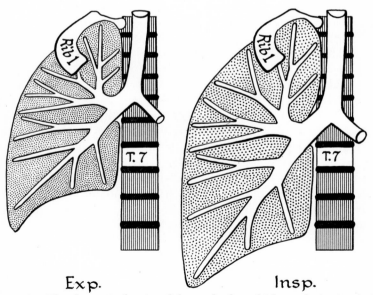

Exp.   Insp.

FIGURE 1.   The change in the size of the tracheobronchial tree during inspiration.

3

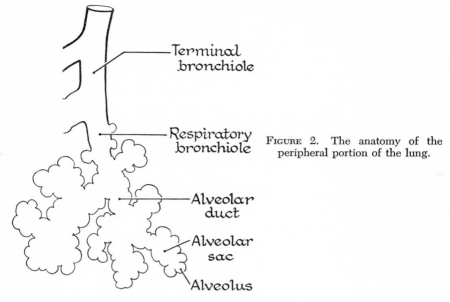

FIGURE 2. The anatomy of the peripheral portion of the lung.

the stretching on inspiration and recoil during expiration of the elastic tissue and smooth muscles of the bronchial walls. It has been suggested that the bronchi widen during inspiration because the smooth muscles in their walls undergo a decrease in tone and that they narrow during expiration because they regain their tone, but no evidence has been presented to substantiate this. Variations in the caliber of the bronchi, in the form of undulations with a very slow rhythm, have also been observed. During a cough, they may take the form of a peristaltic expulsive wave, which originates in the bronchioli and ends in the vocal cords.

The bronchi divide into successively smaller branches, down to the terminal bronchioles and the respiratory bronchioles, which can be recognized by their alveolar outpouchings. As can be seen in Figure 2, the respiratory bronchioles radiate into the alveolar ducts, which in turn give rise to the alveolar sacs. The latter consist of groups of alveoli which have a radius of approximately 55 to 65 microns. It has been estimated that there are three to four billion alveoli in the human lungs and that they occupy an area of 70 to 100 square meters. During inspiration the alveolar ducts become elongated and widen, and the openings into the alveolar sacs increase in size. It has been suggested that there is very little increase in the volume of the alveoli during inspiration.

ACTION OF THE RESPIRATORY MUSCLES

Normally, the inspiratory increase in the lung volume takes place in three dimensions: anteroposterior, transverse and longitudinal. This three-dimensional increase in volume is produced by the elevation of the ribs, resulting from the contraction of the scalene and intercostal muscles as well as from the descent of the diaphragm. The volume of the lung does not increase uniformly in all directions; instead, different portions of the lung expand in varying degrees, because of the anatomical structure and conformation of the thoracic cage. The extent and direction of the anterior movement depends on the relative positions of the ends of the ribs. Because the anterior portion of a rib is always lower than its posterior end, it must move forward when the shaft is elevated, thereby producing an increase in the anteroposterior diameter of the chest. In addition, because the middle portion of the shaft of the rib is situated at a lower level than the two ends of the ribs, the shaft is carried outwards in a lateral direction when it is elevated during inspiration.

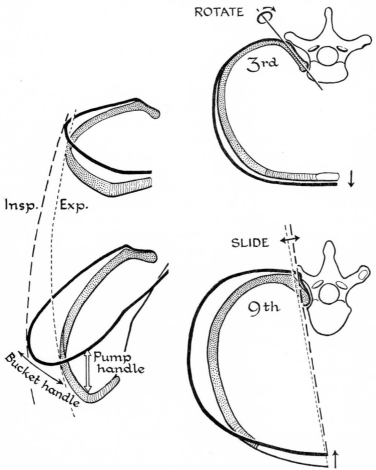

FIGURE 3. Anteroposterior and superior view of an upper and lower rib during inspiration and expiration.

During inspiration, the lower part of the thoracic cage enlarges transversely to a greater extent than does the upper portion. This occurs because when the first rib is fixed, there is a summation of the effect of muscular contraction of the intercostal muscles on each succeeding underlying rib, so that they swing through a greater segment of an arc during inspiration than do the upper ribs. In addition, the lowermost ribs are segments of circles which are larger than those of the upper ribs. All of these aspects are illustrated in Figure 3.

THE SCALENE MUSCLES

The scalene muscles, which arise from the transverse processes of the cervical vertebrae, raise the anterior end of the first rib, together with the manubrium sternum, by their contraction during inspiration. Not only does the contraction of the scalene muscle elevate the first rib, thereby slightly increasing the anteroposterior diameter of the upper outlet of the thorax, but it also stabilizes the upper chest cage, thereby enabling the contraction of the intercostal muscles to elevate the remaining ribs.

THE INTERCOSTAL MUSCLES

The first to the sixth ribs are connected with one another by the intercostal muscles, whose fibers run downward and forward. Since the first rib is fixed by the scalene muscles, contraction of the intercostal muscles results in an upward and forward movement of the remaining five ribs, a movement which has been likened to that of a pump handle. There is very little lateral movement of the first four ribs, which overlie the upper lobes of the lungs. The increase in size of this portion of the chest cage is, therefore, chiefly in an anteroposterior direction.

The fifth and sixth ribs, which are situated approximately over the middle lobe of the right lung and the lingular segment of the left lung, differ from the upper four ribs in having a greater curvature. Because of this, inspiratory elevation of these two ribs increases both the anteroposterior and the transverse diameter of that portion of the thoracic cage.

The seventh to the tenth ribs, which overlie the lower lobes of the lung, differ from the ribs above them in both their shape and the direction of their movement. The anterior ends of these lower four ribs are situated at almost the same level as their posterior ends. In addition, there is considerable bowing of their shafts. The inspiratory movement of these ribs, which has been likened to that of a bucket handle, primarily increases the transverse diameter of this portion of the thoracic cage. At the same time there is a slight decrease in the anteroposterior diameter.

THE DIAPHRAGM

The diaphragm is probably the principal muscle of inspiration. Not only does contraction of this muscular organ increase the volume of the thoracic cage in a vertical direction, but it also tends to increase the transverse diameter of the lower thoracic cage. This increase in the transverse diameter occurs because the muscular fibers of the diaphragm run in a vertical direction from their attachment at the costal margins. Since the diaphragm is normally dome-shaped, contraction of its fibers moves the lower ribs in an upward and lateral direction (Fig. 4). On the other hand, if the diaphragm is flattened and no longer dome-shaped, as in chronic obstructive emphysema, it behaves like a flat sheet of muscle. Under such circumstances, its contraction is less effective in increasing the longitudinal dimension and may actually narrow the transverse diameter of the lower thorax. Apart from its function in normal breathing, the diaphragm also plays an important role in other respiratory acts such as coughing, sniffing and sneezing. In addition, contraction of the diaphragm, in conjunction with the contraction of the abdominal muscles, raises the intra-abdominal pressure. This influences the return of venous blood from the abdomen, and also assists in defecation, vomiting and parturition.

Unlike the intercostal muscles, which are innervated from the corresponding thoracic segments of the spinal cord, the diaphragm derives its nerve supply from the third, fourth and fifth cervical segments via the phrenic nerves. The diaphragm, therefore, continues to function even when the intercostal muscles are paralyzed by either a lesion in the upper thoracic region or the administration of a spinal anesthetic.

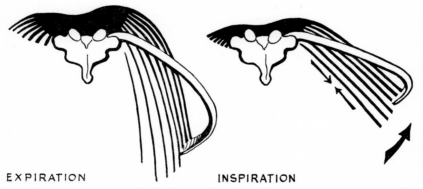

EXPIRATION INSPIRATION

FIGURE 4. Contraction of the diaphragm, because of its dome shape, results in elevation of the ribs with a consequent increase of the transverse diameter of the chest.

ACCESSORY RESPIRATORY MUSCLES

Under normal circumstances the prime function of the scalene and sternomastoid muscles, which serve as accessory respiratory muscles, is to stabilize the upper rib cage. They may act in a more positive manner during a forced inspiration or in cardio-respiratory diseases which are associated with difficulty in breathing. Electromyographic studies have suggested that the scalene muscles may also contract during a vigorous cough or sneeze. It is likely that the purpose of this contraction is to further stabilize the outlet of the rib cage in order to support the apex of the lung and prevent its herniation into the neck.

Although it is generally stated that the intercostal muscles are also active during expiration, there is no evidence to support this premise, and there is some evidence against it. No electromyographic activity has been recorded from the intercostal muscles either during normal expiration or when ventilation has been considerably increased. On the other hand, these muscles, in association with the abdominal muscles, do contract during forced expiratory efforts, as well as during maneuvers which produce an increase in intra-abdominal pressure.

LUNG VOLUMES

The position of the chest cage when the muscles are relaxed, which is the situation at the end of a normal expiration, is called the *resting level* or *mid-position.* The resting level is determined by the balance between the elastic forces of the lungs, which tend to reduce their volume, and the elastic forces of the chest wall, which tend to increase it. Even after various maximal inspiratory and expiratory maneuvers, the lung volume normally returns to its original level. Nevertheless, this equilibrium volume is not constant, but can be influenced by various conditions. For example, the resting level shifts to a more inspiratory position whenever there is obstruction to the expiratory flow of air or when the lung loses its elasticity, as in chronic obstructive emphysema.

The changes in the volume of the lungs that can be produced by the action of the respiratory muscles may be studied by means of a recording spirometer. One generally thinks of the lung volumes as divided into various components. Figure 5 illustrates these subdivisions. They are shown as approximate proportions of the total lung capacity, because their absolute values vary considerably, even in normal persons, being dependent upon the age, sex and size of the person.

Though the lung volume compartments are quantitatively different in persons of different age and size, the proportion of the total lung capacity which each occupies is remarkably similar in different healthy individuals. The resting level or the functional residual capacity is about

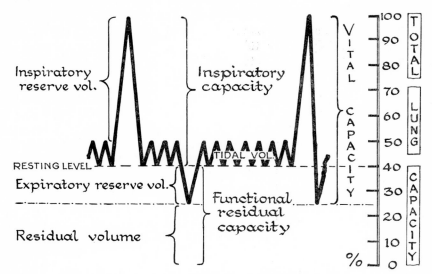

FIGURE 5. The subdivisions of the lung volume.

40 per cent, the vital capacity about 70 to 75 per cent and the residual volume approximately 25 to 30 per cent of the total lung capacity. This principle is illustrated in Table 1, where the values obtained in two males of the same age but of different size are shown.

The *total lung capacity* is the total amount of air that is present in the lungs after a maximal inspiration. The *vital capacity* is the maximal amount of air that a subject is able to expire after a maximal inspiration. This is usually approximately 75 per cent of the total lung capacity. Its absolute value is limited by the strength of the respiratory muscles, as well as by the elastic resistance of the lungs and the chest wall.

Almost all of the remaining lung volumes are estimated with reference to the normal end-expiratory position of the chest or its resting level. The *tidal volume* is the volume of air which is breathed in during inspiration or out during expiration. Its absolute amount varies with the

TABLE 1

LUNG VOLUMES IN TWO MALES OF EQUAL AGE BUT DIFFERENT SIZE

LUNG VOLUME	HT., 180 CM. ml.	% TLC	HT., 150 CM. ml.	% TLC
Total lung capacity.............	7790	100	4680	100
Vital capacity.................	6030	77	3280	70
Inspiratory capacity............	4100	53	2555	51
Functional residual capacity......	3690	47	2115	49
Residual volume...............	1760	23	1400	30
Expiratory reserve volume.......	1930	24	715	19

activity of the subject. It varies from individual to individual, but is usually stated to be about 500 ml. in normal subjects under resting conditions. By multiplying the tidal volume and the respiratory rate, the *minute ventilation* may be determined.

The *inspiratory capacity* is the maximum volume of air which can be inspired from the resting level. It normally averages about 60 per cent of the total lung capacity. Since the tidal volume is included in this measurement, the *inspiratory reserve volume* is the maximal volume of air which can be inspired over and above the tidal volume from the resting level.

The *functional residual capacity* is the quantity of air which remains in the lungs after a normal expiration. Normally, the functional residual capacity is about 40 per cent of the total lung capacity, but this also varies from individual to individual. It is smaller in the supine position. It increases if there is an expiratory obstruction to the flow of air or a loss of lung elasticity. It is composed of two compartments, only one of which, the expiratory reserve volume, can be determined with an ordinary recording spirometer. The other compartment, the residual volume, is estimated by means of dilution techniques.

The *expiratory reserve volume* is the maximal volume of air which can be expired beyond the resting level, when expiration is carried on to its fullest extent. It is limited by several factors: the extent of elevation of the diaphragm during expiration, the strength of the expiratory muscles, the resistance of the chest wall to a further decrease in volume and the tendency for the smaller airways to close during a forced expiration.

The *residual volume* of the lungs is the amount of air which is still in the lungs at the end of a maximal expiration. It is normally approximately 25 per cent of the total lung capacity. Some authorities consider the size of the ratio of the residual volume to the total lung capacity to be significant. A ratio which is greater than 30 per cent is thought to be indicative of chronic obstructive emphysema, but a high ratio is also seen when the lungs are hyperinflated as a result of an expiratory obstruction.

FORCES AND RESISTANCES INVOLVED IN BREATHING

In order to carry out the breathing movements, the respiratory muscles must overcome both elastic and nonelastic resistances of the lung and the chest wall. The essential difference between the elastic and the nonelastic components is that the force which is required to overcome the elastic resistance is stored during deformation, whereas the force which is required to overcome the nonelastic resistance is dissipated as heat because of friction. As will be seen, there are other resistances which are difficult to classify. For instance, in obesity the resistance of the chest wall may be likened to a weight which is lifted against gravity through a distance. On the other hand, if this resistance increases as it moves, it may behave like an elastic resistance; in fact, it is usually regarded to act as an elastic resistance. Elastic resistance is related to the change in the volume of the lung; nonelastic resistance is related to the rate at which the volume changes. The commonly used ventilatory function studies, which are described later, may yield indirect information about these mechanical resistances. However, definitive information can be gained only if the variations in pressure which are involved are measured simultaneously with the volume changes and the rate of air flow.

RESPIRATORY PRESSURES

Normally there is no attachment between the visceral layer of the pleura on the surface of the lung and the parietal layer on the interior surface of the thoracic chamber. These two layers are in close apposition, being separated only by a thin film of fluid which acts as a lubricant. The lungs are held out against the chest wall by the atmospheric pressure, which is being applied both at the surface of the body as well as within the lungs. When the respiratory muscles are relaxed at the resting level, the elastic recoil of the lungs which tends to reduce the lung volume is counterbalanced by the tendency of the elastic forces of the chest wall and extrapulmonary structures to increase it. Because of the pull of these forces in opposite directions, the pressure within the potential pleural space, the *intrathoracic pressure,* is less than that of the atmosphere. During inspiration, the intrathoracic pressure becomes even more negative, because the lung offers resistances to distention. Since the force required to overcome the elastic resistance is stored in the tissues during inspiration, no additional force is necessary during expiration. For this reason, the intrathoracic pressure normally remains subatmospheric even during expiration. If there is active contraction of the expiratory muscles during expiration, however, the intrathoracic pressure becomes greater than that of the atmosphere.

The *intrapulmonary pressure* is difficult to determine, but may be imagined to be that which is measured if a catheter is inserted into the alveoli of the lung. It is the pressure that is required to overcome airway resistance and, unlike the intrathoracic pressure, it varies rhythmically above and below atmospheric pressure during expiration and inspiration. When the airway is open and there is no movement of air, and therefore no airway resistance, the intrapulmonary pressure is equal to that of the atmosphere. This situation exists momentarily at the ends of inspiration and expiration. The relationship between the intrathoracic

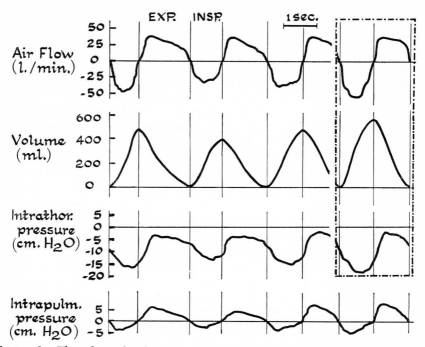

FIGURE 6.   The relationship between the intrathoracic and the intrapulmonary pressures during breathing.

and the intrapulmonary pressures during the breathing cycle is shown in Figure 6. It can be seen that, at end-expiration, the intrathoracic pressure is subatmospheric, becoming even more negative at end-inspiration, whereas the intrapulmonary pressure is at atmospheric levels during these moments.

When air is moving, the intrathoracic pressure is the algebraic sum of the pressure required to overcome the elastic resistance and the pressure required to overcome the nonelastic resistance. At any instant when air is moving, therefore, the difference between the intrathoracic pressure and the pressure which is required to overcome the elastic resistance represents the pressure which is required to overcome the nonelastic resistance.

In order to calculate the resistances overcome by the respiratory muscles during breathing, the pressure variations involved must be separated into those required to overcome both the elastic and the nonelastic resistances of the lung as well as those required to overcome the elastic and the nonelastic resistances of the chest wall. As will be discussed later, the resistances of the chest wall are difficult to measure. On the other hand, the resistances which the lungs offer during breathing may be determined if the changes in the pressure difference across the lung, the flow of air and the tidal volume are measured during breathing.

In order to determine the pressure difference across the lung which is required to overcome the elastic and the nonelastic resistances of the lung during breathing, the intrathoracic pressure must be measured. This can be determined by recording the pressure in either the pleural cavity or the esophagus. The intrapleural pressure probably varies in different areas of the pleural cavity, however, particularly in the dependent parts or over local diseased areas; a single measurement, therefore, does not necessarily reflect the over-all pressure required to overcome the total resistances to breathing. For this reason, as well as the discomfort and inherent danger associated with the insertion of a needle into the pleural cavity, the changes in pressure within the esophagus during respiration have been used as an index of the changes in intrapleural pressure. Although the relationship between the esophageal and intrapleural pressures is not consistent and varies from one individual to another, it may nevertheless yield a better measure of the pressure at the surface of the lungs because it reflects the pressure over a larger area.

Since the act of breathing is a dynamic process, it is essential to record the instantaneous pressure changes across the lung that occur throughout the breathing cycle. This is usually done by connecting the needle or the balloon to tubing which leads to one side of a membrane or diaphragm, such as a strain gauge, in order to record the pressure changes electronically. The other side of the strain gauge is usually connected to a tube which conducts the pressure at the mouth. Since it is presumed that the pressure at the mouth reflects that within the airways, the strain gauge is therefore recording the pressure across the lung.

The flow of air into and out of the lungs can be recorded by having the subject breathe through a wire mesh screen, which offers a slight but definite resistance to the air flow. The drop in pressure which takes place across the screen is proportional to the rate at which the air is flowing through it. This pressure drop is instantaneously recorded by means of a strain gauge similar to that used for measuring pressure.

The changes in volume which occur during breathing can be recorded simultaneously by electronic means either by integrating the air flow curve or by using a recording spirometer.

ELASTIC RESISTANCE

Elastic forces are those which tend to return a tissue to its original size or shape after it has undergone a limited degree of distortion. The elastic resistances which the tissues of both the lungs and the chest wall offer during breathing are perhaps best understood if one imagines the lung-thorax system to be in the form of a two-plate piston within a container, as illustrated in Figure 7, A.

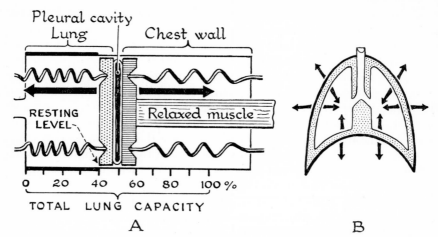

FIGURE 7.   The elastic forces of the lungs and chest wall at the "resting level" in a mechanical analogy (A) and within the thorax (B). The elastic forces are pulling equally in opposite directions.

The opposing surfaces of the two plates are attached to a rubber balloon, the interior of which represents the pleural space. The plates are attached to springs which are pulling in opposite directions. The springs attached to the plate on the left represent the elastic resistance of the lung, and the springs attached to the plate on the right represent that of the chest wall. The total capacity of the container is indicated as 100 per cent (the *total lung capacity*). When the piston is at its resting position, which is 40 per cent of the total lung capacity, the forces exerted by the two sets of springs are equal. This situation is analogous to that at the resting level or mid-position of the lungs and the chest wall, as shown in Figure 7, *B.*

When the piston is pulled out as far as possible, it tends to recoil because the spring representing the elastic force of the lung is stretched. The spring representing the elastic force of the chest wall is compressed and actually attempts to re-expand (Fig. 8, *A*). This situation is analogous to that which exists when a maximum inspiration is made, that is, when the lung volume is at 100 per cent of capacity. The elasticity of the chest wall is exerting a small force in an expiratory direction, thereby assisting the lung elasticity, which is exerting a strong force in the same direction. In this position, both elastic forces are being opposed by the action of the inspiratory muscles.

As the piston is allowed to return to its original position, the stretch on the spring which represents the lung elasticity diminishes (Fig. 8, *B*). The spring which represents the chest wall is no longer compressed, but instead reaches a position at which it is not exerting a force in either direction. Similarly, the force of the lung elasticity in an expiratory direction diminishes when air moves out of the lung following a maximal inspiration. When a lung volume which corresponds to about 67 per cent of the total lung capacity is reached, the chest wall is in its resting position and is exerting no force in either direction.

As the piston is pushed past its resting position, as by the action of the expiratory muscles, the spring representing the pulmonary elasticity exerts even less retractile force, while that of the chest wall increases (Fig. 8, *C*). At a position of maximum expiration, or, in other words, at the residual volume, the elastic force of the chest wall is acting strongly in an inspiratory direction and is only weakly opposed by the elasticity of the lung, which is still acting in an expiratory direction.

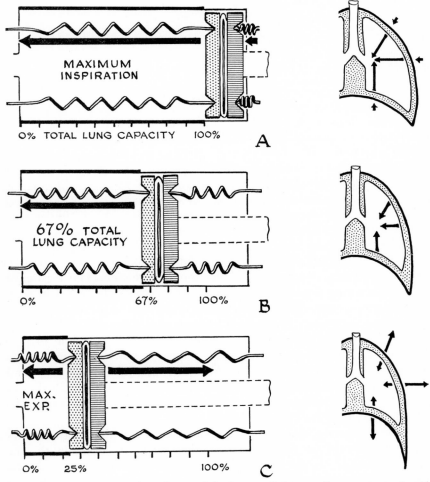

FIGURE 8. The elastic forces of the lung and chest wall at maximum inspiration (A), at approximately 67 per cent of the total lung capacity (B), and at maximum expiration (C).

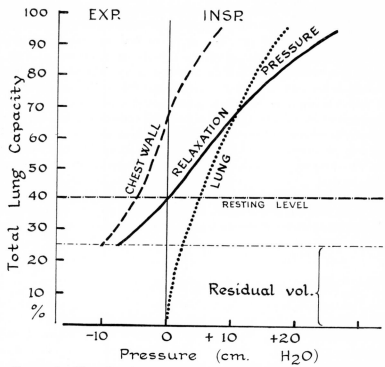

FIGURE 9.   The relaxation pressure curve. The pressure at any lung volume is the resultant of the elastic forces of the lung and chest wall. (From Rahn, H., Otis, A. B., Chadwick, L. E. and Fenn, W. O.: The pressure volume diagram of the thorax and lung. Am. J. Physiol., *146*:161, 1946. By permission.)

The amount of deformation or volume change that the respiratory system undergoes depends upon the applied pressure. The elastic behavior of the respiratory system may be satisfactorily described in terms of its pressure-volume relationship. It can therefore be studied by applying a positive pressure to the upper airway and determining the alteration in volume which results. Similarly, the elastic behavior may be studied by determining the pressure which is exerted against a manometer at different degrees of lung distention, while the flow of air is obstructed at the mouth, and all muscular activity is voluntarily suspended. The pressure readings obtained by this method are called *relaxation pressures.*

The relationship between the elastic forces of the lung and chest wall at different lung volumes, which has been described in the mechanical analogue, is exemplified by the relaxation pressures. At the resting level, the forces being exerted by the lung and chest wall are equal and pulling in opposite directions. The pressure in the airways is therefore the same as atmospheric pressure, and no pressure is recorded on the manometer. When the distention of the lung is greater than that at the resting level, a positive pressure develops against the manometer because the chest tends to collapse when the muscles are relaxed. This pressure is a measure of the inspiratory effort which was previously exerted in order to overcome the elastic resistance of the lungs and the chest wall. On the other hand, a negative pressure develops against the manometer when the lung is deflated below the resting level. The negative pressure which develops then is a measure of the expiratory effort which was previously exerted in order to overcome the elastic resistance. When the pressures obtained at various levels of lung inflation are plotted against the corresponding lung volume, a *relaxation pressure curve* is derived. This pressure curve is the resultant of the elastic forces of the lung and the chest wall. It varies according to the state of expansion of the thorax. Figure 9 shows that the curve is sigmoid in shape but that it is linear near the resting level.

COMPLIANCE

The compliance of the respiratory system, the change in volume which is produced by the application of pressure, defines its elastic resistance to distention. It is usually expressed as the number of liters of distention induced by a change in pressure of one centimeter of water. The pressure change is measured under static conditions when there is no air flowing. The formula for compliance is:

$$\text{Compliance} = \frac{\text{Volume (in l.)}}{\text{Pressure (in cm. H}_2\text{O)}}$$

The separate determination of the compliance of either the lung or the chest wall is carried out by measuring the volume change associated with the difference in the pressure across either the lungs or the chest wall. The compliance of the lungs can therefore be determined by relating the change in volume to the difference between the intrathoracic pressure and that within the air passages. Similarly, the compliance of the chest wall can be determined by relating the change in lung volume to the difference between the intrathoracic pressure and that exterior to the chest wall. It is thus theoretically possible to determine the compliance of the total respiratory system, as well as that of either the lung or the chest wall alone, by the simultaneous recording of the intrathoracic pressure changes and the relaxation pressures. Similarly, the compliance of the total respiratory system and its components can be derived if the respiratory system is inflated by a positive pressure and the distending pressure and the intrathoracic pressure are measured.

Total Respiratory Compliance. The compliance of the total respiratory mechanism is illustrated by the slope of the relaxation pressure curve.

The compliance of the total respiratory system may also be determined by measuring the changes in the resting level which result when a pressure is applied to the external surface of the chest while the subject is breathing spontaneously. Under such circumstances, the compliance of the total respiratory system in normal subjects is approximately 0.12 l./cm. H_2O. It is reduced by any alteration of the compliance of the lung or the chest wall.

Although it would appear to be comparatively simple to determine the total elastic resistances involved in breathing, it should be pointed out that the respiratory muscles must be in a state of either complete relaxation or paralysis. Complete relaxation of the respiratory muscles is extremely difficult to attain except in a well-trained subject, so this method is not always practical. Similarly, although the compliance of the lungs and chest wall, either together or separately, can be measured when the respiratory muscles are paralyzed, one is never certain that the movements of the chest are similar to those which occur in a subject who is breathing spontaneously.

Lung Compliance. The compliance of the lung alone can be assessed in the spontaneously breathing subject by measuring the changes in both the intrathoracic pressure from end-expiration to end-inspiration and the tidal volume. Although either intrapleural or intraesophageal pressure may be measured, it is usually the esophageal pressure which is determined.

Examples of the elastic behavior or the compliance of three different types of lung are plotted in Figure 10. Figure 10, *A*, shows that a change in the intrathoracic pressure of 5 cm. H_2O results in an inspiration of 1 liter of air into the normal lung. Its compliance is therefore 0.20 l./cm. H_2O. When the lung loses its elasticity, as in chronic obstructive emphysema, it becomes easier to distend; in other words, it is more compliant. Figure 10, *B*, illustrates that a change in the intrathoracic pressure of 5 cm. H_2O now results in an inspiration of 2 liters of air. The compliance of these lungs is 0.40 l./cm. H_2O. If the lungs are stiff, as in pulmonary fibrosis or congestion, the same change in the intrathoracic pressure results in a change of volume of only 0.5 liter, so that the compliance is only 0.10 l./cm. H_2O (Fig. 10, *C*).

It would appear to be comparatively simple to determine the compliance of the lung, but it should be pointed out that the determination may be affected by several other factors. An increase in the nonelastic resistance, particularly if it is not uniformly distributed, affects the calculation of the compliance. Local alterations in the mechanical properties of the lungs, such as may occur in unequally distributed bronchial obstruction, can alter the changes in pressure which are necessary to produce a given lung inflation. Figure 11 illustrates the change in the intrathoracic pressure which is normally necessary to bring a liter of air into the lung, as compared to that which is required when there is a local obstruction to air flow. It can be seen that when there is no airway obstruction, the tidal volume is equally distributed to all areas of lung. When an airway obstruction is present, however, there is an increase in the resistance to the flow of air into the lung distal to the obstruction. During very slow breathing it is likely that the air is almost equally distributed, even in the presence of bronchial obstruction, so that the calculated value for the compliance is little altered. During rapid breathing, however, the air tends to move into the areas of the lung which offer the least resistance. In order that the same volume of air may be inspired, a greater intrathoracic pressure must develop, and this results in a fall of the calculated compliance. The compliance deter-

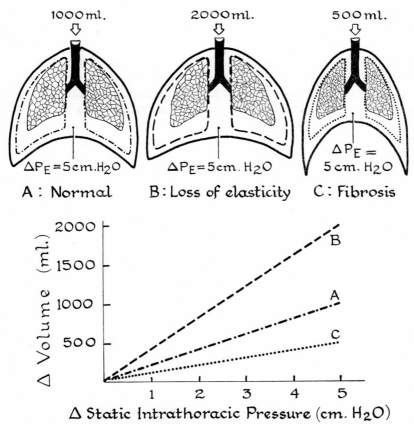

FIGURE 10. The distention produced by a change in intrathoracic pressure of 5 cm. H_2O in a normal lung (A), a lung which has lost elasticity (B), and a lung which has become fibrosed (C).

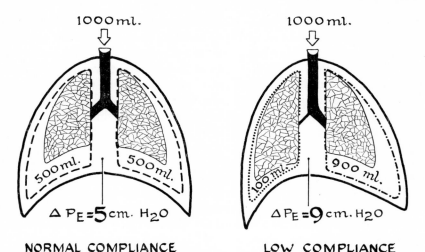

NORMAL COMPLIANCE   **LOW COMPLIANCE**

FIGURE 11.   The effect of a local bronchial obstruction on the pressure-volume relationship of the lungs when 1000 ml. of air is inhaled.

mined under such conditions has been referred to as the *functional
compliance.* When the over-all elastic properties of the lung are studied,
therefore, it is extremely important that all the measurements of pressure
should be truly static, with sufficient time allowed for all areas of the
lung to become inflated. Nevertheless, it should be pointed out that
the functional compliance is important because it indicates that the
elastic resistance that is actually overcome during breathing may be far
greater than that which is reflected in the static measurements. This is
particularly true in obstructive bronchiolar disease.

     Another factor may affect the distensibility of the lungs. It has
been suggested that one-half or more of the elastic recoil of the lungs
is due to the tendency of the moist surfaces of the alveoli to contract
because of surface tension. On the other hand, as has been described
above, the lungs do not normally collapse completely but remain partially
inflated even after a maximal expiration. The parenchyma of normal
lungs has been shown to secrete a surface-active material which lines
the air spaces and has the ability to reduce the effect of surface tension
and therefore the tendency of the alveoli to collapse. This is very important because the smaller bronchioles are liable to become completely
occluded at very low lung volumes or during a forced expiration, especially if small bubbles of fluid should be present in the bronchioles or
if there is increased tone of the bronchial smooth muscle, as in bronchospasm. Once the bronchioles become closed, pressures greater than those
which would normally cause expansion are required to reopen them.

     This effect has been demonstrated by attempts to reinflate col-
lapsed lungs of cats by the introduction of gas or fluid under pressure

into the tracheobronchial tree. Air under pressure failed to inflate these lungs until a critical pressure was reached, but fluid under pressure significantly reduced the critical opening pressure. Since it is likely that there is a much smaller effect of surface tension when fluid is used, these findings suggest that surface tension may have played a role in the resistance to inflation which was offered by the cats' lungs. Similar observations have been made during attempts to inflate the lungs removed from stillborn children.

Examples of difficult re-expansion of collapsed lungs are frequently encountered, particularly in the newborn. Here, the pressure which must develop to produce the initial inspiration may be as great as 50 mm. Hg, whereas subsequent breaths require pressure changes of only 5 to 10 mm. Hg. It is of interest that no surface-active material capable of reducing surface tension is found in the newborn infant who develops the "respiratory distress syndrome."

A similar effect on the distensibility of the lungs is seen in other clinical situations. During thoracic surgery, the anesthetist frequently has to exert large pressures by squeezing the anesthetic bag in order to expand a collapsed portion of a lung. Following the expansion, much smaller pressures are necessary to produce further expansion. In pulmonary edema the presence of fluid or secretions in the tracheobronchial tree increases the resistance to the distention of the lungs; it is likely that surface tension plays a role in increasing this resistance. It has been suggested that surface tension may also be an important factor in producing the shortness of breath experienced by a patient suffering from congestive heart failure while he is lying in the supine position.

Chest Wall Compliance. In order to measure the compliance of the chest wall it is necessary to determine both the total and the lung compliance simultaneously. A technique has recently been described which measures the changes in resting level resulting from a pressure applied to either the upper airway or the external surface of the chest. By measuring the changes in intrathoracic pressure simultaneously, the compliance of the chest wall can be calculated. By means of this technique the compliance of the chest wall in normal subjects is approximately 0.22 l./cm. H_2O. In obese subjects, on the other hand, the compliance of the chest wall has been found to be greatly reduced, averaging 0.077 l./cm. H_2O. Although in this case the extra resistance may be likened to lifting a weight through distance, it is possible that this resistance may be increasing as it moves through greater distances, so that it can be included in the elastic resistance.

NONELASTIC RESISTANCE

In addition to inertia, which is probably produced by constant

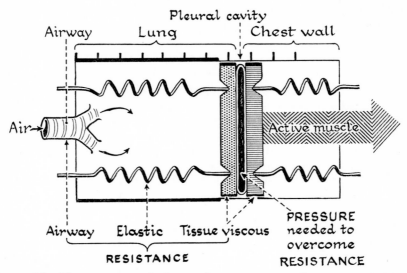

FIGURE 12. The resistances which must be overcome in order to move air into the lungs during breathing.

acceleration and deceleration, but is nevertheless considered to be negligible, there are two types of nonelastic resistance which must be overcome during breathing. There is, first of all, a resistance to the movement of air in the air passages, including the nasal passages, the nasopharynx, the larynx and the trachea, which have been shown to contribute about 20 per cent of the nonelastic resistance at low rates of air flow and as much as 45 per cent at higher rates of flow. The pressure which is necessary to overcome the resistance to the flow of air in the tracheobronchial tree is the intrapulmonary pressure. In addition, there is tissue viscous resistance, which is due to the friction of such tissues as the peribronchial tissues, lung parenchyma and vascular structures sliding over one another during movement of the lungs, and which is presumably influenced by the rate of distention. These resistances are illustrated by the analogy in Figure 12, which demonstrates that both a frictional and an airway resistance must be overcome, in addition to the elastic resistance, while the piston is being pulled out or pushed in.

AIRWAY RESISTANCE

The pressure which is required to overcome the nonelastic resistance is the sum of the pressures which are necessary to overcome the airway resistance and the tissue viscous resistance. The resistance in the airways is the result of two types of airflow resistance—the *laminar re-*

sistance, which is related to the velocity and the viscosity of the respired gas, and the *turbulent resistance,* which is due to changes in direction of the flow of air, such as occurs at the bifurcations of the tracheobronchial tree and in regions of high velocity, as well as to changes in the cross-sectional area of the tracheobronchial tree. The latter type of resistance is related to the velocity of the respired gas as well as to its density. Laminar resistance occurs throughout both the upper and lower respiratory tracts, whereas turbulent resistance appears to be predominant, at least in normal subjects, in the upper respiratory tract. In diseases which affect the tracheobronchial tree, turbulence often plays a major role in producing airway resistance.

TISSUE VISCOUS RESISTANCE

Several attempts have been made to distinguish airway resistance from tissue viscous resistance. Using techniques which measure nonelastic resistance during the inhalation of gases which have a greater or lesser viscosity than that of air, it is possible to calculate by extrapolation the resistance which would be present if a gas possessing no viscosity whatever were being inhaled. The pressure required to overcome the tissue viscous resistance can then be derived. The latter pressure has also been determined by the simultaneous estimation of the pressure required to overcome the airway resistance and that which is necessary to overcome the total nonelastic resistance. The tissue viscous resistance has been found to form only a small part of the total nonelastic resistance, the major resistance being that which occurs in the airways. Therefore, and since these techniques are difficult, it is the total nonelastic resistance which is usually determined clinically. This determination can be obtained from the simultaneous measurements of the changes in the intrathoracic pressure, the tidal volume and the rate of air flow.

One would suppose that the intrathoracic pressure curve could be divided into its elastic and nonelastic components by merely joining the points of end-expiration and end-inspiration with a straight line, as is indicated by the dotted line in Figure 13, which is an excerpt from Figure 6. Since the pressure required to overcome the elastic resistance is linearly related to the change in lung volume, however, a straight line is incorrect, unless the change in lung volume is constant and air is flowing at a constant rate during inspiration. In Figure 13 the dotted line is therefore incorrect. The shape of the line which joins the points of end-expiration and end-inspiration depends upon the rate of the change in the lung volume. The correct line is demonstrated in Figure 13 by the thin solid line. The pressure which is required to overcome the nonelastic resistance at any moment in the respiratory cycle is the difference between the

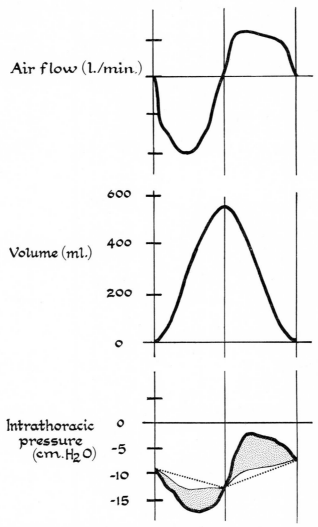

Air flow (l./min.)

Volume (ml.)

600

400

200

0

Intrathoracic
pressure
(cm. H₂O)

0

-5

-10

-15

FIGURE 13.   Excerpt of a breathing cycle from Figure 6. The change in the portion of the intrathoracic pressure which is required to overcome elastic resistance during breathing is indicated by the thin continuous line. The pressure necessary to overcome the nonelastic resistance at any instant is indicated by the shaded portion.

intrathoracic pressure and the pressure required to overcome the elastic
resistance at that time.

THE PRESSURE-VOLUME LOOP

An analysis of the elastic and the nonelastic components of the
intrathoracic pressure curve, such as has been described, is a time-

consuming procedure. In a simpler method, the simultaneous changes of the volume and the intrathoracic pressure are plotted against one another. In this way the time element is removed from the relationship between the two measurements. By this method a loop is formed, its outer boundaries being derived from the intrathoracic pressure changes at different degrees of lung inflation during the respiratory cycle. A pressure-volume loop determined in a normal subject is illustrated in Figure 14, *A*. Since the elastic resistance is linearly related to the state of lung distention, a line joining the points of end-expiration and end-inspiration, when there is no flow of air, represents the pressure which is required to overcome the elastic resistance at any given instant during the breathing cycle. The difference between the intrathoracic pressure and that portion required to overcome the elastic resistance at any given moment during the breathing cycle is, therefore, the pressure necessary to overcome the nonelastic resistance at that particular moment. Similarly, one can see from the pressure-volume loop that if the airway distal to the pressure measurement is suddenly obstructed during breathing so that there is no flow of air, the intrathoracic pressure changes to that which is required to overcome the elastic resistance at that particular lung volume. The change in pressure which occurs is also important. It represents the pressure which was required to overcome the nonelastic resistance which happened to be present just prior to the interruption of air flow.

A pressure-volume loop which was determined in a patient suffering from obstruction of the airway due to bronchospasm is shown in Fig. 14, *B*. When there is airway obstruction, the pressure-volume loop is considerably widened and there is a great increase in the pressure required to overcome the nonelastic resistance during both inspiration and expiration.

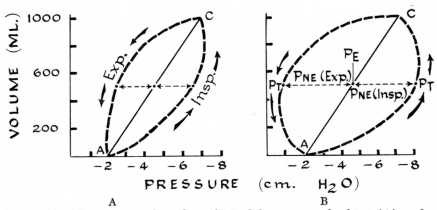

FIGURE 14. The pressure-volume loop obtained from a normal subject (A), and a patient with bronchial obstruction (B).

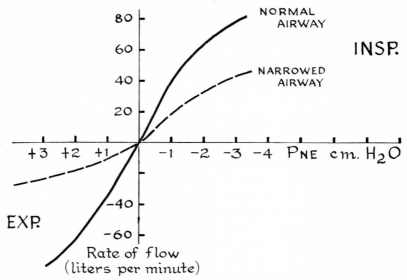

FIGURE 15.   The pressure-flow relationship in a normal subject and a patient with bronchial obstruction.

PRESSURE-FLOW RELATIONSHIP

When the nonelastic component of the intrathoracic pressure is plotted against the simultaneous rate of air flow, a pressure-flow plot is derived. This is illustrated in Figure 15, where the inspiratory air flow is shown in the right upper quadrant and expiration in the left lower quadrant. It can be seen that the pressure change is linearly related to the air flow up to a certain point. After this there is a disproportionate increase in the pressure required to produce a further increase in air flow. The linear portion of the curve is due to the laminar resistance, and the horizontal portion of the curve is due to the addition of turbulent resistance. The total resistance at any particular flow rate, expressed in cm. of H_2O per liter of air flow, can be determined by the formula:

$$\text{Resistance} = \frac{\text{Pressure}}{\text{Flow}}$$

The total nonelastic resistance is approximately 1.8 cm. $H_2O/l./$ sec. of air flow in the normal subject. Only about one-tenth of the resistance at this rate of air flow is due to turbulence.

Figure 15 also shows the pressure-flow plot derived from the pressure-volume loop in Figure 14, which was obtained from a patient suffering from airway obstruction. It can be seen that a given flow of air requires greater than normal pressure, indicating that the resistance to air flow is increased. In patients suffering from obstruction of the airway, the total nonelastic resistance is increased and may be greater than 5 cm. $H_2O/l./min.$ of air flow. In these patients, this resistance is predominantly due to turbulence. When the ventilation is increased above normal, such as during exertion, this turbulent resistance becomes exceedingly high.

WORK OF BREATHING

Work must be performed by the respiratory muscles in order to overcome the resistances which are offered by the lung and the chest wall during breathing. Three aspects of the work of breathing are of extreme importance in understanding pulmonary disability: (1) the total mechanical work which is done during breathing, (2) the relationship between the amount of work that is done and that portion of the total ventilation which is actually taking part in gaseous exchange, or the alveolar ventilation, and (3) the amount of oxygen which is consumed by the respiratory muscles while they are performing this work.

MECHANICAL WORK OF BREATHING

Work is usually expressed in terms of a weight which is moved through a distance. In the respiratory system, the pressure change, which is expressed in cm. H_2O, is the weight, one centimeter of water being equal to one gram of weight. The volume change, which is expressed in cc., is equivalent to the distance over which the weight moves. In order to measure the mechanical work which is done during breathing, it is therefore necessary to obtain simultaneous measurements of both the volume change and the pressure which is exerted across the respiratory system.

TOTAL WORK OF BREATHING

The work which is necessary to overcome the elastic resistance of the total respiratory system may be estimated from the relaxation pressure curve. However, there does not seem to be any method available for measuring the total amount of work being done on the lung, the respired gases, the chest wall, the diaphragm and abdominal contents, while a subject is breathing, because no technique has as yet been devised for the determination of the nonelastic resistance of the chest wall. Nevertheless, there are two techniques which measure indirectly the total amount of mechanical work which is carried out during breathing. In the first method, a respirator is substituted for the respiratory muscles of a paralyzed or "completely relaxed" subject. It is presumed that movements of the chest by the respirator are similar to those which are produced by the action of the respiratory muscles during breathing. In the second method, the total mechanical work is calculated by measuring the oxygen consumption of the respiratory muscles as well as the efficiency with which added respiratory work loads are handled. It is possible to calculate the total work of breathing by the latter technique because the efficiency of the respiratory muscles remains constant over a large range of added work loads, suggesting that their efficiency is the same when there is no added work load. It has been estimated that the total mechanical work during quiet breathing is approximately 0.3 to 0.6 kg. m./min. by the first technique, and 0.8 to 3.0 kg. m./min. by the second. It is of interest that the total mechanical work during quiet breathing is no greater in chronic obstructive emphysema than it is in the normal subject when measured by the second technique.

MECHANICAL WORK DONE ON THE LUNGS

The mechanical work which is carried out solely on the lungs during a breathing cycle can be estimated by simultaneously measuring the changes in the intrathoracic pressure, utilizing either the esophageal or intrapleural pressures, as well as the volume displacement which takes place. When these pressure measurements and volume alterations over the period of a complete breathing cycle are plotted against one another, a pressure-volume loop is obtained, similar to that which has previously been described.

Figure 16 demonstrates the information which can be derived from such a loop. The mechanical work necessary to overcome the elastic resistance is calculated from the area of the trapezoid (O, A, C, D), and the mechanical work required to overcome the nonelastic resistance during both inspiration and expiration is calculated from the area of the loop (A, B_1, C, B_2). The portion of the loop which falls to the right of the line A B C during inspiration represents the mechanical work necessary to overcome the nonelastic resistance during inspiration. That portion which falls to the left of the line A B C represents the mechanical work required to overcome the nonelastic resistance during expiration.

During quiet breathing almost all of the muscular work is carried out during inspiration, since the elastic recoil of the lungs is sufficient to overcome the nonelastic resistance of both the air and the tissues during expiration. The expiratory portion of the nonelastic loop does not usually fill the entire trapezoid representing the elastic work, indicating that some of the elastic energy which was built up during inspiration is dissipated in the form of heat. If the expiratory portion of the nonelastic work loop falls entirely within the trapezoid it indicates that the intrathoracic pressure has been less than that of the atmosphere throughout expiration. If a portion of the expiratory nonelastic work loop falls outside the trapezoid, it signifies that the intrathoracic pressure was greater than that of the atmosphere during expiration and that expiratory muscular work was apparently required for that part of the expiration.

The total mechanical work which is carried out on the lungs during a breath is calculated from the sum of the work necessary to overcome the elastic resistance, the inspiratory nonelastic resistance and the portion of the expiratory nonelastic work loop which falls outside of the elastic work area. The total amount of mechanical work carried out on the lungs per minute may be determined by multiplying the work done during each breath by the respiratory rate.

In normal subjects the total mechanical work performed on the lungs has been estimated to be approximately 0.3 to 0.7 kg. m./min. In a patient suffering from diffuse bronchial obstruction such as bronchial asthma or chronic obstructive emphysema, the mechanical work necessary to overcome the nonelastic resistance is increased so that the pressure-volume loop becomes widened in a manner similar to that illustrated in Figure 14, *B.* In pulmonary fibrosis, the work required to overcome the nonelastic resistance may be only slightly altered. On the other hand, much more work must be performed in order to overcome the high elastic resistance of these "stiff lungs," with the result that the area of the elastic work trapezoid is increased. In addition, in patients suffering from respiratory disease this work may become disproportion-

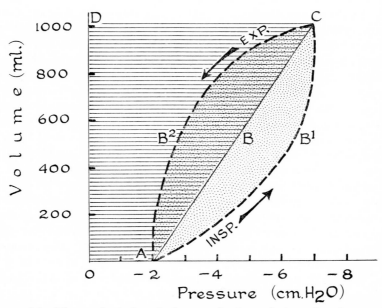

FIGURE 16. The mechanical work done on the lungs during a breathing cycle.

ately greater when the ventilation increases. It is probable that the disturbances in the mechanical properties of the lung and the resultant
increase in mechanical work limit the activity of a patient.

THE RELATIONSHIP BETWEEN MECHANICAL WORK AND ALVEOLAR VENTILATION

There would also appear to be a relationship between the mechanical work of breathing and the rate and depth at which a person
breathes. For any given alveolar ventilation there is an optimum respiratory rate and tidal volume during which the total mechanical work of
breathing is minimal. Both normal subjects and patients with respiratory
disease appear to breathe at a rate and depth at which the work of
breathing is least. When the elastic resistance becomes increased, as in
pulmonary fibrosis or kyphoscoliosis, the respirations tend to become
rapid and shallow, probably because of the increase in mechanical work
which is required to overcome the elastic resistance with even small
increases in tidal volume. On the other hand, when the nonelastic resistance becomes increased, as in diffuse bronchial obstruction, the respirations tend to become slower and deeper, because a faster respiratory
rate leads to an increase in the resistance to air flow.

THE OXYGEN COST OF BREATHING

In order to perform the mechanical work necessary for breathing,
the respiratory muscles require oxygen. During quiet breathing the total
oxygen consumption of the body is between 200 and 300 ml./min. The
oxygen consumption of the respiratory muscles alone has been estimated
by determining the difference in the oxygen consumption during breathing at rest and during increased ventilation (Fig. 17). In such an experi-
ment, the nonrespiratory oxygen consumption is estimated by extending
the calculation backwards to a situation in which there is no ventilation
at all. The difference between the total oxygen consumption and the
nonrespiratory oxygen consumption at any level of ventilation, therefore,
represents the oxygen consumption of the respiratory muscles at that
ventilation. The oxygen cost of breathing at rest varies from 0.3 to 1.9
ml./l. ventilation in the normal subject. This is about 2 per cent of the
total oxygen consumption. In the resting emphysematous subject, on the
other hand, the oxygen cost of breathing is between 3.0 and 18.0 ml./l.
ventilation, which may amount to as much as 50 per cent of the total
oxygen consumption.

Figure 17 illustrates the change in oxygen consumption associated
with increases in ventilation in both a normal subject and a patient with
bronchiolar obstruction. It shows that normal subjects are able to increase

their ventilation considerably without much alteration in the total oxygen consumption. On the other hand, the oxygen consumption rises considerably with small increases in ventilation in patients in whom the resistance to air flow is high. In addition, even in the normal subject, there is a level of ventilation at which the oxygen consumption rises disproportionately when the ventilation is further increased. During moderate increases in ventilation it may amount to about 5 per cent of the total metabolism. During strenuous exercise, when the total oxygen consumption is ten times greater than that at rest, as much as 20 per cent of the oxygen consumed may be required for the respiratory muscles alone. When there is an obstruction to the flow of air, this disproportionate increase in the oxygen consumption occurs at a much lower level of ventilation.

The high oxygen cost of breathing associated with an increased ventilation during severe exercise in normal subjects and in patients suffering from diffuse bronchial obstruction while resting is extremely important clinically. If the oxygen consumption of the respiratory muscles is high, little oxygen is available for the other muscles of the body, particularly during exercise, and this may be a limiting factor, especially for patients suffering from respiratory disease.

In addition, a level of increased ventilation may be reached during which the tendency to lower the alveolar carbon dioxide tension is offset by the increased metabolic production of carbon dioxide by the respiratory muscles. Although a subject could voluntarily increase his ventilation still further, it would serve no useful purpose, greater ventilations merely increasing the tendency towards carbon dioxide retention. This

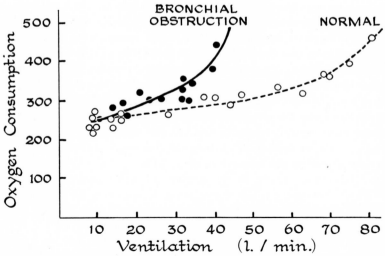

FIGURE 17. The changes in oxygen consumption associated with increases of ventilation in a normal subject and a patient with bronchial obstruction.

has been estimated to occur in normal persons at a ventilation of about 140 l./min. On the other hand, in patients with an increased oxygen cost of breathing, the level of ventilation which is maximally effective in lowering the partial pressure of carbon dioxide may be as low as 15 to 20 l./min.

EFFICIENCY OF THE RESPIRATORY MUSCLES

In order to calculate the efficiency of the respiratory muscles, one must know the total mechanical work of breathing and the oxygen consumption of the respiratory muscles at a given ventilation. The formula for estimating this is:

$$\text{Efficiency (per cent)} = \frac{\text{Mechanical work (kg. m.)}}{\text{Oxygen cost (kg. m.)}} \times 100$$

The total mechanical work of breathing performed on the lungs can be approximately determined by using the esophageal pressure as an index of the intrathoracic pressure. The total work performed in moving the lung, chest wall and abdominal contents, however, cannot be directly measured in the spontaneously breathing subject. On the other hand, the efficiency with which an added respiratory work load is handled may be calculated by measuring the extra oxygen which is consumed while the subject breathes through a known inspiratory resistance. By this method, the efficiency of the respiratory muscles in normal subjects has been found to vary between 5 and 10 per cent. The mechanical efficiency of the respiratory muscles is therefore low, even in the normal person, being much lower than that reported for other forms of muscular work. The respiratory muscles of the patient with chronic obstructive emphysema are not doing more work at rest than are those of a normal subject, but the oxygen cost of performing this work is much greater, indicating that the efficiency of the patient's respiratory muscles is reduced, being between 1 and 3 per cent. Although the mechanism of reduction in efficiency of the respiratory muscles in chronic obstructive emphysema has not been elucidated, it is possibly due to the altered resting level in this condition, the mechanical advantage of the respiratory muscles being reduced in the inspiratory position.

CHAPTER II

The Distribution of Gas and Blood and Gaseous Exchange

DURING inspiration, fresh air enters the respiratory tract, becomes humidified and heated to body temperature, and is mixed with the gas which is already present in the tracheobronchial tree. This gas, in turn, then enters the alveoli and mixes further with the gas which is present in the alveoli. During expiration, the air from the tracheobronchial tree is followed out of the lungs by the mixed gas from the alveoli. In this way, oxygen is added to the air in the alveoli, and the carbon dioxide which has been transferred from the pulmonary capillary blood to the alveoli is then expired into the atmosphere.

THE DISTRIBUTION OF GAS

In young healthy persons, and particularly in older persons, the inspired air is not distributed uniformly throughout the lungs. There are probably several reasons for this. Since the degree of inspiratory movement of the upper part of the chest cage is less than that of the lower part, the amount of inspired air reaching the upper lobes is probably less than that going to the lower lobes. In addition, it has been suggested that there is a sequential distribution of the inspired gas, the gas entering and leaving some areas of the lung before it reaches others.

In addition to the mild nonuniformity of gas distribution, which can be attributed to the unequal movements of different portions of the chest cage, the distribution of the inspired gas is affected by regional alterations in the mechanical resistances offered by the lung, the airways and the extrapulmonary structures. The effect of local airway resistance is illustrated in Figure 18, which represents the moment-to-moment concentration of nitrogen in the expired air following a single inspiration of pure oxygen. Where there is no obstruction (Fig. 18, A), the inspired gas

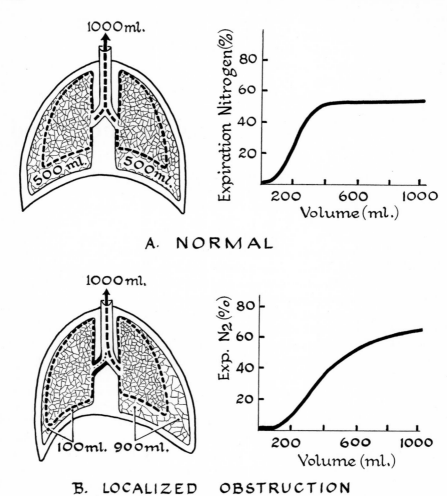

FIGURE 18.   The effect of a localized airway obstruction on the distribution of air.

enters both lungs almost synchronously and equally. Expiration also takes place in the same fashion. The gas from the dead space is washed out initially and is followed by an equal amount from each lung. As a result, there is an almost definite plateau in the curve of the nitrogen concentration. The very slight rise in the plateau is probably due to sequential ventilation of different areas of the lungs. In Figure 18, *B,* the inspired oxygen is asynchronously and unequally distributed because the oxygen moves into and distends those areas of lung which offer the least resistance before it enters the others. The nitrogen in the nonobstructed lung is, therefore, well diluted by the oxygen, but that in the obstructed lung is not. During expiration, air moves out of the unobstructed lung first, but that from the obstructed lung is delayed. The asynchronous delivery of air from the two lungs results in a rising alveolar plateau of the nitrogen concentration curve, and, in addition, the record suggests an enlarged dead space. Regional alterations of the elastic resistance or the tissue viscous resistance alter the distribution of gas in a similar manner.

A change in posture also affects the manner in which inspired air is distributed. Even in a normal subject, the distribution is less uniform in the supine position than it is in the upright position, and it is altered still further when the subject lies with his head lower than the rest of the body. When the subject lies in the lateral recumbent position, the gas distribution has been demonstrated to be more uneven in the upper lung than in the lower one.

Several methods are used to investigate the manner in which the inspired air is distributed within the lung. In general, a relatively insoluble reference gas, such as helium or hydrogen, is inspired so that any variations in the pulmonary blood flow or the diffusion of gas do not influence the measurement. The manner in which the inspired gas is distributed can be estimated by measuring the rate at which the nitrogen in the lung is diluted during the inhalation of oxygen or helium, or the rate at which the lung and a spirometer reach equilibrium with respect to a foreign gas, such as helium or hydrogen.

The simplest technique is the former, in which the elimination of nitrogen is studied by means of an instantaneously recording nitrogen meter while the subject is breathing 100 per cent oxygen for seven minutes. Figure 19 illustrates the types of records which are obtained from a normal subject and a patient suffering from chronic obstructive emphysema when this technique is used. Since pure oxygen is being inhaled, the nitrogen in the lung is progressively diluted, so that the concentration of the expired nitrogen falls with each breath. The rate of fall depends upon the manner in which the oxygen is distributed throughout the lung. In the normal record, the concentration of nitrogen in the expired air drops very quickly immediately after the subject starts to breathe oxygen. It then continues to fall uniformly, but at a much slower rate. At the end of the seven minutes, the nitrogen concentration of the final portion of a maximal expiration is low in a normal subject, indicating that the nitrogen in the lung has become well diluted. The nitrogen concentration of the gas in this alveolar sample is called the *index of intrapulmonary mixing*. If the index is greater than 2 per cent, it is considered to be indicative of an abnormal distribution of inspired gas, because it indicates that the nitrogen within the lung has not been well diluted.

The distribution of inspired air is particularly abnormal in many patients with chronic respiratory disease; poorly ventilated and hyper-

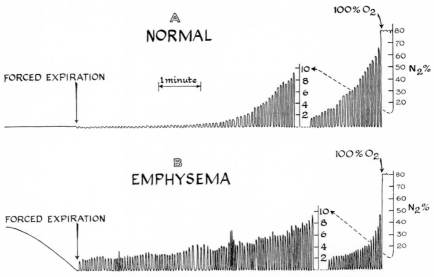

FIGURE 19.   The washout of nitrogen from the lung during the inhalation of
100 per cent oxygen in a normal subject (A) and a patient with chronic obstructive
emphysema (B). The records read from right to left, and the scale is increased fivefold
when the nitrogen concentration has fallen below 10 per cent.

ventilated areas may co-exist side by side. In the record obtained from a
patient with chronic obstructive emphysema, there is also an initial rapid
dilution of the nitrogen after the patient starts to breathe oxygen. This is
followed by a slower rate of dilution which does not take place uniformly.
In addition, the nitrogen concentration of a forced expiration at the end
of seven minutes is very high, indicating that the forced expiration is
squeezing air out of portions of the lung which have not been well diluted
by the pure oxygen. The analysis of these records is discussed further in
Chapter XVIII.

      An abnormal distribution of inspired gas is encountered clinically
in a variety of respiratory defects, such as a regional loss of elasticity
with a resultant inequality of elastic properties in different areas of the
lung, such as occurs in chronic obstructive emphysema; or a regional
increase in resistance to pulmonary distention, such as occurs when
there is pulmonary congestion or exudate in the alveoli or alteration of
the architecture of the lung by fibrosis, tumors or kyphoscoliosis. In addition, the distribution of gas is altered by regional variations in the airway
resistance, as in bronchial asthma, chronic bronchitis, bronchiectasis and
chronic obstructive emphysema, or in the forces applied to the chest wall
by the respiratory muscles, as in muscular dystrophy or local muscular
weakness or paralysis.

GASEOUS EXCHANGE

PROPERTIES OF GASES

Before we discuss the gaseous exchange in the lungs, an explanation of certain physical properties of gases is essential. One of the most important actions of any gas is the exertion of pressure on its surroundings. If a volume of gas is placed in a container, the gas expands until it fills the container, because the gaseous molecules travel at great speed throughout the container. The gas exerts a pressure which is dependent on the amount of bombardment on the walls of the containing vessel by the gaseous molecules. According to Boyle's law, the pressure rises if the capacity of the container is reduced because the molecules of gas are closer together and cause a greater bombardment on the walls of the container. Similarly, according to Gay-Lussac's law, the pressure of a gas is proportionate to its temperature if the volume is kept constant. The pressure rises when the temperature of the gas is elevated, because the speed of molecular movement increases, causing greater bombardment of the molecules on the boundaries of the confining space.

Another faculty possessed by gases is that of diffusion. As the gaseous molecules move about at great speed in all directions, they eventually are evenly distributed throughout the confining space, so that the pressure of the gas is the same throughout. If a mixture of two or more gases is confined within the same space, each gas behaves independently, as if it alone were in that space. The molecules of each gas are uniformly distributed throughout the mixture of gases, and the pressure of each gas depends on its own concentration, regardless of the concentration of the other gases.

The pressure which any one gas exerts, whether alone or mixed with other gases, is called the *partial pressure,* or the *tension,* of that gas. It is indicated by the small letter "p" preceding the symbol for the gas. For example, the partial pressure of oxygen is denoted by pO_2 and that of carbon dioxide by pCO_2. The total pressure exerted by a mixture of gases is the arithmetical sum of the partial pressures of all the different gases which make up the mixture. The total pressure of air at sea level, which is 760 mm. Hg, is the sum of the partial pressures of the oxygen, the carbon dioxide, the nitrogen and the inert gases, such as argon and neon, which it contains. Since there is approximately 20.94 per cent oxygen, 0.04 per cent carbon dioxide and 79 per cent nitrogen in ambient air, their partial pressures are 159, 0.3 and 600 mm. Hg, respectively. The remainder of the atmospheric pressure is due to the traces of inert gases which are present.

When the partial pressure of a gas is different in two parts of a system, a *diffusion gradient* exists between the two parts. The gas, therefore, diffuses from the area in which its partial pressure is high to that in which its partial pressure is low. If the system is left undisturbed, the diffusion of the gas continues until its partial pressure is the same in both parts of the system. The rate at which the gas diffuses depends upon the nature of the barrier between the two parts of the system, the diffusing properties of the gas involved and the steepness of the diffusion gradient.

ALVEOLAR AND ARTERIAL GAS TENSIONS

As the air is inspired into the lungs and is carried toward the alveolar spaces, it becomes saturated with water vapor, which evaporates from the surfaces of the tissues. Water vapor is similar to any other gas, in that it exerts a partial pressure and behaves independently from the other gases in a mixture. On the other hand, since it is in equilibrium with the liquid phase, it behaves differently from other gases in one respect: Its partial pressure depends almost completely on the temperature and is almost independent of the barometric pressure. At normal body temperature, the partial pressure of water vapor is 47 mm. Hg.

The total pressure of the gases in the alveolar air corresponds to that of the ambient barometric pressure. Owing to the presence of water vapor, the total pressure of dry alveolar gas is equal to that of the barometric pressure minus 47 mm. Hg. Whenever alveolar air or expired air is analyzed, it is reported in terms of the dry gas. In other words, in order to determine the partial pressure of an alveolar gas, we multiply its concentration by the barometric pressure minus 47.

Thus, $pA = C_A \times$ (barometric pressure $- 47$)

where p represents the partial pressure, and C the concentration, of the alveolar gas, A.

Since the concentration of oxygen in the alveolar air is approximately 14 per cent, that of carbon dioxide approximately 6 per cent and that of nitrogen approximately 80 per cent, their respective partial pressures are approximately 103, 40 and 570 mm. Hg. It must be pointed out that although the respiratory gases in the alveoli are commonly thought of as having specific concentrations, these concentrations are, in fact, changing from moment to moment, as well as being different in various parts of the lung. The moment-to-moment changes in alveolar gas concentration are related to the different phases of the respiratory cycle, whereas the differences in various parts of the lung are related to variations in the ventilation-perfusion ratios of the different alveoli, which will be discussed later. Any stated value for alveolar gas concentration is some sort of average figure, therefore, and cannot describe the actual situation in all parts of the lung.

Normally the air which enters the alveoli takes part in gaseous exchange with the mixed venous blood in the pulmonary capillaries. In this way, the gas tensions of the blood in the pulmonary veins become approximately equilibrated with the gas tensions of the alveolar air, and "arterialized" blood leaves the alveolus (Fig. 20). The partial pressures of oxygen and carbon dioxide of the blood coming to the pulmonary capillaries are 40 and 46 mm. Hg, respectively, and those of the blood leaving the alveoli and entering the pulmonary veins are 100 and 40 mm. Hg, respectively.

In normal persons, the correlation between ventilation and perfusion is remarkably good throughout the lungs, and the arterial partial pressure of carbon dioxide is approximately the same as the alveolar carbon dioxide tension, as measured by the end-expiration sampling technique. In patients, the alveolar partial pressure of carbon dioxide must be estimated by an indirect method because direct alveolar sampling techniques, such as the collection of end-expiratory samples, cannot be relied upon to give representative values for alveolar air in patients whose alveolar gases vary in different parts of the lungs. Since the arterial blood contains contributions from all the perfused alveoli, and therefore acts as a physiologic integrator, the arterial carbon dioxide tension has been used to estimate the mean alveolar carbon dioxide tension. The assumption that the arterial partial pressure of carbon dioxide is approximately equal to the mean alveolar carbon dioxide tension is justified, provided the alveolar carbon dioxide tension is defined as the mean partial pressure of carbon dioxide of all the alveoli which are perfused.

The alveolar oxygen tension is not the same as that of the systemic

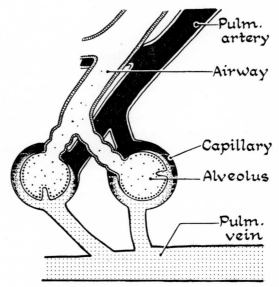

FIGURE 20. The normal distribution of gas and blood.

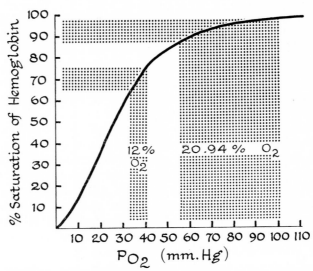

FIGURE 21.   The effect of admixture of venous blood on the arterial partial pressure of oxygen while breathing room air and 12 per cent oxygen.

arterial blood even in normal subjects. The difference in the partial pressure of oxygen between the alveolar air and the arterial blood is the resultant of several factors usually grouped together into two main components. Part of the gradient is due to the difference between the alveolus and the end of the capillary, the *membrane component,* which is the result of a resistance to diffusion. The remainder of the gradient is due to the difference between the end of the capillary and any peripheral artery, the *venous admixture component,* which is due to the admixture of poorly oxygenated blood distal to the end of the capillary. An uneven distribution of gas and blood is included in this component.

It has been shown that the diffusing capacity of oxygen and the gradient for oxygen between the alveoli and the systemic artery are not changed by breathing a hypoxic gas mixture. On the other hand, when this mixture is breathed, the effect of any venous admixture on the arterial oxygen tension is markedly reduced, so that there is an increase in the proportion of that part of the gradient which is due to the difference between the alveoli and the end of the pulmonary capillary. This is explained by the shape of the oxyhemoglobin dissociation curve, which defines the relationship between the partial pressure of oxygen and the oxygen saturation of the hemoglobin. Figure 21 demonstrates that when air is being breathed, a decrease in the arterial oxygen saturation of 10 per cent, resulting from the admixture of venous blood, is associated with a considerable fall in oxygen tension. On the other hand, when 12 per cent oxygen is inhaled, the same amount of venous admixture is associated with only a slight fall in oxygen tension because of the steepness of the dissociation curve. This indicates that the major portion of any difference between the alveolar and arterial oxygen tensions at low levels of oxygenation is due to the membrane component and that the venous admixture component contributes most of the difference at normal or high levels of oxygenation. This information is extremely important, for it is used in the assessment of venous admixture or the diffusing properties of the lungs.

Whenever the gas exchange in the lungs becomes inadequate in a patient suffering from respiratory disease, the arterial partial pressure of oxygen falls. A lower than normal arterial oxygen tension may be due to either one or several different alterations of respiratory function: (1) There may be a hypoventilation of the alveoli in relation to the metabolism. In this situation the hypoxia is associated with carbon dioxide retention, as evidenced by a high partial pressure of carbon dioxide in the arterial blood. (2) There may be uneven ventilation-perfusion ratios in different areas of the lungs. When this occurs, the arterial carbon dioxide tension may be decreased, normal or increased, depending on the ability of the individual to hyperventilate in response to the hypoxia. (3) There may be a shunting of venous blood into the arterial system through either an intrapulmonary or an intracardiac communciation. In these conditions, the arterial carbon dioxide tension is generally normal or decreased because the lungs are usually healthy and capable of compensatory hyperventilation. (4) Finally, there may be an increased barrier to diffusion. In such cases, the arterial carbon dioxide tension is frequently low, because of the easy diffusibility of this gas and the hyperventilation induced by the hypoxia.

ALVEOLAR VENTILATION

Practically, the all-important portion of the air that is inspired is that which is concerned in the exchange of gases with the blood. Gaseous exchange occurs only in the alveoli and not in those parts of the respiratory system which serve as the conducting airway.

DEAD SPACE

The mouth, the nose, the pharynx, the larynx, the trachea, the bronchi and the bronchioles are collectively called the *anatomic dead space.* Functionally, however, the dead space is a physiologic concept, not an anatomic one, and it may be defined as that volume of the inspired gas which does not take part in gaseous exchange. The *physiologic dead space,* therefore, includes the volume of the inspired gas which occupies the anatomic dead space and the volume which ventilates alveoli that are not perfused by capillary blood flow. On the other hand, there really is not such a sharp division between the ventilation of the dead space and the alveoli, because if some areas of lung are overventilated, even though normally perfused, they contribute to the dead space. In addition, some diffusion of gas probably takes place from the tracheobronchial tree into the alveoli.

In healthy persons the volumes of the anatomic and the physiologic dead spaces are almost identical. The physiologic dead space, which is approximately 150 ml. in healthy young males at rest, has been shown to increase with exercise or an increase in the tidal volume. Because of the dead space, a healthy person utilizes only about 70 to 80 per cent of each tidal volume for gaseous exchange. In patients suffering from pulmonary disease, however, there is ventilation of alveoli whose perfusion is inadequate or absent, and hyperventilation of other alveoli which are normally perfused. As a result, the physiologic dead space is increased. In these patients, therefore, a considerably smaller proportion of the inspired air is available for the oxygenation of and removal of carbon dioxide from the pulmonary capillary blood.

Measurements of the physiologic dead space are based on *Bohr's formula,* which states that the expired air consists of a mixture of two components, each with a particular composition: a component from the physiologic dead space, and an alveolar component which has given up oxygen and received carbon dioxide.

$$\text{Thus, } V_T \times C_T = (V_D \times C_D) + (V_A \times C_A)$$

where V represents a gas volume and C a gas concentration, the subscripts signifying the specific gas volume referred to, T being tidal gas, D dead space gas, and A alveolar gas.

For instance, if a tidal volume of 600 ml. of air which contains 20.94 per cent oxygen were inspired, and the concentration of oxygen were 16 per cent and 14 per cent in the expired and alveolar air, respectively, the dead space can be calculated:

$$16\% \ (600) = 20.94\% \ D + 14\% \ (600 - D)$$
$$D = 179 \text{ ml.}$$

From knowledge of the frequency of respiration per minute (f) and the tidal volume (V_T), the minute ventilation (V_E) can be calculated:

$$V_E = V_T \times f$$

The alveolar component of the tidal volume consists of the quantity of air which remains after the dead space volume has been subtracted from the tidal volume. The alveolar ventilation per minute (V_A) can, therefore, be calculated from the formula:

$$V_A = (V_T - V_D) \times f$$

TABLE 2

EFFECT OF RESPIRATORY RATE AND TIDAL VOLUME ON ALVEOLAR VENTILA-
TION, WHEN MINUTE VENTILATION AND DEAD SPACE ARE CONSTANT

V_E (l./min.)	V_D (ml.)	V_T (ml.)	f	V_A (l./min.)
8.0	150	1000	8	6.8
8.0	150	500	16	5.6
8.0	150	250	32	3.2

Even though the minute ventilation is kept constant, the alveolar ventilation is altered by changes in respiratory frequency. This is illustrated in Table 2, representing a subject in whom the dead space is 150 ml. and the ventilation is 8 l./min.

It can be seen that as the respiratory rate increases, the alveolar ventilation decreases. Similarly, the alveolar ventilation falls if the tidal volume diminishes, despite a constant minute ventilation. Clinically, alveolar hypoventilation is found frequently in patients who are breathing shallowly and rapidly, such as those suffering from severe obesity or kyphoscoliosis.

Table 3 demonstrates that the alveolar ventilation per minute also decreases if the dead space is increased and the minute ventilation and the respiratory rate remain constant. This situation arises particularly in patients with chronic obstructive emphysema, in whom the physiologic dead space is large. An increase in the tidal volume would normally compensate for the effect of an enlarged dead space, but the capacity for such an increase is frequently diminished in patients with chronic respiratory disease.

An increase in the dead space or a decrease in the tidal volume, therefore, results in the same net effect, namely, a reduction in the alveolar ventilation, with consequent effects on the arterial blood gas tensions. If an increase in the dead space and a decrease in the tidal volume should occur simultaneously, the situation would, of course, become severely aggravated.

TABLE 3

EFFECT OF INCREASE IN DEAD SPACE ON ALVEOLAR VENTILATION, WHEN
MINUTE VENTILATION AND RESPIRATORY RATE ARE CONSTANT

V_E (l./min.)	V_D (ml.)	V_T (ml.)	f	V_A (l./min.)
8.0	150	500	16	5.6
8.0	200	500	16	4.8
8.0	250	500	16	4.0

Clinically, it is often difficult to estimate the adequacy of alveolar ventilation, but an accurate estimate can be made in the laboratory by measuring the minute ventilation and the concentration of carbon dioxide in the expired and alveolar gases. The alveolar ventilation is also calculated from the Bohr equation. Since the concentration of carbon dioxide in the dead space is zero, the equation becomes:

$$V_E C_E = V_A C_A$$

where V is the volume and C the gas concentration, the subscript E signifying the expired minute ventilation, and A the alveolar ventilation.

For instance, if the minute ventilation is 6 l./min. and the concentrations of carbon dioxide are 4 per cent and 6 per cent in the expired and alveolar gases, the alveolar ventilation is:

$$4\% \ (6) = 6\% \ V_A \text{ or } 4 \text{ l./min.}$$

It should be pointed out that even though the alveolar ventilation may be adequate while at rest, it is frequently inadequate during exercise in patients with respiratory disease.

VENTILATION-PERFUSION RATIOS

Just as it is essential to know the volume and the distribution of the alveolar ventilation, a knowledge of the volume and the distribution of the pulmonary capillary blood flow is equally important. Although the distribution of inspired gas can be measured by using nitrogen or other inert gases which are not affected by perfusion, the distribution of the pulmonary capillary blood flow to the various alveoli cannot be measured. The tests which have been used to measure uneven ventilation are inadequate by themselves, for a uniform ventilation does not necessarily mean that there is a uniform perfusion of the alveoli or that the ratio between ventilation and perfusion of the alveoli is the same in the different areas of the lung. The ratio of the alveolar ventilation to the pulmonary capillary blood flow, or the perfusion, in each part of the lung plays an important role in determining the degree of oxygenation of the pulmonary venous blood. Under basal conditions, the ventilation-perfusion ratio of the whole lung is 0.8; in other words, when the alveolar ventilation is 4 l./min. the pulmonary blood flow is 5 l./min. Nevertheless, the absolute value of this ratio for the whole lung is relatively unimportant, for it is essential to know whether the same ratio exists in all parts of the lung. If it does, the blood is maximally oxygenated. Hypoxia develops if the ratio of the alveolar ventilation to the perfusion is not uniform throughout the lungs, even though the total alveolar ventilation, the total pulmonary blood flow and the diffusion of gases may be normal. As a result of variations in the ventilation-perfusion ratios throughout the lung, there is an increase in the difference between the alveolar and the arterial partial pressures of oxygen, which is called the alveolar-arterial or A-a gradient. This is an increase in the over-all difference between the mixed alveolar gas and the mixed pulmonary capillary blood. There is no essential difference between the partial pressures of a particular alveolus and that of its end-pulmonary capillary blood.

Unfortunately, there are no simple tests of the distribution of pulmonary blood flow, and it can only be indirectly assessed. It is possible, however, to derive a rough estimate of the relationship between the ventilation and the perfusion of the alveoli. Bronchospirometry is a method by which the oxygen uptake of each lung can be determined. Normally, 55 per cent of the total oxygen uptake takes place in the right lung, and the left lung takes up 45 per cent. Since oxygen can be taken up only by the pulmonary capillary blood, deviations from these values with no change in ventilation may signify that the blood flow is uneven. In the lateral recumbent position, there is a rise in the oxygen uptake of the lower lung, presumably because the blood flow increases in the dependent lung. When the body posture is changed from the supine to the erect position, there is a fall in both the ventilation and the perfusion of the upper lobes. The perfusion is particularly affected. It has been estimated that there is practically no blood flow through the upper lobes of the lungs when a person is in the erect position. In this position, the greatest portion of the blood flows through the basal parts of the lungs; in the supine position the maximal blood flow takes place through the dorsal portions of the lungs.

A continuous analysis of the concentration of the carbon dioxide in the expired gas yields valuable information about the ratio of the pulmonary blood flow to the ventilation in the different areas of the lungs. If the last part of the expired alveolar gas contains only a slightly greater concentration of carbon dioxide than its initial portion, the ratios are nearly uniform throughout the lungs. If the last part of the expired alveolar gas contains a much higher content of carbon dioxide than its initial portion, the ventilation-perfusion ratios must vary in the different areas of lung. The early part of the expiration must have come from a region with a high ratio and the late part of expiration from a region with a low ratio.

VENOUS-ADMIXTURE-LIKE PERFUSION

When there is perfusion of inadequately ventilated alveoli, as is illustrated in Figure 22, *A*, or in the extreme case, perfusion of nonventilated alveoli, a low ventilation-perfusion ratio is present. Under such circumstances, a portion of the pulmonary blood is only slightly aerated, if at all. This poorly aerated venous blood leaves the pulmonary capillary and then mixes with fully "arterialized" blood coming from the other pulmonary capillaries. This venous-admixture-like perfusion leads to hypoxia and carbon dioxide retention in the arterial blood. Carbon dioxide retention may not develop, however, if there is sufficient hyperventilation of the remaining well-perfused alveoli. On the other hand, owing to the shape of the oxyhemoglobin dissociation curve, hyperventilation by itself does not correct arterial hypoxia to any significant degree.

DEAD-SPACE-LIKE VENTILATION

Whenever the ventilation of alveoli is maintained but the blood perfusion is limited (Fig. 22, *B*), or in the extreme case, when there is no perfusion, a high ventilation-perfusion ratio is present. The gas entering these alveoli takes little part, if any, in the gaseous exchange. The gas leaving such alveoli, therefore, tends to have the same composition as the gas in the tracheobronchial tree, thus contributing physiologically to the dead space. This is called *dead-space-like ventilation.* The blood that perfuses these alveoli becomes fully oxygenated and probably excessively depleted of carbon dioxide. However, the quantity of blood flowing through the vessels which perfuse these alveoli is so small that the total gas exchange is minimal. A greater than normal burden, there-

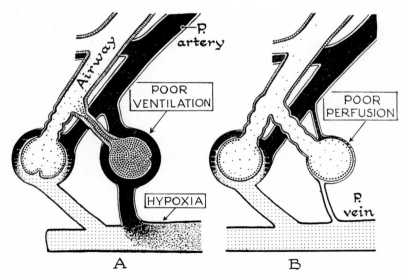

FIGURE 22. The effect of alterations of ventilation-perfusion ratios on gas exchange. Venous-admixture-like perfusion (A) and dead-space-like ventilation (B).

fore, falls on the other alveoli. Adequate oxygenation and carbon dioxide elimination, as evidenced by the presence of normal arterial oxygen and carbon dioxide tensions, may occur in the presence of excessive dead-space-like ventilation, but only if the normally perfused alveoli are hyperventilated. Such a compensatory hyperventilation is observed clinically, probably because of the increased stimulation of the chemo-receptors by the hypoxia and hypercapnia.

Disturbances in the ventilation-perfusion ratios are predominant in patients suffering from chronic obstructive pulmonary emphysema. In the early stages, compensatory hyperventilation may insure an adequate effective alveolar ventilation, so that the arterial carbon dioxide tension may be normal, despite the presence of hypoxia. In the later stages, however, because of the mechanical disturbances in the lungs, the patient is frequently unable to increase his ventilation sufficiently to provide an adequate alveolar ventilation. Under these circumstances, the low arterial partial pressure of oxygen is associated with a high partial pressure of carbon dioxide.

TRUE VENOUS ADMIXTURE

A lower than normal arterial oxygen tension may also occur when mixed venous blood which has not come into contact with alveoli enters and mixes with blood in the pulmonary vein or the systemic circulation. This situation, called *true venous admixture,* is illustrated in Figure 23. Even in normal persons approximately 2.5 per cent of the total pul-

FIGURE 23. The effect of true venous admixture on gas exchange.

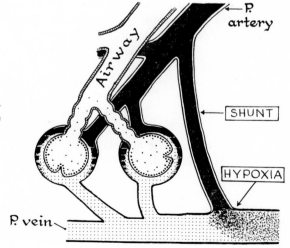

monary blood flow enters the arterialized systemic circulation by means of the thebesian and the bronchial veins which empty into the left side of the heart and the pulmonary veins. There is an increase in the amount of true venous admixture in those congenital heart diseases in which blood is shunted from the right side of the heart to the left side and in pulmonary arteriovenous aneurysm, in which blood is shunted from the pulmonary artery to the pulmonary vein. As a result, considerable arterial hypoxia is present in such situations, but because the lungs themselves are usually healthy, no carbon dioxide retention develops. In fact, the hypoxia frequently leads to hyperventilation with resultant hypocapnia.

The amount of mixed venous blood which is being shunted into the systemic circulation can be assessed by measuring the oxygen saturation of the arterial blood while the subject is breathing 100 per cent oxygen. Under such circumstances, all the blood coming in contact with the alveoli is maximally oxygenated. In the absence of a true venous admixture, the inhalation of pure oxygen results in complete saturation of the arterial blood, whereas if a shunt is present, the saturation remains incomplete despite the fact that pure oxygen is being inhaled. The degree of unsaturation, and therefore the difference between the alveolar and the arterial partial pressures of oxygen, depends upon the amount of true venous admixture.

If the arterial oxygen tension is lowered by the inhalation of gas mixtures which are low in oxygen, the effect of venous admixture on the partial pressure of oxygen is diminished. As was described earlier, this is due to the shape of the oxyhemoglobin dissociation curve, which is flat at high levels of oxygenation and steep at low levels. The difference between the alveolar and arterial partial pressures of oxygen which results from true venous admixture therefore becomes smaller at low levels of oxygenation. A large difference between the alveolar and the arterial oxygen tensions under such circumstances is almost entirely due to a barrier to the diffusion of oxygen.

DIFFUSION OF GAS

Even though the alveolar ventilation and the ventilation-perfusion ratios are both normal, and no venous admixture is present, the arterial oxygen tension may still be low. Under such circumstances, there is probably an abnormal barrier to the diffusion of oxygen from the alveoli into the pulmonary capillary blood, so that the *diffusing capacity* of the lungs is reduced. This is illustrated in Figure 24, which shows that all the blood which is perfusing the alveoli has not become fully oxygenated.

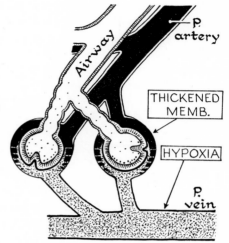

FIGURE 24. The effect of a diffusion
defect on gas exchange.

THE ALVEOLOCAPILLARY MEMBRANE

The tissue fluid barrier across which the respiratory gases diffuse normally includes the alveolar membrane, the capillary endothelium, the blood plasma, the wall of the red cell and the intracellular fluid which separates the molecules of hemoglobin in the red cell. These are usually considered together as a single *alveolocapillary membrane.*

THE DIFFUSING PROPERTIES OF THE GASES

The rate of diffusion of a gas from its gas phase into its liquid phase is directly proportional to its solubility in the liquid and inversely proportional to the square root of its molecular weight. The gases which take part in the gaseous exchange across the alveolocapillary membrane are oxygen and carbon dioxide. Carbon dioxide, which is twenty-five times more soluble than oxygen in saline but has a larger molecular weight, diffuses about twenty times more rapidly through the alveolocapillary membrane than does oxygen.

THE DIFFUSION GRADIENT

The rate at which a gas diffuses across a barrier is also directly proportional to the partial pressure gradient or difference between its partial pressures on either side of the barrier. The difference in partial pressures across the alveolocapillary membrane is greatest at the point where the venous blood enters the capillary and least at the point where the blood leaves the capillary. The size of the partial pressure gradient along the alveolocapillary membrane is dependent on the slope of the

PULMONARY

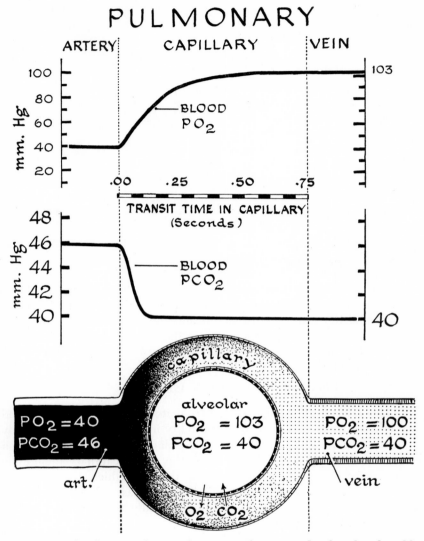

FIGURE 25.   The change in the partial pressures of oxygen and carbon dioxide as blood passes along the pulmonary capillary.

dissociation curve for each gas. This is illustrated in Figure 25, which shows the changes in the partial pressures of oxygen and carbon dioxide in the blood as it passes along the lung capillary, a process which has been estimated to take approximately 0.75 second at rest. The slope of the oxyhemoglobin dissociation curve is steep at low levels of oxygenation and relatively flat at high levels. The exchange of oxygen from the alveolus to the capillary, therefore, takes place first in the steep portion and then in the flat part of the dissociation curve. Since the initial oxygen pressure gradient is very large, oxygen moves rapidly from the alveoli to the capillaries, and about 95 per cent of the diffusion of oxygen takes place before the blood has passed halfway along the capillary. The equilibration of the partial pressure of oxygen on either side of the membrane takes place during the remaining half of the transit time in the capillaries. Very little gradient exists normally at the end of the capillary, so that the partial pressure of oxygen in the pulmonary vein is almost equal to that in the alveolus.

The carbon dioxide dissociation curve is steep at all levels, and it is estimated that the equilibration of carbon dioxide between the alveolus and the capillary takes place in about 0.072 second. Since carbon dioxide diffuses across the alveolocapillary membrane 20 times faster than does oxygen, it is likely that no significant gradient for carbon dioxide ever develops, because an over-all resistance to diffusion which is great enough to cause a significant carbon dioxide gradient would be associated with such a fantastic oxygen diffusion gradient that survival would be impossible.

Oxygen and carbon monoxide, which have a great affinity for hemoglobin, have proved to be most satisfactory for the qualitative estimation of the diffusing capacity of the lungs. In order to calculate the diffusing capacity of the lungs for a specific gas, it is necessary to know the amount of gas which is diffusing across the alveolocapillary membrane per minute as well as the mean gradient of its partial pressures between the alveolus and the pulmonary capillary. This is indicated in the following formulae:

$$D_{O_2} = \frac{\dot{V}_{O_2}}{P_{\overline{A-C}}}$$

and

$$D_{CO} = \frac{\dot{V}_{CO}}{P_{\overline{A-C}}}$$

where D is the diffusing capacity of the particular gas, oxygen or carbon monoxide, in ml./mm. Hg./min.; $\dot{V}$ is the volume of the gas which is diffusing per minute; and $P_{\overline{A-C}}$ is the mean pressure gradient between the alveolus and the capillary of that particular gas.

THE VOLUME OF THE DIFFUSING GAS

The amount of oxygen or carbon monoxide which diffuses across the alveolocapillary membrane in one minute can be determined by estimating the difference between the amount of gas which is inhaled and the amount which is exhaled. The formula for the calculation of the oxygen consumption is:

$$\dot{V}_{O_2} = V_E \left(F_{I_{O_2}} \times \frac{F_{E_{N_2}}}{F_{I_{N_2}}} - F_{E_{O_2}} \right)$$

where $\dot{V}_{O_2}$ is the oxygen consumption per minute, V_E the expired ventilation, and F the concentration of the particular gas in the inspired air (I) and the expired air (E).

Similarly, the amount of carbon monoxide which diffuses across the alveolocapillary membrane is calculated from a knowledge of the volume of gas which is breathed and the concentrations of carbon monoxide and nitrogen in the inspired and expired air. The formula is therefore similar to the one above, except that carbon monoxide is substituted for oxygen:

$$\dot{V}_{CO} = V_E \left(F_{I_{CO}} \times \frac{F_{E_{N_2}}}{F_{I_{N_2}}} - F_{E_{CO}} \right)$$

THE MEAN GRADIENT BETWEEN THE ALVEOLUS AND THE CAPILLARY

The *mean gradient* is a single figure which is the over-all physiological effect of an ever-changing gradient between the alveolus and the pulmonary capillary. The gradient which actually exists varies along the course of the pulmonary capillary. The diffusion gradient for oxygen diminishes from the point at which the venous blood arrives at the alveolus to that point along the course of the capillary where the partial pressures of the gas phase and the blood phase approach equilibrium. Figure 26 illustrates the actual gradients for oxygen, as well as the mean capillary oxygen. The *mean oxygen tension* in the pulmonary capillary has been determined from the shape of the curve representing the change in oxygen tension along the course of the capillary, by means of a planimeter, so that the volumes of the shaded areas represented by X and Y are equal. It is the mean gradient which is used to calculate the diffusing capacity of the lungs for oxygen.

The mean gradient for oxygen is difficult to determine, although it can be estimated by the use of a modification of Bohr's integration technique. In this method, it is necessary to determine the partial pressures of the oxygen in the alveoli, the mixed venous blood and the blood leaving the pulmonary capillaries. The alveolar oxygen tension is derived from the partial pressures of the oxygen in the inspired gas and in the arterial blood, as well as the respiratory quotient. In calculating the alveolo-arterial oxygen tension gradient, advantage is taken of the effect of the inhalation of a hypoxic gas mixture on the venous admixture component of the total gradient (Fig. 21). If that part of the alveolo-arterial gradient due to venous admixture could be completely abolished, the entire difference would then be due to the membrane component. As a result, all the information which is necessary for the calculation of the diffusing capacity would then be available. However, since the effect of venous admixture is not completely nullified while a gas mixture is breathed which is low in oxygen, a trial and error method is used to determine the gradient for oxygen between the alveolus and the end of the pulmonary capillary, at both normal and low levels of oxygenation. The oxygen tension at the end of the pulmonary capillary is calculated from the alveolo-arterial oxygen tension gradient at both of these levels of oxygenation. The value for the partial pressure of oxygen in the mixed venous blood must be assumed.

It is much easier to measure the mean gradient for carbon monoxide because of its remarkable affinity for hemoglobin. Measurable quantities of carbon monoxide can diffuse into the pulmonary capillary blood without producing a significant partial pressure in the plasma. In practice, the partial pressure of carbon monoxide in the pulmonary capillary is considered to be zero. For this reason, the mean gradient between the alveolus and the capillary is the mean alveolar carbon monoxide tension. This is not quite true, however, since it has been shown that the speed of the inter-reaction between carbon monoxide and hemo-

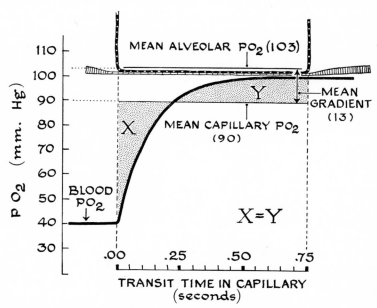

FIGURE 26. The change in the partial pressure of oxygen as blood passes along the pulmonary capillary and the mean alveolocapillary gradient.

globin is slow and therefore interposes a significant resistance to the flow of the gas from the alveolus to the hemoglobin molecule. The same can be presumed to be true for oxygen, although there is little evidence to support this. Nevertheless, this suggests that measurements of the diffusing capacity of the lung are affected by the resistance of the alveolocapillary membrane as well as that within the blood itself.

The diffusing capacity for oxygen falls whenever there is a diminution of the total area of alveolocapillary membrane available for diffusion, such as after the operative removal of a portion of lung. The diffusing capacity for oxygen has been shown to decrease with age and to increase with height. The suggestion has been made that these changes are related to the size of the pulmonary vascular bed. Because of the easy diffusibility of carbon dioxide and the hyperventilation induced by the hypoxia, an alteration of pulmonary function due to a diffusion defect is manifested by a low arterial oxygen tension but a normal or low carbon dioxide tension.

Contrary to general opinion, an impaired diffusion of oxygen from the alveolar air to the pulmonary capillary blood is seldom the primary cause of a low arterial oxygen saturation. With the exception of a relatively rare group of cases which have a specific type of alveolar pathology, arterial hypoxia in pulmonary disease usually results either from an inadequate alveolar ventilation or a poor correlation between ventilation and perfusion. In pulmonary fibrosis, when the blood vessels are surrounded by fibrous tissue, there may be a merging of the effects resulting from diffusion difficulty, poor distribution and venous admixture.

CHAPTER III

The Respiratory Function
of the Blood

THE UPTAKE of oxygen from the alveoli and its distribution to the various organs and tissues of the body are vital functions of the circulation. Equally important is the ability of the blood to take up carbon dioxide from the tissues, and subsequently to release it so that it may be eliminated from the lungs. The transport of these two gases by the blood is referred to as the respiratory function of the blood.

Of the total amount of oxygen and carbon dioxide in the blood less than 5 per cent is present in simple solution. Reversible chemical reactions are responsible for the transport of the remainder of the two gases, and in both cases, hemoglobin plays a major role. The exchange of oxygen and carbon dioxide between the systemic capillaries and the tissues is illustrated in Figure 27, and that which takes place at the alveolocapillary membrane is illustrated in Figure 28.

THE TRANSPORT OF OXYGEN

Since the partial pressure of oxygen is high in the alveoli and low in the mixed venous blood, oxygen diffuses from the alveoli into the pulmonary capillary blood. It is carried in the blood in two ways: as dissolved oxygen in physical solution in the plasma, and combined with the hemoglobin in the erythrocytes. The amount of oxygen which is dissolved and the amount which is combined with hemoglobin both depend upon the partial pressure of oxygen in the arterial blood.

OXYGEN IN PHYSICAL SOLUTION

The amount of oxygen which dissolves in a given volume of plasma is directly proportional to its partial pressure in the gaseous

55

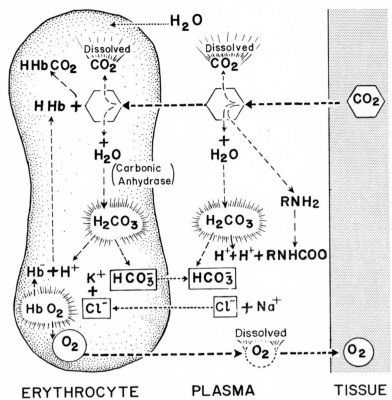

ERYTHROCYTE   PLASMA   TISSUE

FIGURE 27.   Gaseous exchange between the systemic capillaries and the tissues.

phase, which, in turn, is in equilibrium with the oxygen tension in the plasma. The amount of oxygen in physical solution in the plasma of the arterial blood, where the partial pressure of oxygen is normally 100 mm. Hg, is 0.31 vol. per cent. In the venous blood, where the partial pressure of oxygen is about 40 mm. Hg, there is 0.12 vol. per cent. Thus, the oxygen in solution in the plasma diminishes by only 0.19 vol. per cent as the blood passes through the tissues. This means that normally when the blood flow is about 5 l./min., only 9.5 ml. of oxygen would be given off to the tissues in a minute. However, the tissues normally utilize about 250 ml. of oxygen in a minute. If the blood contained only dissolved oxygen, therefore, about 130 l. of blood would have to circulate through the tissues in a minute in order to satisfy their oxygen requirements.

OXYGEN COMBINED WITH HEMOGLOBIN

Most of the oxygen in the blood is carried in the erythrocytes in combination with hemoglobin as oxyhemoglobin (HbO_2). Hemoglobin which is not combined with oxygen is called reduced hemoglobin (Hb).

One gram of hemoglobin is capable of combining chemically with 1.34 ml. of oxygen. In a normal man who has a hemoglobin content of 15 grams/100 ml., the blood is therefore capable of carrying 20.10 vol. per cent of oxygen as oxyhemoglobin, in addition to the comparatively small amount dissolved in the plasma. Although hemoglobin is capable of combining with this amount of oxygen, however, it does not normally do so. The extent to which hemoglobin combines with oxygen is usually expressed as the percentage saturation, and is illustrated in the following formula:

$$\% \text{ saturation} = \frac{\text{oxygen content (HbO}_2)}{\text{oxygen capacity (HbO}_2 + \text{Hb)}} \times 100$$

The oxygen saturation of the arterial blood in a normal person breathing room air is about 97 per cent. The saturation of hemoglobin depends upon the partial pressure of the oxygen in the plasma. When the oxygen tension is high, most or all of the hemoglobin combines with

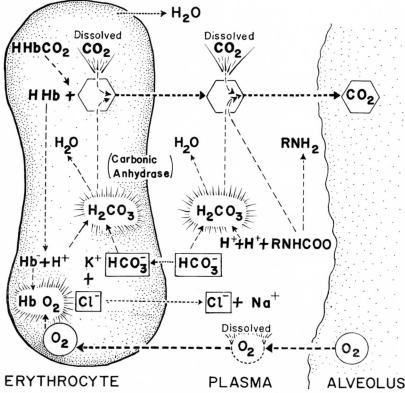

FIGURE 28.   Gaseous exchange between the pulmonary alveoli and the capillaries.

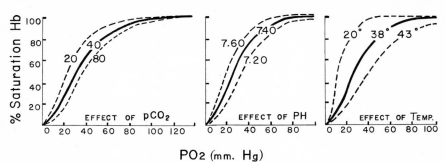

FIGURE 29.   The oxyhemoglobin dissociation curve and the effect of changes in
pCO₂, pH, and temperature.

oxygen; when the oxygen tension is low, as in respiratory disease, only a
small amount of hemoglobin combines with oxygen.

Unlike the amount of dissolved oxygen in the plasma, which is
directly proportional to the partial pressure of oxygen, the amount of
oxyhemoglobin formed in the red cell is not linearly related to the tension. The relationship between the partial pressure of oxygen and the
saturation of hemoglobin is expressed by the *oxyhemoglobin dissociation
curve,* illustrated in Figure 29. The characteristic double bend or S-shape
means that the hemoglobin clings to oxygen over a fairly wide range of
oxygen tension at both extremes of the scale and gives up oxygen readily
at intervening oxygen tensions.

The converse of this is also true, in that hemoglobin takes up
oxygen very readily at the intervening oxygen tensions, but not at both
extremes of the scale. It can be seen from Figure 29 that if the concentration of oxygen in the alveoli were less than 1 per cent, little oxygen
would be absorbed by the hemoglobin in the red cells. If the concentration were increased to 9 per cent, which is equivalent to a partial pressure
of about 60 mm. Hg, a large amount would be absorbed and the hemoglobin would become 90 per cent saturated. If the oxygen concentration
in the alveoli were elevated still further, the oxyhemoglobin would
increase by only a small amount. In other words, a change in the alveolar
oxygen concentration from 9 to 15 per cent, so that the partial pressure
becomes 100 mm. Hg, raises the oxyhemoglobin saturation only to 97
per cent. It is obvious, as well, that even if the alveolar oxygen tension
were raised well above 100 mm. Hg, there would be only a slight further
increase in oxyhemoglobin content.

Oxygen is given up to the tissues from the arterial blood. The
oxygen which is directly available to the tissues is that in physical solution in the plasma. As it is taken up by the tissue cells, the partial pressure of the oxygen in the plasma falls, so that the oxyhemoglobin begins
to dissociate. In this way, oxygen is liberated from the red cells into the
plasma and is then made available to the tissues. The passage of oxygen

from the erythrocytes to the plasma is facilitated by the close apposition of the hemoglobin to the surface of the red cells and the disc shape of the red cells, which increases the surface area available for diffusion.

The oxyhemoglobin dissociation curve illustrates that the hemoglobin relinquishes oxygen readily when the oxygen tension drops below 60 mm. Hg. Since the oxygen tension of the tissue cells is about 40 mm. Hg, the oxygen diffuses rapidly from the blood into the tissue cells. An average of about 5 ml. of oxygen/100 ml. of blood is given up by the blood to the tissues of the body. Even after the tissues have received all their requirements, the venous blood is still 70 to 75 per cent saturated with oxygen under ordinary circumstances. Part of this remainder represents a reserve that can be drawn on by the tissues with only a slight further reduction in oxygen tension.

The amount of oxygen which is given off by the blood to a particular tissue depends not only on the oxygen tension of that tissue but also on the partial pressure of carbon dioxide, the pH and the temperature of the blood. Figure 29 shows that the oxyhemoglobin dissociation curve moves to the right whenever there is a rise in the carbon dioxide tension, the hydrogen ion concentration or the temperature. It is believed that changes in carbon dioxide tension influence the dissociation curve because of the concomitant pH changes.

The influence of these factors on the dissociation of oxyhemoglobin means that, at a given partial pressure of oxygen, the oxyhemoglobin gives up more oxygen under conditions in which there is an elevated carbon dioxide tension, a lowered pH or an elevated temperature. These effects are extremely important, because they act as a safeguard for the welfare of the tissues. A decrease in the oxygen tension in the tissue capillary blood, such as occurs when the activity of the tissues is increased or when the blood flow is decreased, is accompanied by an increase in carbon dioxide tension and hydrogen ion concentration, which, in turn, assist in the unloading of oxygen from the blood to the tissues. Conversely, the fall in blood carbon dioxide tension as the blood passes through the lungs causes the dissociation curve to shift to the left, so that the hemoglobin is capable of taking on an additional quantity of oxygen. The effect of temperature is easily demonstrable in situations in which there is undue cooling of a tissue. When the hands are extremely chilled, for example, they may be red not only because the tissues utilize less oxygen, but also because the oxyhemoglobin has been unable to dissociate.

THE TRANSPORT OF CARBON DIOXIDE

One respiratory function of the blood is the carriage of excess carbon dioxide from the tissues to the lungs and the regulation of the pH. The pH of arterial blood is ordinarily about 7.40, at which time there is about 56 vol. per cent of carbon dioxide in the blood. The carbon dioxide produced in the tissues must be added to this blood at the systemic capillaries and eliminated at the pulmonary capillaries. The carbon dioxide dissociation curve is relatively steep so that, despite a rise in carbon dioxide tension of only 5 or 6 mm. Hg, the blood takes up about 3 to 4 vol. per cent of carbon dioxide as it passes through the systemic capillaries. To understand how this additional carbon dioxide is carried, it is necessary to understand how the carbon dioxide is distributed in the blood. It is present both in the plasma and the erythrocytes in essentially three forms, as dissolved carbon dioxide, as HCO_3^- and as carbamino-carbon dioxide.

TRANSPORT AS DISSOLVED CARBON DIOXIDE

Some of the carbon dioxide is transported in the physically dissolved form in both plasma and erythrocytes. In the plasma, some of this dissolved carbon dioxide reacts with water to produce carbonic acid. This hydration of carbon dioxide takes place according to the equation:

$$CO_2 + H_2O \leftrightarrows H_2CO_3$$

The equilibration of this reaction in the plasma is far to the left, so that the concentration of dissolved carbon dioxide is about 1000 times greater than the concentration of carbonic acid. The amount of dissolved carbon dioxide depends on its solubility coefficient, its partial pressure and the temperature. At body temperature, 0.067 vol. per cent or 0.0301 mM/l. of carbon dioxide is dissolved in plasma for every mm. Hg partial pressure of carbon dioxide. In the arterial blood, where the carbon dioxide tension is normally about 40 mm. Hg, there is approximately 1.2 mM/l. of dissolved carbon dioxide, and in the venous blood, where the tension is about 46 mm. Hg, there is 1.38 mM/l. of dissolved carbon dioxide. This is an increase of only 0.18 mM/l. or 0.4 vol. per cent, however, and the blood transports considerably more carbon dioxide than this. As mentioned earlier, about 4 vol. per cent or 2 mM/l. of carbon dioxide enters the systemic capillary blood as it passes through the tissues. Most of this is carried as bicarbonate.

TRANSPORT AS BICARBONATE

When carbonic acid is formed, it ionizes according to the equation:

$$H_2CO_3 \leftrightarrows H^+ + HCO_3^-$$

Since only a minute amount of H_2CO_3 is formed in the plasma, only a small amount of bicarbonate is formed. On the other hand, the plasma bicarbonate content increases considerably when the blood becomes venous because the red cells are capable of enhancing the ability of the plasma to carry bicarbonate. About 60 per cent of the carbon dioxide that the blood takes up from the tissues is hydrated in the red cells, where the hemoglobin is. It is the strong buffering power of the hemoglobin that is responsible for the considerable increase in plasma bicarbonate.

The Chloride Shift. There must be an equal number of cations and anions in the plasma and in the erythrocytes. The chief cations in the plasma are H^+ and Na^+; in the erythrocytes the chief cation is K^+. The anions in the plasma are HCO_3^-, Cl^-, OH^- and protein$^-$; in the erythrocyte there are Hb^-, HbO_2^-, HCO_3^-, Cl^- and OH^-. The healthy red cell membrane is relatively impermeable to cations or the hemoglobin anion and is permeable to only HCO_3^-, Cl^- and OH^- ions. Since the nondiffusible hemoglobin anion is in the red cell, and since the numbers of anions on either side of the red cell membrane are equal, it follows that at equilibrium the concentrations of the diffusible anions are greater in the plasma than in the red cells. This anion equilibrium between the plasma and the erythrocytes is disturbed whenever diffusible anions are added to the blood or the amount of nondiffusible anion in the erythrocytes changes.

When carbon dioxide enters the blood in the peripheral capillaries, the number of diffusible anions increases because the carbon dioxide combines with water to form carbonic acid, which in turn dissociates to form H^+ and HCO_3^-. At the same time, the number of nondiffusible anions in the erythrocytes decreases for two reasons. When carbon dioxide enters the red cells, the pH drops slightly, and the number of oxyhemoglobin anions (HbO_2^-) decreases because of the formation of oxyhemoglobin molecules ($HHbO_2$). In addition, as the oxyhemoglobin is being reduced, hemoglobin, a weak acid, is formed. It therefore readily combines with H^+ ion to become the undissociated HHb. Because of the increase in diffusible anions in the blood and the reduction in nondiffusible anion within the red cells, the anion equilibrium across the red cell membrane is disturbed. In order to restore the ionic equilibrium between the red cells and the plasma, the diffusible anions must be redistributed. As a result, some Cl^- moves into the red cells and is replaced in the plasma by HCO_3^- which moves out of the red cells. This process of ionic exchange is called the *chloride shift*. In in this way the plasma bicarbonate content increases considerably.

H_2O Shift. The volume of the red cells, as measured by the hematocrit, is a little larger in the venous than in the arterial blood because the entry of carbon dioxide into the red cells results in the ingress of anions, so that the number of osmotically active elements is increased within these cells. Water consequently enters the red cells by osmosis, until a new osmotic equilibrium is reached, with a larger red cell volume.

TRANSPORT AS CARBAMINO-CARBON DIOXIDE

Some of the carbon dioxide is also carried as carbamino-carbon dioxide. In the plasma, an exceedingly small and uncertain amount of carbon dioxide is bound in the carbamino form to the proteins. The change in the plasma carbamino-carbon dioxide content when the blood becomes venous is not considered to be significant. On the other hand, when oxygen is given up to the tissues, the hemoglobin in the erythrocytes combines with about 30 per cent of the additional carbon dioxide and carries it in the form of carbamino-bound carbon dioxide.

As is shown in Figure 28, the reverse of the processes which have been described takes place in the lungs. Because the partial pressure of carbon dioxide is 46 mm. Hg in the mixed venous blood and only about 40 mm. Hg in the alveoli, the blood gives up its excess carbon dioxide to the alveoli. Because of the high solubility of this gas in aqueous media, diffusion is rapid, and equilibrium between the carbon dioxide tensions of the pulmonary capillary and the alveolar air is promptly established. About 30 per cent of all the carbon dioxide which is exchanged is given up from combination with hemoglobin as carbamino-carbon dioxide when oxygen, whose partial pressure in the alveoli is about 100 mm. Hg, passes through the plasma into the red cells and oxygenates the hemoglobin to approximately 97 per cent of its capacity. In contrast to what takes place in the tissues, the amount of diffusible anions decreases and the number of nondiffusible anions in the red cells increases so that the equilibrium for anions between the red cells and the plasma is once again altered. Consequently, the diffusible anions are redistributed and some Cl^- leaves the red cells and HCO_3^- enters it. On entering the red cells, the HCO_3^- combines with H^+ to form H_2CO_3, and this in turn is dehydrated to carbon dioxide and water, the carbon dioxide then passing through the plasma into the alveoli. At the same time, the osmotic equilibrium between the red cells and the plasma is once again maintained by the movement of water out of the red cells into the plasma.

All of the reactions which have been described, with one exception, are very rapid. The exception is the dissociation of carbonic acid into carbon dioxide and water as well as the reverse form of this reaction. This is a slow process and if the elimination of carbon dioxide were to depend on it alone, only 10 per cent of the available carbon dioxide would be removed from the blood during its passage through the pulmonary capillaries. The red blood cells, however, contain a high concentration of an enzyme called carbonic anhydrase, which accelerates the reversible reaction of the formation of carbonic acid from carbon dioxide and water. The rate at which all the reactions involving carbon dioxide proceed has no effect on the equilibrium which is finally reached. However, the rate of the circulation of the blood sets a definite limit within which these reactions must take place. An erythrocyte is present in the lungs for a period of less than a second, and it is during this brief time that the reactions which liberate the carbon dioxide from the mixed venous blood into the alveolar air must take place. The reverse chloride shift is important in this regard, for without it, it would be impossible for the bicarbonate to enter the red cells from the plasma and there be rapidly dehydrated to carbon dioxide by the carbonic anhydrase so that it can be eliminated by the lungs during the brief interval the blood spends in the lung capillaries.

THE pH OF BLOOD

The acidity of a solution depends upon the number of hydrogen ions it contains. The concentration of hydrogen ions in pure water is about 10^{-7} moles per liter. By convention, a solution in which the concentration of hydrogen ions is higher than 10^{-7} moles per liter is called an acid solution, whereas one with a concentration which is lower than 10^{-7} moles per liter is called an alkaline solution. It is customary to express the acidity of a solution in terms of the negative logarithm, to the base 10, of the hydrogen ion concentration. This is called the pH of a solution.

The power by which an acid-salt mixture is able to stabilize the acidity or the pH of a solution against changes which might be caused by adding H^+ or OH^- is called its buffer action, and the acid-salt mixture is called a buffer system. The reaction of any solution which contains both acid and salt can be expressed by the equation:

$$pH = pK + \log \frac{\text{(buffer anion)}}{\text{(undissociated buffer)}}$$

in which pK is a constant which varies, depending on the types of acid and salt involved.

The relationship between carbonic acid and the anion bicarbonate in the plasma is used clinically to establish the existence and the severity of any disturbances in the acid-base balance. In this case, the equation is the Henderson-Hasselbalch equation:

$$pH = pK + \log \frac{HCO_3^-}{H_2CO_3}$$

The pK of this buffer system is 6.11. In addition, the concentration of carbonic acid is proportional to the concentration of dissolved carbon dioxide, which in turn depends upon the partial pressure of carbon dioxide and its solubility coefficient. Since 0.0301 mM/l. of carbon dioxide is in solution for every mm. Hg partial pressure of carbon dioxide, the equation becomes:

$$pH = 6.11 + \log \frac{HCO_3^-}{0.0301 \ pCO_2}$$

All the carbon dioxide in the plasma is present as either bicarbonate or dissolved carbon dioxide, but only the total carbon dioxide content, and not the bicarbonate, can be measured. If the equation is rearranged to include only those components which can be measured, it becomes:

$$pH = 6.11 + \log \frac{total \ CO_2 - 0.0301 \ pCO_2}{0.0301 \ pCO_2}$$

The Henderson-Hasselbalch equation illustrates that the pH of the blood plasma remains unchanged as long as there is a constant ratio between the levels of bicarbonate and dissolved carbon dioxide (or the carbon dioxide tension). The ratio of bicarbonate to dissolved carbon dioxide is normally maintained at 20:1. Whenever this ratio is altered by either respiratory or metabolic conditions, the pH becomes abnormal.

Respiratory causes of disturbances in the acid-base balance result from a primary carbon dioxide excess or deficit. The initial event, as far as the bicarbonate buffer system is concerned, is a change in the carbon dioxide tension and therefore the dissolved carbon dioxide, which alters the pH of the blood in an inverse direction. An elevated arterial carbon dioxide tension, which can be produced by both the inhalation of carbon dioxide or an impaired elimination of the gas, results in an acidosis. Conversely, a fall in arterial carbon dioxide tension, which is produced by hyperventilation, causes an alkalosis.

The development of hypercapnia or hypocapnia indicates a change in the ratio between the rate at which carbon dioxide is produced and the rate at which it is eliminated. The amount of carbon dioxide eliminated from the pulmonary capillary blood is dependent on the alveolar ventilation rate, which in turn is normally governed by the action of the medullary respiratory center. This relationship between carbon dioxide production and elimination is depicted by the formula:

$$P_{A_{CO_2}} = \infty \frac{\dot{V}_{CO_2}}{V_A}$$

where $P_{A_{CO_2}}$ is the alveolar CO_2 tension; $\dot{V}_{CO_2}$ is the carbon dioxide production in ml./min., and V_A is the alveolar ventilation in l./min.

This formula shows that if the alveolar ventilation is doubled while the metabolism remains constant, the alveolar, and therefore the arterial, carbon dioxide tension falls to half its normal value. The converse of this occurs whenever there is a diminution in the alveolar ventilation without a concomitant fall in the metabolism. Alveolar hypoventilation with consequent hypercapnia has a particular clinical importance and is encountered frequently. Hypercapnia develops whenever the total ventilation falls or when the physiologic dead space increases without a proportionate rise in the minute ventilation. The arterial carbon dioxide tension also rises whenever the metabolic production of carbon dioxide rises without a proportionate increase in the alveolar ventilation. This is particularly true when the work of breathing is great, for under such circumstances, increases in ventilation may be associated with the production of more carbon dioxide than can be eliminated by the lungs.

When the arterial carbon dioxide tension rises for any of the above reasons, the amount of bicarbonate and total carbon dioxide also increases. Unfortunately, this acute increase in total carbon dioxide content is not recognizable, for it is still within the normal range. Because of the increase in carbon dioxide tension, the ratio between the bicarbonate and the dissolved carbon dioxide is less than 20:1. As a result, the pH falls, so that the patient is suffering from a condition called *respiratory acidosis.* If this should persist, the kidneys begin to conserve cations in order to combat the acidosis. Bicarbonate anions are exchanged for chloride ions and are conserved with the cations. If bicarbonate continues to be retained, the normal ratio of bicarbonate to dissolved carbon dioxide is almost re-established, and the pH returns towards a normal level.

Hypocapnia due to alveolar hyperventilation is also encountered frequently, particularly in patients with hypoxic hypoxia due to respiratory disease. Other common causes are cerebral damage such as a cerebrovascular accident or the ingestion of a drug, such as salicylate, which is a respiratory stimulant. It is also seen occasionally in highly emotional or apprehensive persons. When the partial pressure of carbon dioxide is lowered, the plasma bicarbonate level also falls, but the ratio of bicarbonate to dissolved carbon dioxide is still greater than 20:1 so that the pH rises, a condition called *respiratory alkalosis.* If the hypocapnia persists, excess cations, and in addition bicarbonate anions, are excreted by the kidneys, while chloride is conserved. If the plasma bicarbonate level falls sufficiently, the ratio of bicarbonate to dissolved carbon dioxide may return towards its normal value, so that the pH may be almost normal.

Disturbances in the acid-base balance may also take place as a result of metabolic disturbances, in which case there is an initial alteration in the bicarbonate concentration of the blood. These "metabolic" disturbances of acid-base balance occur when the relationship between fixed anions and fixed cations in the blood is altered. For instance, in diabetic ketosis excess H^+ ions react with bicarbonate to form carbonic acid so that the bicarbonate level and the pH fall. This is called *metabolic acidosis.* The fall in arterial pH stimulates ventilation so that the arterial pCO_2 is secondarily lowered. In this way, the ratio of bicarbonate to dissolved carbon dioxide tends to return towards normal so that the pH is nearly normal. Conversely, when excess OH^- is present in the blood, it reacts with carbonic acid so that the bicarbonate level and the pH rise, a condition called metabolic alkalosis. The carbon dioxide tension tends to rise secondarily because the elevated arterial pH inhibits respiration. In metabolic conditions, therefore, the respiratory system acts as the compensatory device whereby the arterial carbon dioxide tension is altered secondarily in order to restore the normal ratio of bicarbonate to dissolved carbon dioxide, so that the pH may be maintained at a normal level.

THE LABORATORY ESTIMATION OF ACID-BASE BALANCE

In order to assess any disturbance in acid-base balance, it is essential to measure at least two of the variables in the Henderson-Hasselbalch equation, so that the third may be calculated. For example, if the arterial pH and the carbon dioxide content are measured, the carbon dioxide tension can be calculated. Measurement of only one component is of little value, and, in fact, can frequently be misleading. For instance, the finding of an elevated pH indicates that alkalosis is present, and a low pH indicates acidosis, but these may be due to either a respiratory or a metabolic condition. Similarly, an elevated total carbon dioxide content may be due to either a metabolic alkalosis or a compensated respiratory acidosis, and a low total carbon dioxide content to either a metabolic acidosis or a compensated respiratory alkalosis. In addition, since the amount of dissolved carbon dioxide and bicarbonate do not rise appreciably when carbon dioxide is retained acutely, no recognizable alteration of the total carbon dioxide content may occur in acute respiratory conditions, even though the carbon dioxide tension is considerably abnormal. Finally, a low carbon dioxide tension may be found in respiratory alkalosis or metabolic acidosis, and an elevated carbon dioxide tension is found in both respiratory acidosis and metabolic alkalosis.

The test for the carbon dioxide combining power can be particularly misleading, for it is only an index of the alkali reserve, or the bicarbonate content, of the blood. Like the total carbon dioxide content, the carbon dioxide combining power is often within normal limits in acute respiratory conditions despite marked alterations of the carbon dioxide tension. On the other hand, this test is of value in metabolic disturbances in which the bicarbonate is primarily affected or in chronic respiratory conditions in which the bicarbonate level is secondarily altered. It is apparent, therefore, that the test for the carbon dioxide combining power is a test of some value for following changes in bicarbonate level. Even then, however, it does not yield an absolute measurement of the bicarbonate level and is to be recommended only when facilities are not available to measure directly the components of the Henderson-Hasselbalch equation.

CHAPTER IV

The Regulation of Respiration

Respiration normally takes place rhythmically and unconsciously. As was pointed out earlier, only the diaphragm and the intercostal muscles are active during a normal quiet inspiration, and expiration is not associated with any active muscular contraction. During forced respiration, or in dyspneic states, both the accessory inspiratory and the expiratory muscles are called into play, often without any conscious effort.

It is thought that breathing is ordinarily controlled by respiratory centers within the pons and the medulla. From ablation and transection experiments, it has long been known that neither the cortex, the cerebellum nor the anterior part of the brain stem is necessary for respiration. The localization of the respiratory centers as well as their mode of action has been intensively studied in the experimental animal. The role of these centers in the human is not definitely known, although the results of the animal experiments have been applied to the human. Any discussion of the control of respiration in the human is therefore based on the assumption that the general arrangement is fundamentally the same in all the higher animals, including the human.

On the other hand, the higher centers probably can also control breathing directly and at will, as in circus performers who are able to control respiratory movements and breathe primarily with one hemithorax. Many activities such as crying, laughing, eating and drinking interfere inconsequentially with the normal breathing pattern for short periods of time.

THE RESPIRATORY CENTERS

Studies with minute electrodes, which were used to record action potentials and to stimulate or destroy definite small regions of the brain stem, have shown that the "respiratory centers" are not sharply demarcated structures. Instead, they presumably consist of a number of motor areas scattered throughout the gray reticular formation of the pons and the medulla. Although a clear-cut distinction has not been made, it is generally accepted that there are three main symmetrically paired respiratory centers responsible for the maintenance and the control of rhythmic respiratory movements. These are the inspiratory, the expiratory and the pneumotaxic centers.

INSPIRATORY CENTER

When an area in the ventral reticular formation of the medulla is electrically stimulated, a vigorous and co-ordinated inspiratory movement results. If this stimulus is maintained continuously, it is capable of keeping the chest in a state of deep inspiration even though fatal asphyxia may develop. Such an uninterrupted inspiratory effort is called *apneusis.*

EXPIRATORY CENTER

Electrical stimulation of an area in the dorsal reticular formation of the medulla induces an expiration which persists as long as the stimulation is continued. There is some evidence to suggest that stimulation of the expiratory center inhibits the activity of the inspiratory center.

On the basis of knowledge derived from animal experimentation, it is thought that the medullary respiratory centers possess an automatic rhythm of alternate discharges of impulses from the inspiratory and expiratory components. In the inspiratory center, the rate of discharge of action potentials increases rapidly before inspiration begins. As inspiration begins and proceeds they continue to rise but at a slower rate. Shortly before the end of inspiration, central expiratory activity develops, and the inspiratory action potentials rapidly fall off. When the discharge rate from the expiratory center falls, inspiratory activity begins. As will be discussed later, this inherent rhythmicity is modified by both afferent nerve impulses and chemical influences.

PNEUMOTAXIC CENTER

For many years it was thought that the rhythmicity of the medullary respiratory centers was dependent upon a higher center termed the pneumotaxic center, situated bilaterally in the tegmentum of the pons. This was based on the observation that section of the brain stem immediately above the medullary respiratory centers in the vagotomized animal abolished respiratory movements and resulted in a state of uninterrupted inspiration or apneusis. This concept has had to be modified, however, following the observation that in such animals the respiratory movements are restored by procedures, such as the administration of morphine or section of the nerves from the carotid bodies, which are considered to depress the activity of the inspiratory medullary centers. The present view, therefore, is that section of the brain stem immediately above the medullary respiratory centers interrupts fibers which are more or less continually moderating the activity of the inspiratory center. Apparently fibers on only one side are sufficient to ensure a rhythmic respiration. In the absence of this moderating influence the inspiratory center is continually active, so that the inherent rhythmicity of the medullary centers is abolished. This concept is acceptable not only because it fits the observations but also because it makes the respiratory motor system no different from any of the others in the body, in that removal of the influence of the upper motor neurones renders the lower motor neurones more excitable. Examples of this are seen in the human suffering from hemiplegia, or in an animal with decerebrate rigidity.

It has also been suggested that the pneumotaxic center is intimately concerned with thermal panting in the dog, for panting does not occur when the brain stem is sectioned immediately above the medullary respiratory centers. It is obvious, however, that transection above the medulla cuts fibers coming from almost anywhere above the medulla, and it is just as likely that fibers coming directly from the thalamus have been sectioned by this procedure.

FACTORS WHICH INFLUENCE RESPIRATION

Changes in ventilation may be caused by many factors, some of which act directly on the respiratory centers and some of which act indirectly via nervous activity. The factors which are known to influence respiration by acting directly on the medullary respiratory centers include the arterial blood gases and pH, changes in cerebral blood flow and various pharmacological preparations. Those which influence respiration by acting on the respiratory centers via nervous activity include the arterial blood gases and pH; pulmonary receptors; pressoreceptors; thermoreceptors; nociceptors in the muscles, tendons and joints; the higher centers and certain pharmacological preparations.

FACTORS ACTING DIRECTLY ON THE RESPIRATORY CENTERS

The medullary respiratory centers are affected directly by alterations of the blood gases, particularly the carbon dioxide tension, as well as the pH of the capillary blood which perfuses through them, and are therefore thought to contain chemoreceptors. These chemoreceptors are apparently not stimulated by a fall in the oxygen tension of the blood, but may actually be depressed by a lack of oxygen. It is considered that, under normal circumstances, the arterial carbon dioxide tension and pH are the prime stimuli operative in regulating respiration, and it is possible that other factors which affect respiration do so by potentiating or depressing the response of the respiratory centers to these stimuli.

CARBON DIOXIDE

A rise in arterial carbon dioxide tension is the most outstanding of all the known chemical influences on ventilation. It must be pointed out, however, that an acute change in the carbon dioxide tension of the arterial blood results in a corresponding inverse alteration in the pH. For this reason, it is difficult to decide whether the carbon dioxide tension or the pH is the principal stimulus of respiration. In addition, the changes in the arterial blood may not necessarily give a true picture of what is happening in the cells of the respiratory center. The carbon dioxide tension and the pH within the cells of the respiratory center may differ significantly from those in the arterial blood because the cells of the respiratory center produce carbon dioxide, and its elimination depends on both the rate at which the blood is flowing through these centers and the capacity of the blood to accept carbon dioxide. The arterial carbon dioxide tension normally is about 40 mm. Hg, and if it is gradually raised by inhaling increasing percentages of carbon dioxide in air, the ventilation increases in a relatively linear fashion. Clinically this fact is utilized frequently by having the patient inhale carbon dioxide postoperatively to make him cough or take deep breaths.

Although the inhalation of 5 per cent carbon dioxide is readily tolerated normally, higher percentages become increasingly distressing, and the subject may become disorientated and apprehensive. In general, headache, dizziness and mental changes such as drowsiness and confusion develop at a carbon dioxide tension of about 80 mm. Hg. The inhalation of about 15 per cent carbon dioxide no longer increases the ventilation, the maximal ventilation being approximately 70 to 90 l./min. This may coincide with a loss of consciousness and the onset of muscular rigidity, tremors and generalized convulsions. When 30 per cent carbon dioxide is inspired, deep anesthesia is induced. At a concentration of 40 per cent, the ventilation becomes depressed and death may occur if this concentration is maintained for any length of time.

In patients with respiratory disease and chronic hypercapnia, some tolerance to the narcotic effects of carbon dioxide may develop, so that mental clarity may be present at levels of carbon dioxide tension which produce extreme depression in patients or experimental subjects who are acutely hypercapnic. Nevertheless, if the respiratory centers should become depressed, as in severe hypoxia or when depressant drugs such as morphine or barbiturates have been administered, the narcotic

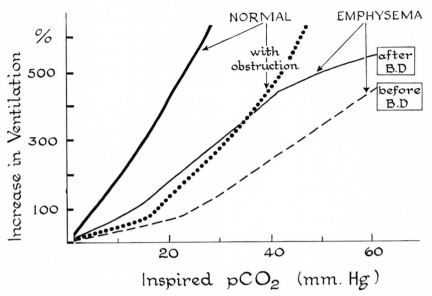

FIGURE 30. The effect of airway resistance on the ventilatory response to carbon dioxide in normal subjects and patients with chronic obstructive emphysema.

and depressant effects of inhaled carbon dioxide may occur at a much lower concentration. In such situations, therefore, the use of carbon dioxide in an attempt to stimulate respiration may actually lead to a further depression of ventilation.

The status of the respiratory center has been assessed clinically by measuring the ventilatory response to inhaled carbon dioxide. Patients who are suffering from severe chronic obstructive emphysema often demonstrate a lower than normal ventilatory response to the inhalation of carbon dioxide. It is likely that chronic elevation of the arterial carbon dioxide tension has reduced the sensitivity of the respiratory center in these patients. A similar situation is seen in normal subjects who have been exposed to an environment of 3 per cent carbon dioxide for some time. The diminished ventilatory response is probably related to an elevated buffering capacity of the blood and intracellular fluid, so that a given change in carbon dioxide tension does not produce the usual increase in hydrogen ion concentration. Another factor which influences the ventilatory response to carbon dioxide in chronic obstructive emphysema is the increased work of breathing. As is shown in Figure 30, the ventilatory response to carbon dioxide is improved when bronchial obstruction is reduced by the use of bronchodilating drugs in patients with chronic obstructive emphysema. Conversely, the ventilatory response of normal subjects falls when they breathe through an artificial airway resistance. These findings indicate that the ventilatory response to carbon dioxide measures the response of the total respiratory system and not just that of the respiratory center; an abnormal response does not necessarily mean that the respiratory center has lost its sensitivity. Thus the ventilatory response to carbon dioxide should not be used to measure the sensitivity of the respiratory system. The desirable measurement is, of course, the number of impulses coming from the respiratory center, but this is obviously unobtainable. On the other hand, measurements of the mechanical work response of the respiratory system may be informative. The mechanical work response of normal subjects is unaltered when they breathe through an artificial airway resistance, but the response of patients with chronic obstructive emphysema and hypercapnia is lower than normal. This suggests that the sensitivity of the respiratory center is indeed reduced in patients suffering from chronic obstructive emphysema and carbon dioxide retention.

The ventilation falls if the carbon dioxide tension of the arterial blood drops acutely below the normal level. At approximately 30 mm. Hg apnea may develop and may persist until the carbon dioxide tension rises again, suggesting that the respiratory centers are inhibited at lower than normal levels of carbon dioxide tension. On the other hand, if low carbon dioxide tensions are maintained for any length of time, as in a patient who is being ventilated in an iron lung, ventilation may be stimulated at lower levels of arterial carbon dioxide, and the response to inhaled carbon dioxide may be greater than it would be normally. Probably a change occurs in the buffering capacity of the blood and intracellular fluid as a result of chronic hypocapnia and increased elimination of base and bicarbonate by the kidneys, so that the change in carbon dioxide tension induces a greater change in pH.

THE ARTERIAL pH

Although the ventilatory response to the inhalation of carbon dioxide is well documented, the fact that it plays the dominant role in the control of normal respiration is not definitely established. Many physiologists are in favor of the reaction theory, which postulates that a rise in the carbon dioxide tension stimulates ventilation because of a concomitant increase in the number of hydrogen ions. Because of this relationship between changes in carbon dioxide tension and the pH, it is difficult to decide which of the two possible stimuli is the essential one. Nevertheless, an alteration in the pH of the arterial blood resulting from a change in the carbon dioxide tension increases ventilation more than it would if the alteration in pH were produced by other acids.

The site of action of the hydrogen ion stimulus is not definitely established as yet, although it is probably situated in the medullary respiratory centers. A striking stimulation of respiration occurs when carbon dioxide or carbon dioxide-bicarbonate solutions are injected into the area of the respiratory center or into the cerebral ventricles. Similar injections of other acids into these sites have no comparable effect. In addition, a vascular area called the area postrema located in the caudal region of the fourth ventricle of the dog has been shown to be sensitive to an increase in the acidity as well as to an elevation of the bicarbonate of the blood perfusing this area when the carbon dioxide tension is being kept constant, although this is a situation in which the pH is high. On the other hand, there is apparently no change in ventilation if the carbon dioxide tension of the blood infused into this area is altered but the bicarbonate level is kept constant, a situation which should also result in a fall in pH and theoretically, therefore, should stimulate ventilation.

When metabolic acidosis develops in a patient, as in uncontrolled diabetes mellitus, it is frequently accompanied by a secondary hyperpnea. In this situation, the hyperpnea continues even though the carbon dioxide tension of the alveoli and the arterial blood is reduced to low levels. This must mean that the respiratory center is being stimulated by some factor other than the arterial carbon dioxide tension, and it suggests that the hydrogen ion may be important in this regard. The maximal respiratory response takes place at a pH of approximately 7.0, at which point there is about a fivefold increase in the ventilation. Below this level, the respirations begin to fail as the toxic manifestations of the acidosis become predominant. Conversely, metabolic alkalosis, such as occurs with excessive vomiting or the administration of alkali, may be accompanied by a moderate reduction in the pulmonary ventilation.

BLOOD FLOW

As was mentioned earlier, respiration may be controlled by the intracellular carbon dioxide tension and pH of the respiratory center. The activity of the center is therefore determined by the rate of elimination of carbon dioxide from the cells of the center, which, in turn, is dependent upon its blood supply. Thus, when there is cerebral vasodilatation, as in hypoxia, there may be excessive removal of carbon dioxide from the respiratory center; consequently the intracellular carbon dioxide tension and H^+ ion concentration fall, and the minute ventilation diminishes. Conversely, cerebral vasoconstriction reduces the rate of elimination of carbon dioxide from the cells of the respiratory center, so that the intracellular carbon dioxide tension and H^+ ion concentration rise, thereby stimulating an increase in ventilation. It has been shown that it is possible to produce rhythmic respiratory activity by alternate constriction and dilatation of the cerebral blood vessels, but it is unlikely that changes in cerebral blood flow affect ventilation under ordinary circumstances. On the other hand, changes in cerebral blood flow may influence respiration considerably under abnormal circumstances, particularly when the blood gases are altered.

THE BUFFERING CAPACITY OF THE BLOOD

As has been indicated previously, a change in the buffering capacity of the blood and the cells of the respiratory center may influence the response of the medullary respiratory center to a change in carbon dioxide tension. Thus a high buffer base such as occurs in a metabolic alkalosis or in a compensated respiratory acidosis may render the center less sensitive to changes in carbon dioxide tension, but a low buffer base such as occurs in a metabolic acidosis or a compensated respiratory alkalosis may increase the sensitivity of the center.

PHARMACOLOGICAL AGENTS

Certain pharmacological agents such as salicylate and amphetamine are known to stimulate respiration, although it is not known whether they stimulate the respiratory centers directly or through the higher centers. This action of salicylates is extremely important, for ingestion of excessive amounts induces a marked hyperventilation which leads to a severe respiratory alkalosis. Conversely, the administration of barbiturates, anesthesia, tranquillizing agents or narcotics such as morphine depresses the respiratory centers so that respiration is diminished. Overdosage of the latter agents is exceedingly dangerous because of the severe hypoxia and respiratory acidosis which may develop.

FACTORS ACTING INDIRECTLY ON THE RESPIRATORY CENTERS

The arterial blood gases also influence respiration by stimulating peripheral receptors which, in turn, send impulses to the respiratory centers. The carotid and aortic bodies, which are innervated by the ninth and tenth cranial nerves, are so constructed that their receptors are exposed to arterial blood.

HYPOXIA

The carotid and aortic bodies are extremely sensitive to changes in the amount of dissolved oxygen in the plasma, a fall in the arterial oxygen tension inducing an increase in ventilation. Under normal conditions, the role of the chemoreceptors of the carotid and aortic bodies in the regulation of ventilation is subordinate to that of the chemoreceptors in the medullary centers. When hypoxia is present, however, they may play an important part in the control of breathing.

If an exceedingly brief period of hypoxia is induced by the inhalation of two breaths of a hypoxic gas mixture, the ventilation is increased as soon as the oxygen tension falls below 93 mm. Hg. On the other hand, marked respiratory stimulation in healthy persons as a result of exposure to longer periods of hypoxia is the exception rather than the rule. There is only a mild increase in ventilation while breathing hypoxic gas mixtures until the concentration of oxygen has been reduced to about 14 per cent. This is equivalent to an altitude of 10,000 feet or an arterial oxygen tension of approximately 60 mm. Hg. During the inhalation of 10 per cent oxygen, which lowers the arterial oxygen tension to approximately 40 mm. Hg, respiration is increased by only about 17 per cent. The maximal response, which is a ventilation of about 40 l./min., occurs during the inhalation of 4 per cent oxygen, but hypoxia of this severity can be tolerated for only a few minutes, and even then, at the risk of acute circulatory failure, unconsciousness and convulsions.

The difference in the responses between the exceedingly brief and the "steady state" periods of hypoxia is probably due to the compensatory mechanisms which take place in the latter situation. In the steady state the initial hyperventilation is not accompanied by a corresponding increase in metabolism. The carbon dioxide tension falls, therefore, and induces a rise in the arterial pH. Both the hypocapnia and the alkalosis inhibit the respiratory center and oppose the stimulation induced by the hypoxia. Because of this extremely mild ventilatory response, hypoxia has been considered to be of little importance in the control of breathing.

In contrast to its effects at sea level, chronic hypoxia is a greater stimulus to ventilation particularly in normal subjects who are maintained at high altitudes or in a pressure chamber for several weeks. In this situation, the buffering capacity of the blood and intracellular fluids is reduced because of the chronic hyperventilation. As has been pointed out previously, this reduction in buffering capacity may increase the sensitivity of the medullary respiratory centers to carbon dioxide, so that it is stimulated at lower carbon dioxide tensions.

In patients with respiratory disease, hypoxia may become an important stimulus to respiration. When there are marked alterations of ventilation/perfusion ratios, true venous admixture or diffusion defect, respiration is stimulated by the resultant hypoxia, so that hypocapnia may be present. Under such circumstances, the hypoxic stimulus to ventilation is, to some extent, defeated by the opposing influence of the hypocapnia and alkalosis. On the other hand, it has been shown that if the carbon dioxide tension is normal or elevated, experimentally induced hypoxia leads to a marked increase in ventilation. This suggests that hypoxia is indeed a powerful stimulus to respiration, as long as the respiratory center is not inhibited by hypocapnia or alkalosis. If the respiratory disease is severe, hypercapnia develops when the alveolar ventilation is inadequate in relation to the carbon dioxide production. If the hypercapnia is severe and has been present for some time, the sensitivity of the medullary respiratory centers may be diminished, a situation which is also encountered in morphine or barbiturate intoxication. Whenever the sensitivity of the respiratory centers is diminished, the peripheral chemoreceptors may become the principal regulators of the respiratory drive, with hypoxia the primary stimulus.

CARBON DIOXIDE TENSION

Although changes in the arterial carbon dioxide tension alone do not appear to stimulate the carotid and the aortic bodies, an increased carbon dioxide tension in the presence of hypoxia causes a stimulation of these centers to increase ventilation. This may be because the two stimuli enhance one another when hypoxia is present, but it is more likely that removal of the inhibitory effect of the hypocapnia and the alkalosis allows the hypoxic stimulus to be maximally effective.

It has recently been suggested that there may be another chemoreceptor in the neighborhood of the pulmonary artery which is responsive to changes in the carbon dioxide tension of mixed venous blood, although the presence of such a chemoreceptor has not been confirmed. Because an excellent relationship between the level of mixed venous carbon dioxide tension and ventilation has been demonstrated during exercise, it has been proposed that the mixed venous carbon dioxide tension may be the prime regulator of ventilation during exercise, but there is no definite evidence that the relationship is one of cause and effect.

ARTERIAL pH

The carotid and aortic bodies are also stimulated by an increase in acidity. These reflexes probably are not essential to the production of hyperpnea by an acidosis, however, because the respiratory response to an experimentally induced acidosis is not abolished by denervation of the carotid and the aortic bodies.

PHARMACOLOGICAL AGENTS

A number of drugs and poisons such as lobeline, nicotine and the cyanides initiate reflexes to stimulate ventilation through the carotid and aortic chemoreceptors. It has been suggested, therefore, that there are two types of chemoreceptors in the carotid and aortic bodies, namely, those which are stimulated by hypoxia and those which are directly stimulated by various drugs.

PULMONARY RECEPTORS

It was demonstrated almost a hundred years ago that contraction of a slip of diaphragmatic muscle was inhibited by inflation of the lung, and it was suggested that the reflex restriction of the amplitude of the tidal breaths was evoked from stretch receptors in the bronchi and the lungs. The converse situation was also described, in that expiration was inhibited by deflation of the lungs, so that inspiration began. These reflexes, which are called the *Hering-Breuer reflexes,* operate through the vagus nerves. If the vagus nerves are sectioned in the experimental animal, the amplitude of breathing increases greatly, and the respiratory rate falls, but the minute ventilation remains essentially unchanged. The change in the rate and depth of respiration after vagal section is not related to the concomitant closure of the glottis, for this change in the respiratory pattern takes place even when the animal is breathing through a tracheostomy.

One might expect that only two sets of receptors and fibers would be involved in the Hering-Breuer reflexes, one activated by inflation of the lungs and the other by deflation, but several kinds of pulmonary receptors have been described. Some receptors in the visceral pleura or close by in the lungs are stimulated by a moderate inflation; others, which are probably smooth muscle spindles in the walls of the tracheo-bronchial tree, are stimulated by a strong inflation or deflation. It would appear, therefore, that information about the degree of stretch of the lungs is conveyed to the respiratory centers not only by the number of impulses but also by the participation of different fibers as the lung inflation is increased.

There are also probably subepithelial nerve endings in the tracheobronchial tree which are receptors for the cough reflex. When stimulated by mechanical irritants, they usually initiate the cough reflex.

The fibers which transmit the impulses from the stretch receptors of the lungs as well as from the cough reflex reach the solitary tract in the brain stem via the vagus nerve. From the solitary tract, fibers are continually given off to the reticular formation, where the impulses either curtail or stimulate the inspiratory center. Apparently curtailment is due to excitation of the expiratory center, which in turn inhibits the inspiratory center.

It has recently been suggested that although the human lung probably contains stretch receptors, their action on the respiratory cycle is much weaker than in animals. Although the role of the Hering-Breuer reflex in the human has been questioned, it is tempting to incriminate an alteration in the normal activity of this reflex as the basis for at least some of the disturbances of respiration seen in respiratory disease. It has been postulated that the reflexes are rendered more sensitive by pathological processes in the lung parenchyma such as congestive heart failure, atelectasis and pneumonia. As a result, they interrupt the inspiratory discharge from the respiratory center and thereby increase the respiratory rate, so that rapid shallow breathing, or tachypnea, is a clinical feature in these conditions.

PRESSORECEPTORS

Receptors in the adventitial coat of the aortic arch and the carotid sinus which are sensitive to alterations in the blood pressure chiefly influence the cardiovascular system, although they also affect respiration to a lesser extent. Impulses arising from these receptors are inhibitory, so that an increase in the systemic blood pressure inhibits pulmonary ventilation. On the other hand, a fall in the blood pressure leads to an increase in ventilation, presumably by reducing a pre-existing inhibitory influence. These responses are only moderate in degree, and their actual role in the human control of respiration is not clear.

RECEPTORS IN MUSCLES AND JOINTS

Afferent activity from any receptor, particularly those involved in muscle activity, influences the tone or level of excitability of many if not all of the anterior horn cells. It would not be surprising, therefore, to find that the respiratory movements are influenced by tension and stretch receptors in the muscles and joints of the extremities, or, for that matter, anywhere in the body. The change in ventilation associated with passive movements has been attributed to some such mechanism. In addition, it is believed that these receptors in the muscles, tendons and joints of the extremities reflexly contribute to the hyperpnea of exercise. However, such afferents are difficult to demonstrate and their importance is difficult to evaluate because of the effect of the other factors, such as carbon dioxide tension, which control respiration and limit the degree of hyperventilation which can be brought about. It is possible that ventilation is stimulated during exercise by the same centers that stimulate muscular activity.

THERMORECEPTORS

Some special receptors sensitive to variations in blood temperature are located centrally in the hypothalamus, and others which respond to alterations in surface temperature are located peripherally in the skin. The principal thermoregulatory centers receiving impulses from the thermoreceptors are situated in the hypothalamus. These centers discharge the appropriate impulses over the somatic and visceral motor nerves to control the production and elimination of heat. It is assumed, at least in animals, that there are connections between the thermoregulatory centers and the respiratory centers. The activity of the carotid bodies is influenced by temperature changes, regardless of the existing gas tension or the pH of the blood. In dogs, the respiratory passages constitute a very important means of heat elimination. In these animals, stimulation of either the peripheral or the central thermoreceptors produces panting. This mechanism for temperature regulation is relatively unimportant in man, but artificial elevation of body temperature does lead to hyperventilation.

The relationship between respiratory activity and blood temperature change in an abnormality of the temperature regulatory centers, such as may occur in fever, is difficult to evaluate, particularly while the temperature is rising. Nevertheless, during sustained fevers the pulmonary ventilation is increased by an amount which is out of proportion to the associated elevation in the metabolic rate. This ventilatory response to an increase in temperature in the human is complicated. Since the pH and the solubility of carbon dioxide in the body fluids are both directly affected by changes in temperature, it may be these factors which are influencing the respiration.

INFLUENCE OF HIGHER CENTERS

As mentioned earlier, animal experiments suggest that the respiratory centers are continually under the influence of higher centers which moderate their activity. In addition, there are many nonspecific reflexes which presumably involve the higher centers to influence respiration. Examples of these are a pain stimulus, apprehension and excitement, all of which tend to augment respiration. Breathing can be altered voluntarily as well, as is exemplified by voluntary hyperventilation or breath-holding. The influence of the higher centers is lessened during sleep when the ventilation is reduced.

It is likely that the higher centers play a role in the hyperpnea of exercise; in fact, it has been shown that the ventilation increases before exercise is begun. Similarly, in respiratory disease the development of apprehension no doubt increases ventilation and further aggravates any hyperpnea that is present.

THE WORK OF BREATHING AND THE CONTROL OF RESPIRATION

It would appear that whenever the work of breathing or the effort required to do this work is increased, the activity of the respiratory centers may be modified and ventilation may be limited. This can be illustrated by healthy subjects whose ventilation is decreased when they breathe through an artificial airway obstruction. It has been suggested that the body tolerates the resultant hypercapnia rather than expend the effort that would be required to keep the arterial carbon dioxide tension at a normal level. This may actually be beneficial, for it has been pointed out that a further increase in ventilation in an attempt to lower the arterial carbon dioxide tension would require so much oxygen that little would be available for nonventilatory muscular work. Just how the body is able to accomplish this feat, however, has never been demonstrated. Nevertheless, these considerations suggest that hypercapnia is not as potent a stimulus to respiration when the work of breathing is increased.

In addition, the work of breathing influences the pattern of

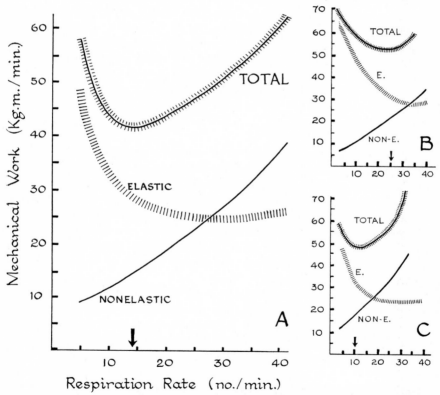

FIGURE 31.   The effect of respiratory rate on the mechanical work of breathing for a particular alveolar ventilation normally (A), when the elastic work is increased (B), and when the nonelastic work is increased (C). The arrows indicate the respiratory rate at which the total work is minimal. (Redrawn and modified, from Otis, A. B., Fenn, W. O. and Rahn, H.: Mechanics of breathing in man. J. Appl. Physiol., 2:592, 1950. By permission.)

respiration. For a particular alveolar ventilation it has been shown that there is an optimal rate and depth at which the work of breathing is minimal. Figure 31, *A*, illustrates that this minimal level occurs for two reasons. When the frequency is too slow, much work is required in order to overcome the great elastic resistance associated with large tidal volumes. In contrast to this, when the frequency is too high, much work is required in order to overcome the nonelastic resistance.

This optimal rate of breathing is altered in disease states. When there is an increase in the work required to overcome elastic resistance the respirations are rapid and shallow. This occurs in such conditions as pneumonia, in which the elastic resistance of the lungs is increased, or in obesity or kyphoscoliosis, in which the elastic resistance of the chest wall is increased. As is shown in Figure 31, *B*, the breathing is rapid and shallow in order to minimize the effect of the increased elastic resistance. On the other hand, as is shown in Figure 31, *C*, the respirations are usually slow and deep when the nonelastic resistance is increased because a faster respiratory rate would necessitate a great increase in the work required to overcome the nonelastic resistance.

THE REGULATION OF VENTILATION IN RESPIRATORY DISEASE

From the above discussion, it is apparent that there are many factors involved in the regulation of breathing. When respiratory function is altered, the minute ventilation may be elevated because of either stimulation of the central or peripheral chemoreceptors by abnormal blood gas tensions or an increased sensitivity of the Hering-Breuer reflexes. If the work of breathing is particularly great, the response to the other stimuli may be modified. Under such circumstances, the pattern of breathing for any particular alveolar ventilation may depend upon the work of breathing.

Aside from laboratory experimentation, it is unusual to find only a single chemical stimulus altered in patients with respiratory disease. Table 4 demonstrates that when the ventilation changes in response to a stimulus, other respiratory stimuli are also affected, and each makes a contribution to the final respiratory response. On occasion, the major chemical agents may work together in stimulating ventilation; in other situations, some may excite and others may inhibit the respiratory centers. For instance, the stimulant effect of hypoxia may be counteracted by the depressant effect of the hypocapnia and the alkalosis which develop secondarily because of the hyperventilation.

In patients with a congenital pulmonary arteriovenous aneurysm, in which there is true venous admixture, or in such conditions as pul-

TABLE 4

THE ALTERATIONS IN CHEMICAL AGENTS DURING VARIOUS CONDITIONS

CONDITION	pH	ARTERIAL pCO_2	pO_2
Inhalation of 5% CO_2 in oxygen	↓	↑	↑
Inhalation of 10% O_2 in nitrogen	↑	↓	↓
Voluntary hyperventilation	↑	↓	↑
Acute alveolar hypoventilation	↓	↑	↓

monary consolidation, atelectasis, congestion or fibrosis, in which there is venous-admixture-like perfusion or a diffusion defect, the ventilation increases because of stimulation of the peripheral chemoreceptors in the carotid and aortic bodies. As a result of the increased ventilation, the patient may have a persistent hypocapnia as well as an alkalosis, both of which would tend to depress ventilation.

When there is "dead-space-like" ventilation, and in some cases of true venous admixture or venous admixture-like perfusion, a tendency towards hypercapnia stimulates the chemosensitive cells of the medullary respiratory center to increase ventilation. If a reduced ventilatory capacity limits or prevents hyperventilation, however, alveolar hypoventilation may result, so that carbon dioxide accumulates in the blood. This hypercapnia does not necessarily produce the expected increase in ventilation, and it has been suggested that the body tolerates hypercapnia rather than expend the energy necessary to increase the ventilation sufficiently to bring the carbon dioxide tension to normal levels. Chronic hypercapnia is followed by an increase of the buffering capacity of the blood and cellular fluids, so that a marked change in the carbon dioxide tension may elicit only a minimal ventilatory response. Under such circumstances, the control of ventilation may depend predominantly on the action of the hypoxic stimulus on the chemoreceptors of the carotid and the aortic bodies.

PERIODIC BREATHING

The regularity of the breathing pattern depends on rapid and precise control of respiratory movements by the factors which influence respiration, so that, under conditions of constant carbon dioxide production, the respiratory center is held at a constant level of activity. If there are variations in the time taken for the feed-back of information to the respiratory centers, or if the elimination of carbon dioxide from the cells in the center is inconstant because of variations in blood flow, the breathing pattern may become uneven. Unevenness might also develop if the center were less responsive than normal and particularly if its responses were fluctuating. Under any of the above circumstances, therefore, one might find an irregular pattern of breathing, in which the respiratory rate and depth vary from moment to moment.

Variations in the pattern of breathing may be made to develop experimentally. For instance, this may occur when a subject breathes oxygen through a long dead space. Initially the inhalation of carbon dioxide which has accumulated in the dead space stimulates an increase in ventilation. As a result, carbon dioxide is washed out of the dead space, so that ventilation is stimulated less. This "hunting" process continues until the subject comes into equilibrium with the expired carbon dioxide in the dead space, and has reached a "steady state." An irregular pattern of breathing is particularly evident if the subject breathes room air through the dead space. Under such circumstances the ventilation waxes and wanes because the respiratory centers are alternately stimulated first by hypoxia alone and then by hypoxia and hypercapnia. This alternate waxing and waning of ventilation is also produced if the circulation time to the brain is reduced by increasing the distance through which blood travels on its way to the brain from the heart.

In view of the many inter-related factors which affect respiration and their variability, one wonders how regular breathing ever occurs. Nevertheless, periodic breathing in which the respiratory pattern is markedly irregular and a series of respiratory efforts are interrupted by periods of apnea occurs in only a small number of clinical conditions. Irregular respirations also occur occasionally in residents at a high altitude, or even at sea level in relatively healthy persons during sleep.

CHEYNE-STOKES RESPIRATION

The commonest form of periodic breathing encountered clinically is known as Cheyne-Stokes respiration. As illustrated in Figure 32, this is a series of respirations which wax and wane, each sequence of breaths being interrupted by a period of apnea. It is possible that this type of breathing is indicative of cerebral ischemia, although the exact mechanism of its development has not been adequately elucidated. A decrease in the rate of blood flow to the brain has been implicated because Cheyne-Stokes respirations have been produced experimentally in the dog by increasing the distance through which the blood must travel on its way to the brain from the heart, and also because it is encountered clinically in patients with congestive heart failure. This breathing pattern is also seen in patients who have cerebral damage due to trauma or disease or in whom the cerebrospinal fluid pressure is increased. Although the presence of this type of breathing is considered to be an ominous sign, it need not be, for it can be reversed, particularly if it is caused by congestive heart failure. In such patients, the administration of oxygen frequently abolishes the periodic breathing.

The mechanism of Cheyne-Stokes respiration is apparently similar to that which develops when air is breathed through a dead space, except that depression of the respiratory center by severe hypoxia is also implicated. This leads to a fall in the oxygen tension and a rise in the carbon dioxide tension, both of which are potent enough to stimulate the sluggish chemoreceptors so that breathing begins again. The respirations which ensue lead to oxygenation of the blood with a consequent relief of the cerebral hypoxia. As a result, the function of the respiratory center improves and the respirations become stronger, so that the arterial oxygen tension rises and the carbon dioxide tension falls. Respirations cease temporarily because the rise in the oxygen tension removes any stimulus to the peripheral chemoreceptors, while the simultaneous fall in the carbon dioxide tension removes the stimulus to the central chemoreceptors. It is possible that the effect of these changes in gas tensions on the cerebral circulation may play a role in the production of Cheyne-Stokes respiration as well. When the arterial carbon dioxide tension rises or the oxygen tension falls, there is a marked decrease in the tone of the cerebral blood vessels, so that they dilate and more carbon dioxide is eliminated from the cells of the respiratory centers. Conversely, they constrict when the oxygen tension is high and the carbon dioxide tension low, so that less carbon dioxide is eliminated from the center. As was pointed out earlier, rhythmic variations in respiration can be brought about by alternate cerebral vasoconstriction and vasodilatation.

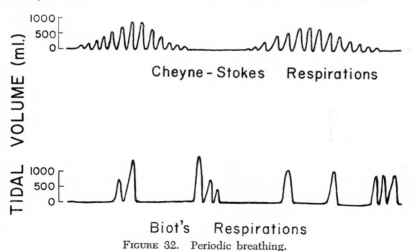

FIGURE 32. Periodic breathing.

BIOT'S RESPIRATION

In another type of periodic breathing, which is most frequently associated with brain damage, there may be one or more respiratory efforts of varying depth with prolonged unequal pauses in between sequences of breaths. This is known as Biot's respiration (Fig. 32). The mechanism by which it develops is not understood, but it is possibly due to a reduction in the inhibitory effect of the higher centers on the inspiratory center, so that the inspiratory center periodically "breaks through" and produces inspirations of varying size.

THE MANIFESTATIONS OF

RESPIRATORY DISEASE

THE SYMPTOMS OF RESPIRATORY DISEASE

THE SIGNS OF RESPIRATORY DISEASE

CHAPTER V

The Symptoms of
Respiratory Disease

THE "SYMPTOMS" of a disease are the abnormal subjective sensations produced by disordered physical or psychical functions in the body. The physical "signs" of a disease are the objective evidences of a pathological process which may be discovered by the observer. It is not always possible to make a sharp distinction between symptoms and physical signs, for some findings, such as dyspnea, cough and cyanosis, may be both subjective and objective. One can generally say, however, that symptoms are what the patient feels, and signs are what the examiner discovers during the course of the physical examination.

Although many factors may cause respiratory disease, only a relatively small group of symptoms are produced. Before we discuss the symptoms of respiratory disease, it is important to understand the function of the upper respiratory tract and the important role it plays in the protection of the tracheobronchial tree and the delicate lung parenchyma.

THE UPPER RESPIRATORY TRACT

The upper respiratory tract protects the tracheobronchial tree and lung parenchyma by warming, humidifying and filtering the air as it is inspired through the nasal passages. No matter how cold or dry the atmospheric air may be, it normally becomes practically saturated and is warmed to almost 37°C. by the time it reaches the trachea. The ciliated epithelium in the tracheobronchial tree, the layer of mucus covering it and the alveoli are unable to function properly unless the temperature is kept close to that of the body and the air which reaches them is humidified. The nasal turbinates, which are highly vascular structures

89

with large amounts of blood flowing through them, act as radiators of heat and warm the inspired air as it flows past them.

Moistening of the inspired air is predominantly carried out by the mucous glands of the nasal mucosa. These glands normally supply about a pint of water daily in order to accomplish this feat. A further slight degree of humidification is probably carried out by the mucous glands of the trachea and bronchi. In disease or old age the nasal mucosa may not be able to deliver this much fluid, so that if bronchial secretions develop, they may be thick and viscid. In patients with a tracheostomy, crusting of secretions is a common occurrence because the inspired air enters directly into the trachea without being properly humidified and warmed by the upper tract.

In addition to their warming and humidifying functions, the nose and nasopharynx prevent the entrance of foreign particles into the deeper portions of the respiratory tract by filtering the inspired air before it reaches the lungs. The larger particles are trapped by the coarse hairs in the vestibule of the nose, and the finer particles which escape past the external nares are frequently trapped in the mucus which coats the nasal mucous membrane. These particles are then either evacuated by a sneeze or are swept backward by the cilia of the epithelial cells of the nasal mucosa towards the nasopharynx and are swallowed.

THE SNEEZE REFLEX

Sneezing is a defense mechanism against irritant materials in the upper respiratory tract. The nervous impulses responsible for this reflex are elicited by irritation of the nasal mucous membrane and stimulation of the sensory receptors of the trigeminal nerves. It is characterized by a deep inspiration which is followed by a violent expiration with the mouth closed, so that the expiratory blast is discharged through the nose.

Infection of the upper respiratory tract or irritants which induce an allergic response characteristically produce congestion of the nasal mucosa, an outpouring of mucus and frequent sneezing. If the irritation is due to infection, the nasal mucosa is hyperemic, and the nasal discharge is usually purulent. In allergic states, the mucosa is pale and boggy and frequently obstructs the passageway, and the discharge is thin and watery. If the paranasal sinuses become involved by the infection, pain may be felt over the corresponding areas of the face and scalp. In both the allergic and infectious forms of rhinitis, as well as in chronic sinusitis, a postnasal discharge is frequently encountered. If this becomes excessive, it may be a precursor to many of the other manifestations of respiratory disease, particularly if there is an alteration of the normal defense mechanisms of the respiratory tract.

THE DEFENSES OF THE RESPIRATORY TRACT

It was formerly believed that it was extremely difficult for foreign material to gain entrance into the lung. The larynx was regarded as a vigilant watch-dog which went into spasm with the slightest irritation, inducing a cough which rejected the foreign material. It is now known that this process applies only to foreign material which irritates the mucous membrane of the respiratory tract. Experiments with nonirritating radiopaque oils containing iodine, such as lipiodol, have shown that foreign material can be readily aspirated into the depths of the lungs even by a normal unanesthetized person. It is evident that secretions from the upper respiratory tract can follow the same course, especially during sleep. Since the upper respiratory tract is not sterile, it is obvious that the lung may be continually contaminated by a great variety of bacteria, fungi and viruses. When one considers the complexity and tortuosity of the whole tract, which invites trapping and pocketing, it is a marvel that the lung is not a cesspool of constant suppuration. That the normal lung is not is due to the operation of very active and effective defense mechanisms which normally protect the tracheobronchial tree from aspiration of foreign substances or accumulation of secretions.

THE LARYNX

Indirect inspection of the glottis with a laryngeal mirror reveals that it widens during inspiration and narrows during expiration. Closure of the larynx protects the respiratory tract from the aspiration of foreign substances. For instance, during swallowing, closure of the glottis prevents food from entering the trachea. Closure of the larynx is essential for the development of positive pressure within the thorax or abdomen, such as during a cough or defecation. Laryngospasm creating strong resistance to air flow may develop reflexly to stimuli applied to non-respiratory organs such as the esophagus. If closure of the larynx persists for a long period, such as during severe paroxysms of coughing, deleterious effects may be produced, because the greatly prolonged increase in intrathoracic pressure may interfere with the venous return to the heart and lead to circulatory collapse and syncope.

Foreign material which manages to evade the defense barriers of the nasopharynx and the larynx and enters the tracheobronchial tree can be removed by other defense mechanisms. These are the action of the cilia, the peristaltic movement of the bronchi and the cough mechanism.

CILIARY ACTIVITY

Ciliated cells are present in all parts of the nasal fossae, the paranasal sinuses, the posterior pharynx and the bronchi as far as the respiratory bronchioles. The ciliated epithelium helps to protect the tracheobronchial tree from invasion by bacteria or other foreign material. Cilia do not act directly on bacteria or foreign particles but only on the mucus to which they have become adherent. The waving cilia carry the layer of mucus upward in a conveyor-belt fashion. There are no cilia in the larynx, so that secretions are conveyed from the trachea to the interarytenoid region, where they are frequently tipped over into the pharynx and swallowed. The ciliary activity of the cells of the upper respiratory tract propels the layer of mucus backwards through the nasal passages into the nasopharynx, whence it may be expectorated or swallowed.

The cilia themselves may be readily destroyed by any inflammation of the mucous membranes except perhaps the most superficial kind. Fortunately, they can also readily regenerate, provided the inflammation has not extended into the deeper layer of the mucous membrane. Ciliary activity may become impaired also by a lack of humidity or the presence of tenacious secretions. When proper drainage from the tracheobronchial tree is impaired, mucus accumulates. This may be expelled by coughing, but it can also be aspirated deeper into the most dependent parts of the lungs, where it may occlude the smaller bronchioles. The commonest example of this state is "hypostatic pneumonia" or "hypostatic congestion," which is especially likely to occur in elderly bedridden invalids. Complete occlusion of some of the smaller bronchioles may occur even in healthy persons, especially during sleep. Ordinarily this may have no ill effects because the lung parenchyma distal to the obstructed bronchioles may be collaterally ventilated and subsequent coughing may expel the plugs.

COLLATERAL VENTILATION

It has been demonstrated that the alveoli receive some of their ventilation from adjacent alveoli through interconnections about 40 millimicrons in diameter, called "alveolar pores." Recently, direct communications between bronchioles and adjacent alveoli have also been demonstrated. These pores have a practical value, for they may prevent the development of lobular atelectasis in instances of bronchiolar obstruction. Thus, occlusion of a secondary bronchus need not necessarily lead to atelectasis, presumably because of the transfer of air through the collateral route from adjacent alveoli to those denied direct ventilation. In addition, these pores may serve as avenues of escape for air which might otherwise be trapped in the peripheral airways and alveoli, particularly in a check-valve type of bronchiolar obstruction.

If these communications are not patent, the air entering the alveoli may be unable to leave, so that the alveoli become distended. Recurrent inspiratory overdistention of the already stretched alveolar walls, particularly during coughing paroxysms, may eventually cause rupture of the alveolar walls and bulla formation. It has, therefore, been suggested that disruption of the alveolar pores is the basis for the air trapping in chronic obstructive emphysema.

Finally, the intra-alveolar connections may be harmful because they are potential pathways for the spread of fluids, cellular exudates, infecting organisms, phagocytes and neoplastic cells.

THE COUGH REFLEX

A cough is a violent expiratory blast which takes place against a partially closed glottis. It differs from a sneeze in that it is less explosive and is perhaps easier to control voluntarily. It protects the tracheobronchial tree from the entry of foreign substances or the accumulation of bronchopulmonary secretions.

A cough is induced by an irritation of the afferent fibers of the pharyngeal distribution of the glossopharyngeal nerve, as well as the sensory endings of the vagus nerve in the larynx, trachea and larger bronchi. The smaller bronchioles are relatively insensitive to irritants; it has been shown that if a radio-opaque fluid is inserted into a bronchopleural fistula, a cough reflex is not elicited until the fluid reaches the larger bronchi. It may also be stimulated by impulses which arise from nerve endings located in the mucous membrane of the pharynx, the esophagus and the pleural surfaces as well as the external auditory canal. The impulses are transmitted to the "cough center" in the medulla, which is probably situated near the respiratory center. Impulses from the cough center are then sent to the muscular systems of the chest and the larynx, and a cough results. The stimuli may be inflammatory, such as an infection; mechanical, such as smoke, dust or foreign bodies; chemical, such as irritating gases; or thermal, such as cold atmospheric air. Thermal stimulation, however, generally occurs only if the tracheobronchial tree has already been affected by other irritants.

The act of coughing, which is illustrated in Figure 33, comprises four separate and distinct phases. The first phase, the initial irritation, induces the second phase, which is a deep inspiration. The third and fourth components comprise the expiratory act. During the short third stage, the glottis is quickly and tightly closed, while the expiratory intercostal and the abdominal muscles contract forcibly, so that the intrathoracic and intra-abdominal pressures rise; this may be called the "compressive phase." After the intrathoracic pressure has reached a very high level, the glottis suddenly opens slightly. Since the intra-abdominal pressure is now higher than the intrathoracic pressure, the diaphragm is pushed up, producing a violent, explosive movement of air from the

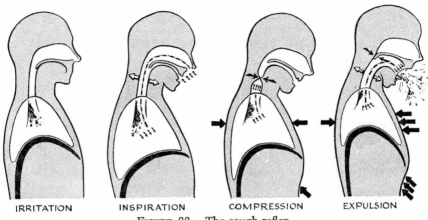

IRRITATION   INSPIRATION   COMPRESSION   EXPULSION

FIGURE 33.   The cough reflex.

lower to the upper respiratory tract. This fourth stage is the "expulsive phase." As soon as the glottis opens, the soft palate rises and closes off the nasopharynx. Consequently, any foreign material expelled from the respiratory tract by the force of the cough enters the mouth and may be expectorated.

Through the use of radio-opaque oils, it has been demonstrated that the intrathoracic airways are compressed concurrently with the onset of the expiratory blast of air. Because of this narrowing, the airflow velocity becomes exceedingly great and jet-like, and any foreign material is expelled in a manner similar to that of a bullet from the barrel of a pistol. In addition, it has been shown that the bronchi, which vary in size in an undulatory manner during normal breathing, may actually develop peristaltic expulsive waves originating in the finer bronchi and travelling upwards during a cough. The bronchial undulations of normal breathing and the peristaltic waves of a cough are probably additional protective mechanisms by which foreign material is moved from the lower respiratory tract to higher levels.

In the smaller bronchioles and in the lung parenchyma, the air blast of the expulsive phase is so feeble that there may be little effect on any foreign material lying in these areas. Instead, this must be moved upwards into the larger bronchi by the continuous action of the cilia. In addition, the foreign material may be forced into the larger bronchi by the normal undulating peristalsis of the bronchial tree, as well as by the squeeze of the chest which occurs during the expulsive phase of a cough. Expulsion of this material may then be completed by the expiratory blast of a succeeding cough.

The diaphragm also plays an active role in coughing. During the initial deep inspiration, it contracts and descends. It remains fixed in this low position as long as the glottis is closed because the elevations of both the intrapulmonary and the intra-abdominal pressures are approximately equal. When the glottis opens during the expulsive phase the intrapulmonary pressure falls, and the diaphragm sharply ascends, being pushed up by the greatly increased intra-abdominal pressure produced by the violently contracting abdominal muscles. It is likely that the diaphragm rises passively during this phase of the cough, but it is also possible that the diaphragm regulates the expulsive force of the cough by controlling the upward push of the abdominal viscera.

Although the cough reflex is one of the prime defenders of the tracheobronchial tree, it has certain inherent features which may be detrimental to the patient. It is possible that the deep inspiration which precedes the expiratory blast may occasionally drag secretions deeper into the more peripheral portions of the lungs. In addition, the expulsive force of the cough may be considerably hampered by the excessive narrowing and shortening of the bronchi which occur during expulsion. Another complication of coughing which must be considered is the possibility that purulent secretions may be splattered throughout the lungs during the expulsive phase and then inhaled into new areas during the next inspiration.

Cough. No one goes through life without an occasional cough, and almost everyone develops a cough each winter. Many adults always cough a few times on first arising in the morning because of the accumulation of postnasal secretions in the posterior pharynx and trachea.

A cough may signify anything from a nervous habit to a serious pulmonary disease. It always deserves a thorough investigation to elucidate the cause. It is one of the commonest symptoms in patients suffering from bronchopulmonary disease. It is important to remember that, although the cough reflex is usually initiated in the tracheobronchial tree, the primary cause of the cough may be nonrespiratory. An example of this is pulmonary congestion due to left ventricular failure. It is important to remember also that excessive secretions in the tracheobronchial tree need not necessarily produce a cough, particularly if some disease process has altered the sensitivity of the nerve endings, and that the peripheral portions of the lung parenchyma may be diseased without necessarily inducing the cough reflex.

Since the cough reflex is the chief protection against stagnation of abnormal secretion in the lungs, it is important that coughing be encouraged whenever there are excessive secretions in the bronchi. Sedatives, particularly morphine and heroin, not only suppress the cough but frequently allow the patient to drown in his own secretions. In general, the cough reflex is the physician's strongest ally; it should not be considered to be a bad symptom which must be drugged out of existence. When the ability to produce a lusty cough becomes impaired, as may occur in certain cases of pulmonary or extrapulmonary disease or when the respiratory center is depressed, the patient is in constant danger of stagnation of the bronchial secretions, which may result in atelectasis and infection.

In spite of the protection offered by the ciliary action and the cough reflex, the natural methods of emptying the tracheobronchial tree may be inefficient if a great strain is placed on them, such as when there are excessive secretions. Secretions from the upper respiratory tract may continually drain into the trachea when a person is in the upright position, and this is particularly true during sleep in the supine position. Although blood-borne abscesses of the lungs are fairly common, most cases of suppurative pneumonia and lung abscess are due to the inhalation of infected material into the bronchi. Even in health, a person spends about eight hours asleep, but during and after general anesthesia, a patient may be in a recumbent position for a long period of time. Under these circumstances, the most dependent parts of the lungs are not the bases of the lower lobes but the posterior segment of the upper lobe and the superior segment of the lower lobe. The aspiration type of pulmonary abscess, therefore, usually develops in these segments.

The Cough Syndrome.   The elevated intrapulmonary pressure which occurs during the compressive phase of the cough may interfere with the venous return to the thorax, resulting in a fall in cardiac output. If the elevated intrapulmonary pressure is maintained for any length of time, such as during the Valsalva maneuver, it may lead to cerebral ischemia and syncope. Similarly, in patients suffering from respiratory disease, particularly those who are subject to severe paroxysms of coughing, the intrapulmonary pressure may be considerably elevated for a long period of time, so that the cardiac output falls and cerebral ischemia and syncope may occur. This sequence of events leading to a loss of consciousness is known as the "cough syndrome."

THE EXPECTORATION OF SPUTUM

As has been mentioned, a considerable portion of the bronchial secretions is delivered to the pharynx by drainage forces other than the cough, and a considerable amount of sputum is automatically swallowed. Young children or animals never spit except as a defensive or offensive gesture, and even in adults who have not been well trained in the social conventions, it is certain that most of the sputum finds its way into the gastrointestinal tract. One should not assume that no abnormal secretions are being formed just because no sputum is expectorated.

The sound of a cough frequently indicates whether it is associated with abnormal secretions. Some coughs are obviously "dry," and the gurgling of abnormal moisture is distinctly heard in others.

Whenever a patient produces sputum it is of the greatest importance to determine its source. The search for the source of the sputum is often the search for a diagnosis, since the production of sputum reflects the reaction of the lung to any persistent irritant, be it atmospheric pollution such as cigarette smoke or smog, a foreign body or infection. Assistance can sometimes be derived from the history obtained from the patient. If most of the sputum is cleared from the throat and is associated with a nasal discharge, it is likely that the secretions are originating from the nose or the paranasal sinuses rather than from the bronchial tree. Occasionally, the patient is able to localize the source of his sputum. Such evidence, however, is not necessarily reliable, and the actual site of origin of the sputum should be determined by a more searching investigation.

The amount of sputum that is produced plays an important role in the establishment of a diagnosis. Very profuse, purulent expectoration suggests gross pulmonary suppuration. If it is abundant in amount and has appeared suddenly following an illness of a few days' or weeks' duration, the diagnosis of a lung abscess is almost certain. If it has gradually increased in amount over a period of years, the diagnosis is very likely chronic bronchitis or bronchiectasis.

The character of the sputum may also yield useful information. Pneumococcic infection is often characterized by scanty, extremely tenacious, blood-stained sputum. A foul odor is practically always indicative of a putrid lung abscess or bronchiectasis. Mucoid sputum which is stained a deep pink color throughout, the so-called "currant jelly" sputum, may occur with a pulmonary neoplasm. A profuse, frothy, pink, watery material which is blown through the lips is characteristic of pulmonary edema. Frankly bloody sputum may be a feature of such serious diseases as pulmonary tuberculosis or bronchogenic carcinoma.

HEMOPTYSIS

Bleeding may originate in any part of the respiratory tract, but the term "hemoptysis," meaning the spitting of blood, is used traditionally only when it can be demonstrated that the blood originates from the lower respiratory tract. This symptom is exceedingly important and always warrants careful investigation. A history of expectoration of blood should, therefore, be amplified along certain lines. Blood in the sputum results from many causes. Simply to say, "The patient saw blood in his sputum," means nothing except that there is probably some abnormality in his respiratory tract. If the statement is analyzed and qualified, however, it then becomes of great value and can make a considerable contribution towards establishing the diagnosis.

Bloody sputum loses much of its significance as far as the lungs are concerned if it is found to be associated with bleeding from a non-pulmonary source. If there is a history of bleeding from the nose or the gums or of the vomiting of blood, it is likely that some of the blood found in the sputum may have been aspirated into the larger bronchi and later expectorated. Abnormal bleeding in other parts of the body suggests that the hemoptysis may be an additional indication of a generalized hematologic disorder. Streaks and specks of blood mixed in the sputum are not usually of great consequence; they occur commonly in acute respiratory infections, probably as a result of congestion of the bronchial mucosa.

Elucidation of all of the associated symptoms and signs is important, and this requires a complete history and physical examination. An important fact to remember, in this connection, is that the more innocuous the patient's story sounds, the more important a full investigation becomes. For instance, the blood spitting of tuberculosis is at first very commonly unassociated with other symptoms. Unless the amount of blood has been large, patients frequently tend to discount it. Likewise, there may be very few, if any, abnormal physical signs elicited following the first hemorrhage due to tuberculosis.

Aside from tuberculosis, the commonest causes of hemoptysis are pulmonary infarction, bronchiectasis, mitral stenosis, bronchogenic carcinoma and pulmonary abscess. Some blood is also frequently expectorated during acute lobar pneumonia; this is usually mixed with very tenacious sputum, and is dark in color. Frank hemorrhages only occasionally accompany pneumonia.

DYSPNEA

Dyspnea may be defined as an awareness of difficult breathing. A person is not usually aware of his breathing, unless he consciously directs his attention to it, except under circumstances in which the ventilation has increased considerably or the effort required for a particular level of ventilation has increased. Strictly speaking, when one says, "The patient complains of dyspnea," one means, "The consciousness of needing air is produced in this patient under circumstances which would not produce such a sensation in a normal person."

Dyspnea during heavy exertion may be relatively normal in elderly people, especially if they are accustomed to sedentary habits or if they are obese. It may also occur in healthy young people during severe exercise. When estimating the significance of the presence of dyspnea, it is important to determine how quickly it has developed. A sudden change in exercise tolerance is of different significance than a change that has taken place gradually over a number of years.

In practice it is wise to define the severity of dyspnea. The patient may initially complain of dyspnea on exertion such as running a short distance or climbing stairs. Later, the disability may progress to the point at which it is present while he is walking quickly, or even while he is walking slowly. At a later stage, dyspnea may be present while the patient is lying in the recumbent position, a condition known as "orthopnea." Finally, the symptoms may increase in severity to the point of being present even while he is sitting at rest.

THE MECHANISM OF DYSPNEA

Although the following discussion presents a possible mechanism for the development of dyspnea, it must be emphasized that it is not based on any scientific evidence. Since dyspnea, like pain, is a subjective complaint, the precise mechanism leading to its development is difficult to establish. It becomes especially so when one tries to formulate a single mechanism for its production. Nevertheless, it is likely that an increased awareness of the act of breathing involves certain central cortical or thalamic areas as well as stimulation of peripheral sensory receptors.

Awareness of the act of breathing varies in degree from person to person and may even exist in a normal person if he "puts his mind to it." The rate and depth of respiration are relatively constant during rest, and it is likely that any one can become accustomed to his own particular respiratory pattern. It appears that the particular rate and depth of respiration which are "selected" are the ones at which the work of breathing is minimal. In any one case, awareness of the breathing act depends, to a large extent, upon past performances. For instance, a person who exercises regularly becomes accustomed to the respiratory effort required for such activity and he normally experiences no dyspnea. On the other hand, a less active person may experience dyspnea when he is called upon to perform an equivalent amount of exercise.

Little is known about the anatomical form or location of the peripheral receptors involved in the sensation of dyspnea. It is possible that they include tension as well as pain receptors in the muscles of breathing. When the muscles of breathing are required to perform an increased amount of work, or when their ability to operate is decreased because of unfavorable circumstances, these receptors send impulses to the "centers of awareness" and dyspnea results.

Dyspnea is experienced by patients with both organic or psychogenic disease. The description of the symptom is usually different in the two groups, and it is likely that the mechanisms are also.

DYSPNEA IN ORGANIC DISEASE

Table 5 presents the factors which are conducive to the subjective sensation of dyspnea. When the respiratory muscles have to perform an increased amount of work, dyspnea may be experienced. This occurs when the ventilation itself is increased or when the resistances to breathing are high. Thus, an acute change in the rate or the depth of respiration resulting from hypoxia, hypercapnia, metabolic acidosis, increased sensitivity of the Hering-Breuer reflexes or the increased ventilation associated with exercise cause one to become aware of his breathing. The change in ventilation results in an increase in the work of breathing, which in turn leads to the subjective feeling of dyspnea. Similarly, dyspnea is a prevalent symptom in diseases of the tracheobronchial tree, the lung parenchyma, the pleural space or the chest wall, in which the mechanical work of breathing is increased. On the other hand, in chronic respiratory conditions in which the respiratory rate and its depth have been altered for a long period of time, a person may be so accustomed to the changed pattern of breathing that the sensation of dyspnea is absent.

Dyspnea may also be experienced if the ability of the respiratory

TABLE 5

ORGANIC FACTORS CONDUCIVE TO DYSPNEA

A. INCREASED WORK OF THE RESPIRATORY MUSCLES
  1. Increased ventilation
     a. Exercise
     b. Carbon dioxide
     c. Hypoxic hypoxia
     d. Metabolic acidosis
  2. Altered physical properties
     a. Increased lung elastic resistance, e.g., pneumonia, congestion, atelectasis, pneumothorax, pleural effusion
     b. Increased chest wall elastic resistance, e.g., kyphoscoliosis, obesity
     c. Increased bronchial nonelastic resistance, e.g., chronic obstructive emphysema, chronic bronchitis, asthma

B. DECREASED ABILITY OF THE RESPIRATORY MUSCLES
  1. Muscular disease
     a. Muscular weakness, e.g., myasthenia gravis, thyrotoxicosis
     b. Muscular paralysis, e.g., poliomyelitis, Guillain-Barré syndrome
     c. Muscular wasting, e.g., muscular dystrophy
  2. Reduced mechanical advantage of muscles
     a. Marked inspiratory position, e.g., chronic obstructive emphysema
     b. Marked expiratory position, e.g., obesity
  3. Hypoxia
     a. Hypoxic hypoxia
     b. Anemic hypoxia
     c. Circulatory hypoxia
     d. Histotoxic hypoxia

muscles to perform work is decreased. Under such circumstances the effort required to perform a given amount of mechanical work may be increased. This occurs when the muscles are weak, paralyzed or wasted, when breathing takes place in an inspiratory or expiratory position or when the muscles are required to function under hypoxic or ischemic conditions. The metabolism of the respiratory muscles may be altered, and this in turn may affect the activity of the receptors. This is really a common occurrence in other muscles of the body, in that we become aware of fatigue and discomfort when they are exercised in hypoxic states. In fact, during severe ischemia, the pain may be excruciating. Under these circumstances, it is likely that there is an accumulation of acid metabolites in the respiratory muscles which are responsible for the stimulation of the receptors and the sensation of dyspnea. Thus, in addition to patients suffering from respiratory disease, dyspnea may also be a complaint of those suffering from neuromuscular disease or anemia.

DYSPNEA IN PSYCHOGENIC DISEASES

Many complaints are often manifestations of underlying psychoneuroses and may include a great variety of subjective sensations. Patients often complain of "shortness of breath" even though there may be no organic reason for it. It must be presumed that, in these individuals, the level of awareness of the breathing act has become increased. It is not surprising that respiratory irregularities and sensations should arise from emotional states, since one of the chief subsidiary functions of the organs of respiration and their accessory muscles is the expression of emotion. Weeping, sobbing, laughing, sighing and groaning are all produced by distortion of the respiratory rhythm. Minor respiratory effects of emotion are seen in the breathlessness of fear or wonder, the shout of elation, the sigh of satisfaction, the gasp of exasperation and the rapid breathing of anger. Variations of these psychophysical effects sometimes occur as symptoms in patients who are emotionally unstable. In addition, various types of functional nervous symptoms can be associated with the respiratory distress which may be described by the patient as "shortness of breath." Usually there is a sensation of suffocation, choking or oppression in the chest and it is often accompanied by other evidences of fear.

A very common complaint is that a full, satisfactory, deep breath cannot be accomplished—in other words, that a satisfactory depth of inspiration cannot be attained. Introspective people worry about this and keep trying to take deep breaths, with the result that they execute a series of imperfect sighs. The complaint is rarely related to organic disease, and it can almost always be readily cured by the simple explanation that it is a habit arising from paying too close attention to a function that should be unconscious and automatic. Nevertheless, such people sometimes spend so much of their time being obsessed by this difficulty that dizziness is induced by the resulting hyperventilation and alkalosis.

The Hyperventilation Syndrome. The hyperventilation syndrome consists of numbness and tingling in the extremities as well as faintness. In severe or prolonged cases there may be associated tetany as a result of the depletion of carbon dioxide with consequent alkalosis. This syndrome occurs most commonly in neurotic women and should be suspected if a resting patient, who is not acutely ill, is breathing at a rate of 30 or more breaths per minute. The diagnosis may be corroborated by the absence of any signs pointing to organic disease of the heart, lungs, blood or nervous system, and especially by the finding of a respiratory alkalosis in the presence of a normal oxygen tension in the arterial blood.

THE CLINICAL ASSESSMENT OF DYSPNEA

As has been pointed out, dyspnea is a subjective complaint, extremely variable between individuals, so that it is extremely difficult to evaluate. It is even more difficult to quantitate, despite numerous reported attempts to correlate dyspnea with every possible measurement of pulmonary function. As there undoubtedly are many factors active in the production of dyspnea, it is obviously fallacious to attempt to correlate dyspnea with any one measurement. It is likely, however, that if any single study would correlate well with dyspnea, it is a measurement of the energy consumed by the respiratory muscles, since dyspnea increases when the mechanical work of breathing becomes greater than normal or when the efficiency of the respiratory muscles is less than normal.

Except in advanced cases, dyspnea should be assessed while the patient is undergoing some type of stress. The most direct and generally the most satisfactory approach is made as the patient performs some form of exercise, such as climbing stairs, walking on a treadmill or pedalling a bicycle, which should be carried out for several minutes, in order to allow the patient to reach a steady state. A rough estimate of the amount of disability that is present can be obtained by the close observation of the patient while he is exercising. Obviously, however, this does not yield an objective measurement.

CHEST PAIN

Pain in the chest is a very common complaint. It often produces great apprehension on the part of the patient because he usually considers it to indicate some sort of disease of the lungs or the heart. In most cases, no such disease exists. It is true that any disease of the lungs may produce pain or discomfort in the chest, but there are many other causes of pain in this region. Consequently, it is important that the actual anatomic source of a chest pain should be searched for and discovered. In order to arrive at a proper evaluation, it is necessary to understand the distribution of the nerve dermatomes over the chest wall and to consider the many possible sources of chest pain.

THE DERMATOMES

If nerve roots are irritated as a result of mechanical pressure or infection, pain is frequently felt over the corresponding areas of the skin of the thoracic and abdominal walls supplied by the dorsal roots of the spinal cord. These areas are known as *dermatomes*. Such pain is frequently accompanied by hyperalgesia over the corresponding area of skin. Pain which is caused by irritation of the nerve roots must be distinguished from that produced by disease in the underlying viscera.

There is a divergence of opinion regarding the exact distribution of dermatomes. Figure 34 illustrates one mode of distribution which has been described. There is no doubt some overlapping of the individual dermatomes; they have been simplified in the illustration.

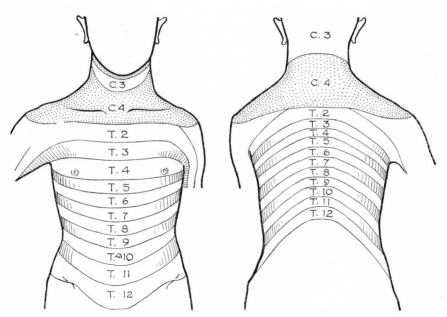

FIGURE 34. The distribution of the dermatomes.

The supraclavicular and the infraclavicular areas of the chest wall, down to the level of the second rib, are supplied by the fourth cervical dermatome. The remaining areas of the thoracic wall are supplied by the second to the sixth thoracic dermatomes. Each dermatome characteristically runs in a horizontal direction to the level of the anterior end of the corresponding intercostal space. They do not run parallel to the intercostal spaces themselves, but actually cross over them. The seventh thoracic dermatome lies at the level of the xiphoid cartilage, and the tenth thoracic dermatome is situated at the level of the umbilicus; the eighth and ninth dermatomes, therefore, occupy areas between them. The eleventh and twelfth thoracic dermatomes supply the lower abdominal wall, the lower level of the twelfth dermatome lying two inches above the level of the pubis. The seventh to the twelfth thoracic dermatomes, therefore, run in an increasingly oblique direction. The missing dermatomes of the fifth to the eighth cervical and first thoracic dorsal roots constitute the brachial plexus. The corresponding dermatomes are located over the shoulder, the arm and the hand.

THE SOURCES OF CHEST PAIN

In determining the source of any chest pain, it is well to suspect and, as far as possible, to examine each component part of the chest from the skin inwards. In the following discussion, trauma and other obvious surgical lesions are not considered.

The Skin.   Pain is not uncommonly localized in the skin of the chest. The cause may be obvious if the pain is caused by a bruise, a boil or a carbuncle. If it is caused by an inflammation of a posterior root ganglion (herpes zoster), it may develop long before the appearance of the characteristic vesicular rash.

The Ribs and Cartilages.   Osteomyelitis of the ribs, of either tuberculous or pyogenic origin, and malignant tumors in the ribs which are usually secondary to cancer of the prostate or the lung are rare causes of chest pain. They are diagnosed by the presence of tenderness, redness or swelling immediately over a rib. Occasionally a rib may be fractured by a paroxysm of coughing resulting in localized pain and tenderness over the affected area. Similarly, a rib cartilage may be fractured or dislocated during a severe bout of coughing and may produce exquisite pain which is accentuated by breathing or coughing.

The Nerves.   Actual disease of the intercostal nerves as a cause of pain is hard to demonstrate, although the diagnosis of "intercostal neuralgia" is a very common one. Most of these cases are now called "myalgia" or "fibrositis," because the pain probably arises from either the muscle or the connective tissue.

Several diseases do involve the posterior roots and lead to chest pain. Herpes zoster, a viral infection of the posterior root ganglions, is characterized by an exquisite hyperesthesia in the area of the distribution of the intercostal nerves or the nerve dermatomes. An eruption consisting of clusters of small vesicles in the same area usually appears a few days after the onset of pain. The pain, together with the hyperesthesia, may persist for a period of time after the rash has healed, although the diagnosis may still be established by the recognition of the brownish discoloration of the skin which is characteristic of a healed herpes infection.

Chest pain may also result from pressure on the posterior nerve root or on the nerve trunk by some disease process. This "root pain" is usually referred to its peripheral distribution or dermatome. The pressure on the nerve root is usually due to some manifest organic disease, such as tuberculous caries, arthritis or neoplasm of the vertebrae.

A profound deficiency disease which involves the central nervous system, such as pellagra, may also give rise to chest pain. This characteristically radiates around the middle and upper thirds of the chest, sometimes referred to as the "pellagra belt." In this disease, the pain is most likely due to degenerative changes in the spinal roots and the posterior columns of the spinal cord. Such gross vitamin deficiencies are now practically nonexistent in civilized countries.

The Muscles. Pain originating in the thoracic muscles is often confused with pleurisy, since it is generally aggravated by deep breathing. Unfortunately, this type of pain is frequently attributed to the heart, with the inevitable devastating results on the mind of the patient. This mistake occurs largely because the site of the muscular pain is most often in the region of the lower left costochondral junctions, which is precisely where most patients think the heart is located.

Fibrositis should be suspected as the cause of a chest pain whenever tenderness on deep pressure is found at the site of the pain, or if it can be reproduced by putting the involved muscle groups into action against resistance. If the pectoral muscles are affected, pain can be produced by having the patient press his hands together while the arms are extended in a horizontal position. This condition is not usually associated with constitutional symptoms.

The Pleura. Like the parietal layer of the peritoneum, the parietal layer of the pleura is the only layer which is sensitive to pain. Irritation of pain fibers in the parietal pleura is conveyed through the chest wall by fine twigs of the intercostal nerves, and results in pain over the chest wall. Characteristically, pleural pain is sharply localized, superficial, knife-like or "catching," is aggravated by respiratory movements, particularly those of deep inspiration, coughing, sneezing and yawning, and is usually associated with constitutional symptoms, such as fever. Suspicion of a pleural origin for the pain is confirmed if a pleural rub can be detected or if fluid is present in the pleural space. The diagnosis of primary pleural pain on less definite evidence is not justified. Pleural pain may be associated with any severe disease within the thorax. When no underlying condition can be detected to account for the pain, it should be assumed that it is due to inflammation involving the pleura itself. Such a "primary" or "idiopathic" pleurisy must be considered to be tuberculous in origin until it is proved otherwise. The diagnosis of pleural pain as an isolated condition is, therefore, almost equivalent to a diagnosis of a tuberculous infection and should be made only after careful circumspection. In doubtful cases, judgment should be withheld during a period of observation, for if a real pleurisy exists, convincing evidence will usually make its appearance in the course of time. In some cases, pleural pain antedates other evidence of pleurisy by many days or weeks.

It must be emphasized that pleural pain can occur in conditions other than inflammation of the pleura and that inflammation of the pleura does not necessarily always produce pain. Pleural pain may also be caused by an abnormal tension within the pleural space, such as that produced by a pneumothorax or a massive collapse of the lung, particularly when adhesions are present. The pain is most likely due to traction on the parietal pleura by adhesions attached to the moving visceral pleura. Patients who are suffering from far advanced chronic obstructive emphysema often complain of a pain or a sensation of pressure across the anterior aspect of the chest which is aggravated by deep breathing. It is usually situated in the sternal area, as well as along the costal margins. This pain appears from time to time, chiefly in response to exertion and coughing and is frequently associated with moderately severe bronchial obstruction. It is possible that it is due to tension on the pleurae by an overdistended lung.

The Diaphragm. Pain arising from the diaphragmatic pleura is mediated through the phrenic and the intercostal nerves. The central portion of the diaphragm is innervated by the third, fourth and fifth cervical nerves so that irritation of this area results in a sharp pain which is referred to the superior ridge of the trapezius muscle on the same side. The pain fibers from the peripheral portions of the diaphragm and its posterior third travel via the fifth and sixth intercostal nerves. Irritation of these areas results in pain along the costal margins, and it may also project into the epigastrium, the subchondral and the lumbar regions.

The Lung Parenchyma. The lungs are usually regarded as insensitive organs. If a pulmonary disease is accompanied by pain, it is likely that the parietal pleura is secondarily involved. There are, however, exceptions to this rule. For instance, a pulmonary neoplasm which does not appear to be involving the pleura sometimes gives rise to a deep aching pain. An acute atelectasis may produce a sudden violent pain, even though it is not associated with a pleural rub or an effusion.

The Tracheobronchial Tree. Acute inflammation of the trachea results in a discomfort under the upper portion of the sternum which is frequently described as a raw, burning sensation. A mild sensation of substernal burning discomfort aggravated by breathing and coughing often occurs in persons suffering from bronchitis.

The Aorta. A dissecting aortic aneurysm produces a tearing retrosternal pain which is sudden in onset and rapidly becomes severe and agonizing. The presence of such an aneurysm may be recognized by an inequality of the level of the blood pressure in the two arms as well as by the extreme restlessness of the patient. This is in marked contrast to the appearance of a patient who is suffering from an acute myocardial infarction, who usually lies quietly and exhibits evidence of peripheral vascular collapse.

The Heart. Pain due to cardiac disease need rarely be confused with pleural or pulmonary pain if the details of the pain are carefully studied. Pain originating in the myocardium is due to ischemia or hypoxia. It is believed that ischemia results in the formation of an excess amount of acid metabolites by the myocardium through anaerobic tissue metabolism, and that these tissue metabolites stimulate the nerve endings in the myocardium. Most of the resulting impulses are sent through the cardiac plexus to the upper five or six thoracic sympathetic ganglia, and then through the white rami of the second to fifth thoracic nerve roots into the spinal cord, from which they reach the skeletal nerves via their respective posterior roots.

Cardiac pain is typically substernal and is brought on by exertion. "Angina of effort," a pain resulting from ischemia of the myocardium due to an inadequate coronary blood flow, is characteristically induced by exertion. It is a squeezing pain which is often described as a heavy or vise-like sensation. The pain frequently radiates and is referred mainly to the base of the neck and the jaw, over the shoulders, the pectoral muscles and down the arms. For some reason the pain is more frequently referred down the left arm rather than the right. Relief of this referred cardiac pain can frequently be accomplished by the surgical excision of the second to the fifth thoracic ganglia of the sympathetic chain, or by severing the nerve fibers as they pass through the sympathetic chain into the spinal cord. The pain of angina usually forces the patient to rest, and it is frequently relieved or prevented by nitroglycerin. The pain has been attributed to the stimulation of nerve endings in the myocardium of the left side of the heart by acid metabolites.

The pain caused by a coronary occlusion has the same distribution as that of angina of effort, but it is usually much more severe and "crushing." It may develop without exertion, and usually is present while the patient is resting. In contrast to angina of effort, it does not disappear during rest, and it may continue for periods varying from minutes to many hours, often requiring powerful analgesics for its relief.

The Pericardium.   When the pericardium is affected by disease, pain may be present in either the substernal area or the left mammary region. The pain may vary in intensity from that of a dull, burning discomfort to a severe pressure, and may actually simulate a myocardial infarction. It frequently becomes aggravated if the patient lies in the supine position or extends his neck. The explanation for this phenomenon is not apparent. Pericardial involvement may be confirmed by the detection of a friction rub which is localized to the precordium.

Neither the visceral pericardium nor the internal surface of the parietal pericardium contains any pain fibers, only the lower part of the external surface of the parietal layer of the pericardium being sensitive. The adjacent diaphragm and pleura are frequently involved by any lesion affecting the lower part of the pericardium. In addition to the characteristic substernal pain of pericarditis, pain may also be felt in the neck and shoulder and the proximal portion of the arms because the affected central portion of the hemidiaphragm receives its sensory supply from the phrenic nerve, and therefore from the middle cervical segments of the spinal cord.

The Pulmonary Vessels.   Patients suffering from pulmonary hypertension may, on exertion, develop chest pain which is similar in many respects to that of angina of effort. The reason for this is not apparent, but it has been suggested that it is due to either dilatation of the pulmonary artery or ischemia of the myocardium of the right ventricle. In contrast to the usual changes which are found in coronary insufficiency, electrocardiographic changes involving the right ventricle are frequently demonstrated when pulmonary hypertension is present. In addition, pulmonary embolism may produce pain which is similar to that of a myocardial infarction, because it produces a fall in the cardiac output so that myocardial ischemia develops.

The Esophagus.   It is presumed that the sensory innervation of the esophagus is derived from the vagus nerves and the visceral sympathetic nerves arising from the inferior cervical and the upper nine thoracic ganglia. The pain which occurs in esophageal lesions is probably produced by tension of the esophageal musculature. It is burning in quality and is occasionally localized to an area of the sternum which overlies the affected portion of the esophagus. It is usually referred to the pharynx, the lower neck, and the arms, and may radiate around the chest cage along the dermatomes corresponding to the spinal segment innervating the involved area of the esophagus.

The commonest symptom which arises from an esophageal lesion is "heartburn." This is a hot, burning, substernal discomfort, which usually develops after a meal and is commonly accompanied by belching. It is apparently brought about by regurgitation of acid gastric contents which produces constriction of the lower part of the esophagus.

The Abdominal Organs. When an esophageal hiatus hernia is present, there may be symptoms of esophagitis and also a severe squeezing substernal pain caused by distention of the herniated gastric pouch within the thorax. This pain characteristically increases whenever the herniation is aggravated by an increased intra-abdominal pressure or assumption of the supine position.

Diseases of the stomach and colon produce pain which is frequently referred to the surface of the abdominal wall, although it may also radiate to the lower anterior chest wall.

Psychogenic Disease. Despite a lack of obvious organic disease, a patient may complain of a nondescript chest pain or of one which, in many respects, simulates that produced by organic disease. Lancinating pains in the chest wall are also very common among anxious patients. These are sharp and fleeting and are often described by the patient as "stabbing." They are probably caused by muscle spasm and can usually be dismissed as inconsequential. Many patients complaining of nondescript chest pain are really apprehensive about the possibility of cardiac or pulmonary disease. It is possible that the consequent nervous tension leads to an undue awareness of the respiratory muscles, for such patients usually do well with reassurance after a careful examination has convinced them that they are free from organic disease.

CONSTITUTIONAL SYMPTOMS

In addition to the cardinal symptoms of respiratory disease which have just been described, patients may complain of various constitutional symptoms such as fever, sweating, anorexia, weakness and loss of weight. The first two symptoms are usually the result of either an infection or tissue destruction, the sweating being caused by sympathetic overactivity. Weakness and loss of weight are probably related to an energy expenditure which is not balanced by an equivalent increase in the caloric intake. The anorexia is difficult to explain.

FEVER

Fever is an elevation of the body temperature due to disease. It is associated with respiratory disease whenever there is infection, degeneration of tissue or extensive trauma. The fever may be continuous, remittent and oscillating, or intermittent with a normal temperature for varying lengths of time. It is not definitely known why a fever occurs during a disease process. It has been stated that the high temperature is a reaction on the part of the organism which enables it to combat the infection. It is possible that the fever causes destruction of some bacteria as well as an increase in cellular metabolism which may lead to the production of immune bodies and an increased ability to phagocytize foreign bodies or bacteria.

Under most circumstances, the body temperature represents a balance between the heat produced by the body and that which is lost. The fever in infectious processes probably results from both an increase in the production of heat and a reduction in the amount of heat that is lost.

It has been suggested that there are two thermoregulatory centers in the hypothalamus, one which is situated in the anterior hypothalamus and prevents overheating and one in the posterior hypothalamus which protects the body from chilling. Abundant neural interconnections have been demonstrated between these two areas, and it is probable that activity of one center tends to inhibit that of the other.

A protein product called "pyrexin" has recently been isolated from degenerating tissues as well as from neutrophilic leukocytes. When this substance is injected into an animal it causes an increase in the body temperature. It has, therefore, been postulated that fever develops in disease whenever this substance is liberated by an injury to either tissue cells or leukocytes. It has also been suggested that the thermoregulatory centers in the hypothalamus respond to this stimulus by raising the level at which the body temperature is normally regulated. Since the body temperature is normal at a time when the hypothalamic thermostat level has been increased, the situation resembles that of exposure to cold. Consequently, the center institutes certain measures to increase the body temperature. These measures are the same as those which take place during exposure to cold, namely, an intense vasoconstriction, pilo-erection or goose pimples, secretion of epinephrine and shivering. The patient may feel cold even though his body temperature is normal or even above normal. He may develop a "chill" during which he shivers so violently that he shakes the bed. The skin feels cold because of peripheral vasoconstriction and a diminished peripheral blood flow. Vasoconstriction reduces the amount of heat which is lost through radiation, and heat production is increased by the greater tone of the muscles and the muscular activity associated with shivering.

SWEATING

Under ordinary or basal conditions, no sweat is secreted, except possibly a small amount from special glands in the skin of the feet, hands and axillae. Nevertheless, about 600 ml. of fluid may be lost in 24 hours from these areas and the moist surfaces of the respiratory tract. This is termed *insensible perspiration.* Under normal conditions, the heat loss by this means constitutes about one-fifth to one-quarter of the total loss of heat from the body.

When the loss of heat by radiation, convection and insensible perspiration is no longer adequate to prevent a rise in the body temperature, a further loss of heat from the skin is dependent upon activation of the sweat glands and the consequent evaporation of sweat. The stimulus to an increase in sweating is thought to be mainly the elevated blood temperature. It has been suggested that when the temperature of the blood increases, the center in the posterior hypothalamus inhibits the tonic discharge of impulses over sympathetic vasoconstrictor fibers, so that a cutaneous vasodilatation occurs, and the thermoregulatory center in the anterior hypothalamus sends impulses to the sweat glands through the cholinergic, postganglionic fibers.

Since overactivity of the sympathetic nervous system leads to sweating, patients suffering from a respiratory disease who are anxious and worried about their breathing difficulty may sweat profusely. Occasionally, drenching "night sweats" may occur, in which the nightclothes become thoroughly soaked. The explanation of this phenomenon is unknown, although if the body temperature is elevated, it might initiate the corrective measures for heat loss. If the body temperature is not abnormally elevated at this time, it may be that the hypothalamic thermostat is set at a lower level during the night, so that measures which are designed to increase the loss of heat are instituted. The possibility of overactivity of the sympathetic nervous system for some unknown reason during the night must also be considered.

ANOREXIA, WEAKNESS, FATIGUE AND WEIGHT LOSS

Anorexia, weakness, easy fatigability and weight loss are frequent complaints of patients suffering from some types of chronic respiratory disease. These symptoms may also be encountered during acute pulmonary infections.

Weakness and loss of weight occur when the expenditure of energy is greater than that which is derived from the combustion of ingested food. This imbalance may occur whenever the total metabolism of the body is increased, thus necessitating a greater than normal supply of nutrient materials. In patients suffering from respiratory disease, the elevated expenditure of energy is frequently a result of either high consumption of oxygen by the respiratory muscles because of increased work of breathing or the elevated metabolism which occurs during a fever. In addition to the increase in the metabolic rate, there may be an excessive loss of protein because of infection, tissue destruction, malignancy or trauma. Finally, an elevated body temperature, by itself, increases the caloric requirements of the body. It has been shown that the need for calories increases at a rate of about 7 per cent for each degree Fahrenheit above the normal body temperature. It is obvious, therefore, that weakness and loss of weight may be encountered in acute or chronic respiratory diseases if the caloric intake does not increase concomitantly with the expenditure of energy.

The anorexia is difficult to explain. If the respiratory disease is severe, the mere act of eating may be so tiring and energy-consuming that the patient may lose all desire to eat. Consequently, a relative anorexia may exist simply because of the effort required for eating.

Chapter VI

The Signs of Respiratory Disease

IN CONTRAST to symptoms, which are the subjective complaints of a patient, physical signs are the objective evidences of a pathological process which are discovered by an observer. When certain properties of the lung and thorax are altered by disease processes, characteristic physical signs indicative of these alterations can be elicited by the clinician during the physical examination of the respiratory system. These signs assist him in arriving at an accurate diagnosis of the disease process. The following discussion deals with the mechanisms involved in the production of the more important of these physical signs.

DEFORMITIES OF THE CHEST

DEFORMITIES DUE TO ABNORMALITIES OF THE THORACIC VERTEBRAE

Since the lungs are enclosed in the semirigid thoracic cage, alterations in the contour of the chest can lead to disturbances within the lung. There is a wide variation in the general contour of the thoracic cage, but the bony structure of the chest cage is normally symmetrical (Fig. 35, A). The symmetry of the chest cage is largely related to a normally straight thoracic spine. Any abnormality of the thoracic vertebrae usually distorts the configuration of the chest. Thus, bizarre distortions of the thoracic cage can result from paralysis of the back muscles due to poliomyelitis, from tuberculous osteomyelitis of the vertebrae and from traumatic injury of the spine. All grades of spinal deformities can occur and the lesser forms may be easily overlooked unless the thoracic spine is routinely examined, both by inspection and by palpation of the spinous processes.

Several types of spinal deformity may be encountered: scoliosis, kyphosis and kyphoscoliosis.

Scoliosis. The commonest deformity of the thoracic spine is scoliosis, a gradual lateral curvature of the thoracic spine which is

113

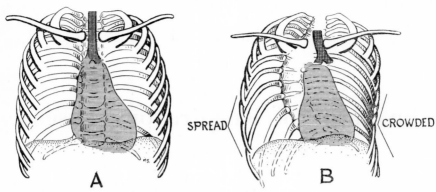

FIGURE 35.   The normal contour of the chest cage (A) and that seen in kypho-scoliosis (B).

usually associated with some degree of rotation or torsion of the verte-brae in their longitudinal axes. It frequently results from improper postural habits. If the person constantly shifts his body weight to one leg while standing, the body tends to be bent laterally, and one shoulder assumes a higher position than the other. This causes an unequal tension on the muscles which are attached to the thoracic vertebrae, resulting in a lateral curvature of the thoracic spine. At the same time, the asym-metrical pull on the transverse spinous processes of the thoracic verte-brae also causes a rotation of the vertebral bodies in the direction of the convexity of the lateral curvature. For reasons which are unknown, 75 to 80 per cent of the cases of scoliosis have a convexity to the right. Initially, this deformity can be corrected by voluntarily straightening the spine, but if the faulty posture is maintained for long periods of time, a permanent deformity may result.

The rib cage becomes distorted in a characteristic fashion by scoliosis of the thoracic spine. On the convex side of the scoliotic spine, the ribs are widely separated because of the lateral deviation of the thoracic vertebrae, while the rotation of the vertebrae produces an angulation of the ribs on their posterior aspect. The altered position and shape of the ribs result in a bulging of the posterior aspect of the rib cage on the convex side, while its anterior aspect is flattened. On the concave side of the spine the ribs become crowded together, and their insertions into the vertebrae are rotated, so that the anterior aspect of the rib cage bulges, while its posterior aspect is flattened.

Kyphosis.   Kyphosis is a relatively acute angular curvature of the thoracic spine, with the convexity directed posteriorly. When it exists as an isolated lesion because of vertebral body destruction, deformity and dwarfing result. In thoracic kyphosis, there is a characteristic hump made up solely of the spine. The ribs are crowded together, causing the anterior portion of the chest and the sternum to bulge forward in a pigeon-breast type of deformity.

Kyphoscoliosis. The deformity of the thoracic spine called kyphoscoliosis is a combination of kyphosis and scoliosis. About 1 per cent of the population are affected by some degree of kyphoscoliosis, although the deformity is usually so mild that no medical attention is required. In most cases the cause of kyphoscoliosis is unknown, although postural abnormalities have been implicated and there is apparently a hereditary tendency in about 25 per cent of cases. Poliomyelitis often leads to kyphoscoliosis because of involvement and weakening of the spinal muscles.

In a severe form of kyphoscoliosis, retraction of one side of the chest may cause extensive compression of the underlying lung, and protrusion of the opposite side may cause overdistention of the lung on that side. This condition, which is illustrated in Figure 35, *B*, is discussed in greater detail in Chapter XIII.

CONGENITAL DEFORMITIES OF THE ANTERIOR CHEST WALL

Certain deformities of the anterior aspect of the thoracic cage have been fairly conclusively shown to be hereditary, as chest deformities may appear in a family over several generations. Two factors seem to be involved in the production of these deformities—an abnormal pull of the diaphragm on the anterior chest wall, and a disproportionate elongation of the ribs. The type of deformity which develops depends on which factor is predominant. All such deformities arise because of impaired development in the embryo of the septum transversum, which later forms the anterior portion of the diaphragm.

Funnel-Chest Depression Deformity. In an infant, the cartilages and bony structure of the chest cage are softer and more mobile than those of the adult, and a congenitally shortened anterior portion of the diaphragm usually causes retraction of the lower anterior chest wall during the inspiratory phase. The apex of the inspiratory depression is situated at the xiphisternal junction. As a child develops, its thoracic bony structure becomes more rigid, so that this sternal depression becomes fixed. The body of the sternum is curved backwards in the fully developed funnel-chest deformity, forming a deep depression on the anterior chest wall which is centered around the xiphisternal junction and resulting in a longer and narrower chest cage than normal.

In the infant, the inspiratory sternal depression produces no symptoms unless there is an associated congenital cardiac lesion. In the adult, the body of the sternum may be depressed so deeply as to be in actual contact with the vertebral column. In such cases, the heart may be distorted and displaced into the left hemithorax and there may be compression of the left lung. In the more severe forms of funnel-chest, there may be symptoms due to compression of the heart or lungs, such as dyspnea, palpitation and cough. In addition, compression of the esophagus may cause dysphagia and other digestive disturbances. These symptoms are very likely produced by pressure on the heart and restriction of its movements, an abnormal rotation of the mediastinum, and compression of the lungs so that they offer an increased resistance to distention. The resulting distortion of the bronchi may also increase the nonelastic resistance and may impair their drainage, so that the person becomes more susceptible to respiratory infections.

Pigeon-Breast Protrusion Deformity. Protrusion deformities of the anterior chest wall occur much less frequently than funnel-chest. In the pigeon-breast deformity, both the sternum and the costal cartilage are projected anteriorly so that there is a resemblance to the breast of a pigeon. This condition is usually associated with a depression of both sides of the chest, so that the transverse diameter of the thoracic cage is narrowed. In some cases, the whole sternum protrudes forward in an oblique direction, so that its lowest part becomes the most prominent part of the chest. In both types of sternal protrusion, the costal cartilages which are attached to the sternum extend forward obliquely.

Another type of protrusion deformity involves the costochondral cartilages alone, the sternum retaining its normal position. This may involve several successive cartilages on only one side, so that a ridge is formed just lateral to the sternum. If these protrusions are present bilaterally, they usually occur at different levels on the anterior chest wall. If the lower costal cartilages are involved bilaterally, the costal arch flares outwards.

The etiology of protrusion deformities is obscure. They may be due to an abnormal overgrowth and lengthening of some of the ribs so that angulation results at their costochondral junctions. If this should occur bilaterally, the sternum becomes protruded. The type of protrusion which results is determined by the growth of the diaphragm. If the growth of the child's diaphragm keeps pace with the increase in the anteroposterior diameter of the chest, the sternum is protruded in an oblique direction. If the diaphragm remains small in comparison with the chest cage, however, the increased tension on the central tendon restrains the xiphoid, and the pigeon-breast deformity of the upper part of the sternum results.

Harrison's Grooves. Harrison's grooves, named for the English physician who first described them approximately 120 years ago, are horizontal depressions on the chest wall at situations corresponding to the attachments of the diaphragm. They extend laterally along the sixth and seventh costal cartilages from the xiphoid process to the axilla. They may be either unilateral or bilateral and are often seen in combination with other congenital chest deformities, such as the funnel-chest and the pigeon-breast. Although it most commonly occurs in children who have suffered from rickets, the condition may also develop in infants suffering from any pulmonary disease associated with a lower than normal intrapleural pressure, such as bronchial asthma, and in children who are free from rickets or pulmonary disease. Many diseases associated with lowered intrapleural pressure may occur in infancy, however, without the development of Harrison's grooves.

It has been suggested that Harrison's grooves may develop because of a deficiency in that part of the anterior segment of the diaphragm which is attached to the costal cartilages of the sixth and seventh ribs. As a result there is an unequal pull on the costal margin so that these costal cartilages and ribs are pulled inward by strong inspiratory contractions of the remaining parts of the hemi-diaphragm. The inward pull may become particularly strong if increased respiratory efforts are necessary to overcome bronchial obstruction.

CLUBBING OF THE DIGITS

Clubbing consists of a painless, nontender enlargement of the terminal phalanges of the fingers and toes and is usually a bilateral condition. It is an important manifestation of certain types of pulmonary disease and is, therefore, of great diagnostic significance.

When clubbing develops, certain changes take place. Initially there is hypertrophy of the soft tissues covering the root of the nail, and the skin overlying the nail bed becomes stretched and glistening. The nail gradually thickens, becoming curved and developing longitudinal ridges, while the pulp of the terminal phalanx enlarges and creates a bulbous appearance. In the advanced stages the nail is thickened, ridged

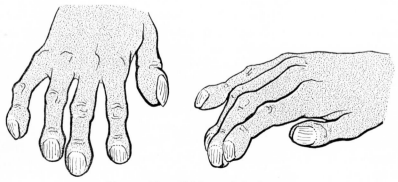

FIGURE 36. Clubbing of the fingers.

and curved, and its distal end overrides the end of the finger. An example of advanced clubbing of the fingers is illustrated in Figure 36.

Clubbing usually progresses slowly, often taking months or years to develop. Occasionally it develops acutely in the course of a week or so when the underlying intrathoracic lesion is an acute septic process. Regression and even disappearance of digital clubbing may take place if the underlying lesion is eradicated by medical or surgical treatment.

HYPERTROPHIC PULMONARY OSTEOARTHROPATHY

Clubbing of the digits may progress to a condition called hypertrophic pulmonary osteoarthropathy. When osteoarthropathy is present, the gross, bulbous, enlarged terminal digital phalanges are associated with a painful, tender thickening of the wrists, the ankles and the long bones of the forearms and legs. This thickening is produced both by new bone formation in the subperiosteal area of the long bones and by thickening of the connective tissue.

PATHOGENESIS OF CLUBBING

This condition is usually acquired, although there is also a rare hereditary form. The acquired form of digital clubbing occurs most frequently in association with serious intrathoracic disease. It is found in association with suppurative disease such as a lung abscess, empyema and bronchiectasis, as well as with malignant conditions such as bronchogenic carcinoma. Digital clubbing may accompany certain congenital lesions of the heart or pulmonary vasculature in which there is a right-to-left shunt, and it is also a frequent manifestation of subacute bacterial endocarditis. In addition, about 5 per cent of the cases of digital clubbing are associated with diseases of the gastrointestinal tract, including those of the liver. This is particularly true of the diseases characterized by chronic diarrhea, such as ulcerative colitis and steatorrhea.

The hereditary form of bilateral digital clubbing, which is also called "familial clubbing," is transmitted as a mendelian dominant and is not related to any disease process. It usually becomes evident at puberty and reaches its most advanced stage during middle age. The benign nature of this type of clubbing is recognized by the fact that it is present in other members of the family, as well as by the absence of any organic disease known to produce the condition.

Unilateral clubbing occurs only in association with diseases which develop either at the upper outlet of the thoracic cage or in the axilla. A syphilitic aneurysm of the arch of the aorta which also affects the innominate artery or a bronchogenic carcinoma involving the brachial plexus may be associated with finger clubbing of the hand on the same side as the lesion. Clubbing of only one finger is extremely rare. It has been described after an injury to the affected finger.

The histological changes are constant in all types of digital clubbing, no matter what the underlying cause. There is evidence of proliferation of the fibro-elastic tissue, interstitial edema, and dilatation and engorgement of the arterioles and venules. There is an increased blood flow through dilated arteriovenous anastomoses, which are very prevalent in the pulp of the terminal phalanges.

Although several theories have been advanced, the exact mechanism leading to clubbing in apparently unrelated diseases is as yet unexplained and is still open to conjecture. Digital clubbing and even hypertrophic pulmonary osteoarthropathy are believed by some investigators to occur whenever the left ventricle delivers more blood than is necessary to meet the needs of the tissues. As a result, the blood pressure and the blood flow in the digits is elevated, so that the growth of the digital tissues and later the periosteum of the bones, particularly the long ones, is increased. The capillary dilatation and the increase or retardation of the tissue metabolism which may be produced by tissue hypoxia further tend to complicate this mechanism.

Until recently, the most attractive explanation for the development of digital clubbing was that tissue hypoxia causes an increase in the number of arteriovenous anastomoses in the digits. This is supported by the fact that when a right-to-left shunt is experimentally produced in animals, changes similar to clubbing may develop in their digits. Although tissue hypoxia may be the mechanism by which clubbing develops in pulmonary conditions or in those associated with a right-to-left vascular shunt, it is difficult to imagine how such hypoxia could occur in patients with steatorrhea or ulcerative colitis. In addition, digital clubbing is rarely associated with a severe chronic anemia, which should lead to considerable tissue hypoxia.

Toxemia has also been proposed as one of the factors in the development of clubbing, but again, this does not explain the development of all cases. Toxemia may be present in certain suppurative pulmonary diseases such as bronchiectasis, lung abscess and empyema. These conditions are usually associated with an elevation of both the sedimentation rate and the plasma globulins, which frequently results in rouleaux formation of the erythrocytes. Because of peripheral vasodilatation and increased blood flow and because the erythrocytes in the rouleaux may not have time to release their oxygen to the tissues, tissue hypoxia may result.

Another hypothesis is based on the ability of reduced ferritin to inhibit the vasoconstricting action of circulating epinephrine, a property which oxidized ferritin apparently does not possess. Reduced ferritin is apparently present in venous blood, but it becomes oxidized in the lungs while passing through alveoli which are normally aerated. In certain pulmonary diseases and in congenital cyanotic heart disease the mixed venous blood may by-pass normal lung alveoli. As a result, the reduced ferritin which it contains may not become oxidized, so that it appears in the peripheral arterial blood. It has been suggested that this leads to vasodilatation of the peripheral arteriovenous anastomoses and the subsequent development of digital clubbing. This theory does not explain the clubbing which develops in diseases which are not cardiorespiratory in origin.

The possibility has also been advanced that digital clubbing may be dependent upon some pathologic nervous reflex. This theory has been considered because surgical removal of a pulmonary tumor often leads to a lessening in the degree of digital clubbing. It is obvious, however, that such an operative procedure may also result in a reduction of any venous admixture and therefore of any hypoxia, so that improvement could easily be explained by such a mechanism. Here again, a reflex such as this would not explain the clubbing which develops in other cardiorespiratory diseases.

SIGNS OF INADEQUATE GASEOUS EXCHANGE

When the gaseous exchange becomes inadequate, hypoxia develops, either alone or in combination with hypercapnia. Both hypoxia and hypercapnia frequently produce signs which should indicate that the gaseous exchange is inadequate. Once it is suspected, confirmation of the inadequacy can be obtained only by an analysis of the oxygen and carbon dioxide tensions and contents in the arterial blood.

HYPOXIA

The term "hypoxemia" means that there is a diminution in the oxygen content of the arterial blood, but it does not differentiate between a diminution due to a reduced partial pressure of oxygen, a diminution due to a lowered oxygen carrying capacity of the hemoglobin, and a diminution due to both. The term "hypoxia" means that there is a lower than normal amount of oxygen in the body, regardless of the cause or the location. Hypoxia may be present even though both the arterial oxygen tension and content are normal. It has been classified into four main types: hypoxic, anemic, circulatory and histotoxic.

Hypoxic Hypoxia. In hypoxic hypoxia the tissues are supplied by arterial blood whose oxygen tension is lower than normal; that is, the hemoglobin is incompletely saturated with oxygen. This condition occurs in patients who are suffering from respiratory or cardiac diseases in which there is alveolar hypoventilation, altered ventilation-perfusion ratios, a diffusion defect or true venous admixture. This type of hypoxia is also present when the concentration of oxygen in the inspired air is lower than normal, e.g., at a high altitude.

Anemic Hypoxia. In anemic hypoxia the tissues are supplied by arterial blood whose oxygen tension is normal and whose hemoglobin is almost completely saturated with oxygen. Since the hemoglobin content is low, however, both the oxygen content and the oxygen capacity of the blood are lower than normal. As a result, the tissues may not receive sufficient oxygen. This variety of hypoxia may be encountered in all the anemic states as well as in certain conditions in which toxic substances combine with hemoglobin, such as carbon monoxide poisoning and methemoglobinemia. This combination prevents the uptake of oxygen by the hemoglobin, so that the oxygen content falls.

Circulatory Hypoxia. This condition may be encountered in cases of generalized circulatory insufficiency, such as shock or congestive heart failure, or when there is a localized obstruction to arterial blood flow. Similarly, a localized venous occlusion produces local hypoxia because it impedes the flow of blood into and out of the capillaries. It may also develop when the tissue utilization of oxygen increases to an extent which is greater than the available supply of oxygen, as in violent exercise or in thyrotoxicosis. The blood which arrives at the tissues may have a normal oxygen tension and content, but the quantity of blood and, therefore, the oxygen supply to the particular organ may be too small for its metabolic demands.

Histotoxic Hypoxia. Some toxic substances, such as cyanide, interfere with the ability of the tissues to utilize the oxygen. Under such circumstances the tissues may become exceedingly hypoxic even though the partial pressure and content of oxygen in the arterial blood are normal.

The Clinical Manifestations of Hypoxia. Hypoxia does not produce a characteristic clinical picture. The signs and symptoms which result from a lack of oxygen vary considerably, and they are largely dependent on the type of hypoxia which is present. The common form of hypoxia in respiratory diseases is hypoxic hypoxia. In this type of hypoxia the severity of the symptoms depends on the degree of the oxygen deficiency as well as its duration. In some patients, mental confusion, hyperpnea, dyspnea and cyanosis may be the dominant features, but in others these findings may be minimal or absent.

HYPOXIA AND CYANOSIS. Cyanosis is a diffuse bluish discoloration of the skin and mucous membranes due to an increase in the absolute concentration of reduced or otherwise unoxygenated hemoglobin in the capillaries. It is best detected where the coverings over the capillaries of the skin or mucous membrane are thinnest and most transparent.

There are normally approximately 2.5 grams of reduced hemoglobin per 100 ml. of blood in the capillary. It has been suggested that cyanosis does not become perceptible until the mean concentration of reduced hemoglobin in the capillaries is almost double the normal value. For example, in a normal person whose hemoglobin content is 15 grams per cent, and whose arteriovenous oxygen difference is 5 vol. per cent, the arterial and venous oxygen saturations are 97 and 74 per cent. This means that there is 0.45 gram of reduced hemoglobin in the arterial blood, and 3.90 grams in the venous blood. Since the blood has been continually giving up oxygen to the tissues during its passage through the capillaries, the average amount of reduced hemoglobin in the capillaries is considered to be the mean of the sum of the arterial and venous values. There are therefore $\dfrac{0.45 + 3.90}{2}$ or 2.18 grams of reduced hemoglobin per 100 ml. of blood in the capillaries.

If pulmonary insufficiency is present, so that the oxygen saturation is reduced to 80 and 50 per cent in the arterial and venous bloods, there are 3.0 grams of reduced hemoglobin in the arterial blood and 7.50 grams in the venous blood. The reduced hemoglobin content in the capillaries at this time is $\dfrac{3.0 + 7.50}{2}$ or 5.25 grams per 100 ml. of blood.

These calculations indicate that cyanosis develops when the oxygen saturation of the arterial blood falls to approximately 80 per cent. This means that cyanosis cannot be perceived until the arterial oxygen tension is approximately 50 mm. Hg, which is similar to that present when 12 per cent oxygen is inhaled.

When cyanosis occurs in patients suffering from respiratory disease, it is usually a manifestation of hypoxic hypoxia. Too great a reliance is placed on the presence of this sign, however, many physicians regarding it as the most characteristic sign of hypoxia. This opinion is just as erroneous as the belief by many that dyspnea is the only characteristic symptom of hypoxia. The presence of cyanosis does not necessarily indicate the existence of hypoxic hypoxia, and, even more important, hypoxic states do not necessarily produce cyanosis. In addition, as has been stated, the hypoxia may already be very severe before cyanosis can be detected.

The problem becomes even more serious when it is realized that the clinical assessment of the degree of cyanosis is notoriously difficult even for an observer with an artistic eye; the detection of a slight degree of cyanosis is extremely difficult. Most examiners, although able to recognize a well-developed cyanosis, are usually inconsistent in their judgment of the presence of cyanosis in different patients, or even in the same patient on separate occasions. The recognition of cyanosis depends on color perception, which is subject to wide variations from one observer to another. In addition, cyanosis becomes more difficult to detect if the skin overlying the capillaries is thickened and pigmented or if the number and size of the capillaries are reduced.

All of these considerations point to the many pitfalls that would exist if the judgment of arterial hypoxemia were to depend entirely on the criterion of cyanosis. It is, therefore, important to realize that although the detection of cyanosis may mean that hypoxia is present, its absence does not necessarily mean that there is no hypoxia. The presence of hypoxia can be established only by an analysis of the oxygen saturation and oxygen tension in the arterial blood. This is especially true in anemic patients, who may have hypoxia severe enough to threaten life without the clinical development of cyanosis. The severity of cyanosis increases with the amount of hemoglobin in the blood, for at a given oxygen saturation there is a greater amount of reduced hemoglobin if the hemoglobin level is high. Thus a patient who is suffering from polycythemia and whose hemoglobin concentration is greater than 20 grams per cent develops cyanosis at a lesser degree of oxygen desaturation than that which is necessary in a normal person. Conversely, in anemia cyanosis would not develop until severe oxygen desaturation were present.

There are other conditions in which grave tissue hypoxia may be present without the warning sign of cyanosis. For instance, it is difficult to detect cyanosis in a patient who has developed a circulatory hypoxia due to peripheral vascular collapse, presumably because of the severe constriction of the surface vessels, which decreases the amount of blood in the capillaries. In carbon monoxide poisoning, in which a non-oxygen-carrying hemoglobin is formed, severe tissue hypoxia may be present even though the skin remains pink and the blood is bright red. This is the situation in cyanide poisoning as well, in which the tissues are unable to utilize the oxygen which is brought to them.

Cyanosis may develop in the absence of any associated underlying disease. This is true particularly in the extremities if the cutaneous arterioles become narrowed as a result of either a cold environment or nervous influences. Vasoconstriction slows the flow of blood through the capillaries, so that the major part of its oxygen is extracted by the tissues and the amount of reduced hemoglobin in the blood is increased.

Since local cyanosis can be present even though the oxygen tension of the arterial blood is normal, clinicians have classified cyanosis according to the mechanism producing it. They have suggested that cyanosis may be either central, in which case there is a central cause such as a disturbance of pulmonary or cardiac function, or peripheral, in which case there is a local cause such as a slowing of the peripheral circulation by cold or increased vasomotor activity. Inspection of the undersurface of the tongue helps to differentiate these two types, for cyanosis which is peripheral in origin is unlikely to occur there. It must be stressed that this is an etiological classification and not anatomical, as is so often assumed, particularly by students. It is obvious that the peripheral portions of the body, such as the fingers and the tip of the nose, become cyanosed in both the central and the peripheral types of cyanosis. It is probably better to classify cyanosis according to whether it occurs in the presence of reduced arterial oxygen tension or normal arterial oxygen tension.

HYPOXIA AND DYSPNEA.   Some clinicians use the presence or absence of dyspnea as a criterion for the diagnosis of hypoxia. Since dyspnea is a purely subjective sensation and can be caused by a variety of factors, its presence or absence cannot be used as an indication of whether hypoxia is present or not. Some clinicians deduce whether hypoxia is present by the presence or absence of an increased ventilation. However, the ventilatory response to hypoxia varies considerably in different individuals. Breathing a low-oxygen mixture may even fail to produce any measurable increase in respiration in some subjects. This relative lack of response is probably related to the inhibiting effect of the associated hypocapnia and alkalosis on the respiratory center. In addition, the peripheral chemoreceptors are not stimulated by arterial blood which has a low oxygen content but a normal oxygen tension, such as may occur in hemorrhage, anemia, carbon monoxide poisoning, methemoglobinemia or sulphemoglobinemia, so that the ventilation does not increase even though there is severe hypoxia of the rapidly metabolizing cells in such organs as the heart and brain.

HYPOXIA AND TACHYCARDIA.   An increase in pulse rate is often used clinically as a guide to the diagnosis of hypoxia, and it is likely that this is a much more reliable index than are the changes in respiration. An acute reduction in the arterial oxygen tension may produce an increase in the pulse rate, even though it does not stimulate respiration. The pulse rate may also increase in those conditions in which the oxygen content is reduced but the arterial oxygen tension is normal, even though the respiratory rate does not. Unfortunately, from the diagnostic point of view, there are many other conditions besides hypoxia which tend to increase the pulse rate. Factors such as fever, hypotension, pain, venous congestion and even drugs make it difficult to assess the rather small changes in pulse rate that may develop because of a moderate degree of hypoxia. Furthermore, in some cases of prolonged hypoxia, the pulse rate may diminish rather than accelerate. It is, however, probably correct to suspect that hypoxia is present if the pulse rate decreases by ten or more beats per minute within a few minutes after starting the administration of 100 per cent oxygen.

The mechanism by which hypoxia produces tachycardia is not very clear. It is not likely that the low arterial oxygen tension stimulates end-organs in the aortic and carotid chemoreceptors to produce a reflex tachycardia, as well as a reflex hyperpnea, because the heart rate falls when a dog's carotid bodies are perfused with hypoxic blood. It has been suggested that the cardio-accelerator response is due to a stretch reflex from the lungs, for it is abolished by section of the pulmonary branches of the vagus nerves. In addition, a low oxygen content may directly stimulate the vasomotor center to produce the tachycardia, and other factors may be operative as well.

HYPOXIA AND HYPERTENSION. A slight increase in the systolic blood pressure and a fall in the diastolic pressure may occur when mild hypoxia is present. At the same time, there is usually an increase in cardiac output. The peripheral blood flow increases in hypoxia as a result of both peripheral vasodilatation and the increase in cardiac output. A progressively rising blood pressure in a patient with severe respiratory insufficiency frequently indicates that the hypoxia is increasing. On the other hand, a rapid drop in blood pressure may occur in some patients if the hypoxia develops acutely or if hypercapnia is severe.

HYPOXIA AND CEREBRAL FUNCTION. In normal persons, the inhalation of 10 per cent oxygen causes a reduction in the cerebral vascular resistance. This results in an increase in the cerebral blood flow, thereby elevating the oxygen tension of the cerebral tissues. Nevertheless, symptoms related to cerebral dysfunction are the commonest manifestations of hypoxia, whether it is acute or chronic. Although these symptoms occur very frequently, they cannot be used as reliable evidence of the presence of hypoxia.

When a patient becomes acutely hypoxic, he may exhibit either somnolence and lassitude or a sense of comfort, well-being and self-satisfaction which is often associated with outbursts of hilarity or obstreperousness. Judgment may become impaired to such an extent that the entire clinical picture resembles one of drunkenness. The neuromuscular co-ordination frequently suffers, as evidenced by clumsiness and a slowed reaction time.

Acclimatization at Altitude. Most of the information regarding acclimatization to hypoxia has been gleaned from studies on subjects who have resided at high altitudes for long periods of time. In these subjects, hyperventilation is a characteristic finding. As a result of this, the alveolar carbon dioxide tension is decreased and the alveolar oxygen tension is a little higher than would be expected. The arterial carbon dioxide tension is also decreased and there is a proportionate fall in the bicarbonate content, so that the pH remains at an approximately normal level. On the other hand, the rate of the formation of red blood cells increases as a consequence of the lowered arterial oxygen tension. The equilibrium between the formation and the destruction of erythrocytes is apparently maintained, but it now exists at a higher level. Since the hemoglobin content rises as well, the oxygen capacity of the arterial blood is elevated. The effects of acclimatization to altitude on the cardio-vascular system are difficult to evaluate. The cardiac output is increased considerably if there is a moderately brief exposure to high altitude, but the cardiac output is normal in persons who have resided at a high altitude for a long period of time.

Acclimatization at Sea Level. In patients who are chronically hypoxic at sea level, particularly those suffering from cyanotic heart disease, the ventilation tends to increase as the arterial saturation de-creases, but there is a wide variation among different subjects. For a given degree of hypoxia, the ventilation increases less in a person who resides at sea level than it does in one who has become acclimatized to a high altitude. In hypoxic persons at sea level the bicarbonate content of the arterial blood tends to be reduced in proportion to the degree of hypoxia, but this occurs to a lesser extent and for a different reason than it does in dwellers at high altitudes. In contrast to the hypocapnia which the latter exhibit, the arterial carbon dioxide tension is usually within normal limits in patients with congenital heart disease. On the other hand, patients with a congenital right-to-left cardiac shunt tend to be in a state of metabolic acidosis. This may be an advantage, since the acidosis shifts the oxyhemoglobin dissociation curve, thereby assisting in the unloading of oxygen to the tissues.

Just as in those who reside at a high altitude, there is an increased formation of erythrocytes in patients who are hypoxic due to respiratory insufficiency. This secondary polycythemia results from stimulation of the kidney to produce erythropoietin, which in turn stimulates the bone marrow. This increases the oxygen carrying capacity of the blood, and therefore its oxygen content, at a particular partial pressure of oxygen. Consequently, the required amount of oxygen is given off to the tissues without producing too great a fall in the partial pressure of the oxygen in the blood.

In patients who are suffering from both chronic hypoxia and hypercapnia, the hematologic response is variable. A good correlation has, as yet, not been made between the hematologic response and the blood gas tensions. Nevertheless, it has been suggested that at a given level of hypoxia, the red cell mass does not increase as much in these patients as it would in an equally hypoxic healthy subject at a high altitude. The role which either infection or hypercapnia plays in altering this response has not been adequately elucidated.

HYPERCAPNIA

Although patients suffering from a chronic respiratory disease tolerate mild elevations of the carbon dioxide tension for long periods of time, severe retention of carbon dioxide leads to the development of a vicious circle which may have serious consequences. The carbon dioxide retention may reduce the sensitivity of the respiratory center so that ventilation falls, leading to further carbon dioxide retention, a further fall in ventilation with its consequent additional carbon dioxide retention and eventually the development of coma and even death.

Hypercapnia is always associated with hypoxia, unless the person is inhaling a concentration of oxygen greater than that in room air. When present, hypercapnia is the consequence of inadequate alveolar ventilation. The alveolar, and therefore the arterial, carbon dioxide tension is intimately related to and dependent upon both the alveolar ventilation and the level of metabolism. For any given level of metabolism, and therefore of carbon dioxide production, a change in the alveolar ventilation results in an inverse alteration of both the alveolar and the arterial carbon dioxide tensions. A decrease in the alveolar ventilation with no change in the output of carbon dioxide, therefore, results in a rise of the arterial carbon dioxide tension. Similarly, the arterial carbon dioxide tension rises when the production of carbon dioxide increases without a proportionate increase in the alveolar ventilation. It is obvious, therefore, that any respiratory condition in which the general body metabolism or the work of breathing is increased may be associated with carbon dioxide retention.

The Clinical Manifestations of Hypercapnia. The manifestations of acute carbon dioxide retention are frequently precipitated in patients suffering from respiratory disease either by the development of an infection or heart failure or by the administration of oxygen or sedatives.

Acute retention of carbon dioxide may also occur in previously healthy persons if the alveolar ventilation is inadequate because the respiratory center is depressed, as in head injuries, cerebrovascular accidents or excessive amounts of barbiturates, tranquilizing agents or anesthetics. Acute hypercapnia due to alveolar hypoventilation may develop when the chest wall or its neuromuscular components become affected by disease, as in acute poliomyelitis or tetanus, or by traumatic thoracic injuries.

The clinical findings indicative of hypercapnia are predominantly neurological and cardiovascular, their severity depending upon the level of the hypercapnia which is present.

NEUROLOGICAL MANIFESTATIONS. Headache is a very common symptom of chronic hypercapnia and it is frequently accompanied by disturbances of consciousness. The patient may become depressed or may show evidence of confusion and hypomanic activity, with hallucinations or catatonia. Extreme lassitude and drowsiness are common, and somnolence and coma may eventually develop.

Muscular movements, such as fine tremors of the facial muscles and intermittent jerking of the fingers and arms, are a characteristic feature of carbon dioxide narcosis. There may be coarse myoclonic jerking of the trunk and arms and occasionally generalized convulsions. In severe states, the limbs are flaccid and the tendon reflexes cannot be elicited. The plantar responses are either flexor or equivocal, although an extensor plantar response can occasionally be elicited if the carbon dioxide narcosis is very deep, a finding which may lead to the suspicion of an expanding intracranial lesion.

The pathophysiology of the neurological manifestations of hypercapnia has not been adequately explained. The cause of the mental changes is uncertain, although both hypoxia and the narcotic effect of carbon dioxide probably play a role. The headache and some of the mental changes may be related to the increase in cerebral blood flow which occurs when the arterial carbon dioxide tension rises. The cerebrospinal fluid pressure is elevated in patients with carbon dioxide retention, and it increases still further when the elevated carbon dioxide tension leads to the retention of sodium and water. Papilledema may also develop; the mechanism for this is uncertain.

CARDIOVASCULAR MANIFESTATIONS. An elevated arterial carbon dioxide tension apparently has two effects on the blood vessels, that of reflex vasoconstriction and that of peripheral vasodilatation. In severe pulmonary disease, it is common to encounter vasodilatation of the peripheral vessels as well as those in the retina. On the other hand, hypercapnia causes vasoconstriction of the pulmonary vessels, thereby aggravating and increasing the level of pulmonary hypertension which may be present. There is frequently definite tachycardia, while the blood pressure may be high, low or normal. Hypotension with generalized peripheral vasodilatation is a common occurrence when the carbon dioxide retention is severe; this is the picture usually seen before death.

SIGNS OF ALTERED PHYSICAL PROPERTIES OF THE THORAX

When a pathological process involves either the lung or the chest cage, certain properties possessed by the thorax and its contents become altered, producing characteristic clinical signs which help the examiner to arrive at a correct diagnosis and to establish the extent of the disease process. These properties are the size, the distensibility and the density of the lungs and chest wall, and the vascular resistance of the pulmonary vessels.

THE SIZE OF THE LUNGS

Any alteration in the size of a lung is reflected by a shift of the mediastinum from its normal midline position within the thorax. The mediastinum shifts because it is normally mobile. If it should be fibrosed, however, and therefore fixed in position, the shift may not occur. When a shift does occur, it is best indicated by an alteration in the position of the trachea and the apex beat of the heart.

The mediastinum may be shifted from its normal midline position by distortion of the bony thoracic cage, a lesion of the lung parenchyma, a disease affecting the pleural space or an abnormality of the diaphragm. Distortion of the chest cage, as in severe kyphoscoliosis of the thoracic spine, generally causes displacement of the mediastinum towards the side of the lung which is compressed (Fig. 35, *B*). When a lung becomes affected by either fibrosis or atelectasis, the mediastinum shifts towards the affected side, because there is not a proportionate reduction in the size of the thoracic cage. As a result, the end-expiratory intrapleural pressure is lowered on that side and the mediastinum is drawn over (Fig. 37). In contrast to this, when a portion of the lung becomes consolidated there is no change in the size of the affected lung and the end-expiratory intrapleural pressure remains the same on both sides. Therefore, as is shown in Figure 38, the mediastinum remains in its normal midline position. If fluid or air collects in a pleural space, the mediastinum becomes displaced towards the opposite normal side (Fig. 39) because of the relative difference in pressure between the two pleural spaces. The end-expiratory pressure in the affected pleural space rises and may even reach the level of atmospheric pressure, so that the pressure in the opposite normal pleural space is considerably lower. The mediastinum therefore shifts to the side which has the lower pressure. If the abdominal contents herniate into the thoracic cavity through

FIGURE 37. The mechanism of the shift of the mediastinum in atelectasis.

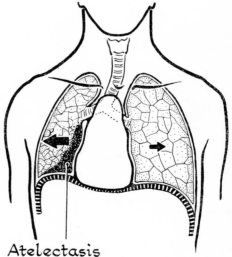

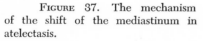

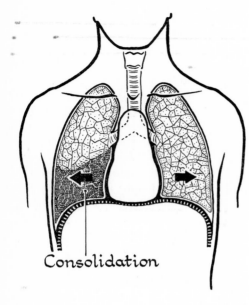

FIGURE 38.   The position of the mediastinum in consolidation.

Consolidation

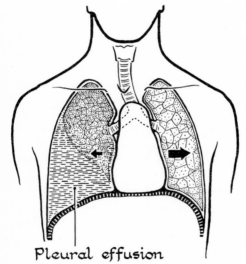

FIGURE 39.   The mechanism of the shift of the mediastinum in a pleural effusion.

Pleural effusion

one of the foramina of the diaphragm, the mediastinum may be displaced to the opposite side. This presumably happens because the intraabdominal pressure, which is normally greater than the intrapleural pressure, is transmitted into the affected hemithorax, so that the pressure on the unaffected normal side is lower. As a result, the mediastinum shifts to the side in which the intrapleural pressure is lower. This is illustrated in Figure 40.

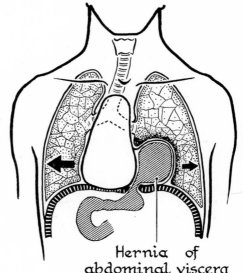

FIGURE 40. The mechanism of the shift of the mediastinum in herniation of the stomach.

Hernia of abdominal viscera

THE DISTENSIBILITY OF THE LUNGS AND THORACIC CAGE

The distensibility of the lungs and thoracic cage is altered in all disease processes affecting the lung parenchyma, the pleural spaces or the chest cage. One of the earliest manifestations of bronchopulmonary disease is consequently a diminished movement of that part of the chest wall which overlies the diseased area.

Chest movement is diminished when there are regional variations in the forces applied to the chest wall by the respiratory muscles, as in muscular dystrophy or poliomyelitis, or when the chest wall itself offers an increased resistance to distention, as in obesity or kyphoscoliosis. Diminished distensibility of the lung, and consequently diminished movement of the chest, is also encountered when there is a regional increase in the resistance to distention of the lung, as in consolidation, fibrosis or atelectasis, or when the lung is compressed by fluid or air in the pleural space.

THE DENSITY OF THE LUNGS AND THORACIC CAGE

Several physical signs indicate an alteration in the density of an area of lung parenchyma. These are alterations in the pitch of the sounds produced by percussion of the overlying chest cage, the quality of the breath sounds or the intensity of vocal fremitus, and the presence of adventitious sounds.

Percussion. Percussion of the chest produces vibrations of the

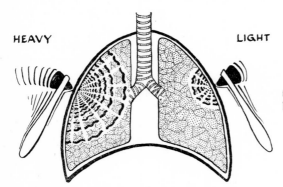

HEAVY   LIGHT

FIGURE 41. The vibrations produced by light and heavy percussion.

chest wall and the underlying lung parenchyma. As is shown in Figure 41, these vibrations not only penetrate medially into the thoracic cavity, but also radiate laterally over the chest wall. The heavier the percussion stroke, the deeper the penetration and lateral radiation of these vibrations, so that ultimately the whole thoracic cavity can be made to vibrate.

On the basis of the pitch of the sound produced by percussion, the examiner is able to determine the ratio that exists between air-containing tissue and solid tissue in the area underlying the percussing finger. Percussion over normal air-containing lung tissue produces slow vibrations, so that the resultant sound has a low pitch and is of a relatively long duration. If the ratio of air to solid tissue is increased, a sound with a lower than normal pitch is produced by percussion. This is the sound heard over a large collection of air in the pleural space or in chronic obstructive emphysema, in which there is a generalized overdistention of air-containing alveoli. On the other hand, if the air to solid tissue ratio is lower than normal, as in atelectasis or consolidation, percussion produces rapid vibrations which quickly disappear. The note is therefore higher in pitch and shorter in duration so that it sounds dull or flat. Thickening of the pleura also produces a dull note on percussion, the pitch of the sound depending on the thickness of the pleura. Similarly, percussion over pleural fluid produces a high-pitched note of varying degrees of flatness, depending on the quantity of fluid present.

The thickness of the musculature and the obesity of the chest wall also affect the number of vibrations and the pitch of the sound produced by percussion. With light percussion, the vibrations penetrate only about two and one-half inches into the thoracic cavity. Assuming that the thickness of a normal chest wall is approximately one inch, the vibrations of light percussion penetrate about one and one-half inches into lung tissue. Under such circumstances, any pulmonary lesion deeper than this does not produce an abnormal sound on percussion. If the thickness of the chest wall is increased, the ratio of air to solid tissue beneath the percussing finger is decreased, so that a higher pitched sound is produced. This obviously has no clinical significance.

The Transmission of Sound. Changes in the density of the thoracic cage and its contents also affect the transmission of sound, which consists of rapidly moving vibrations in the air. In order that sound may be heard, the rate of the vibrations must be within a certain range and above a certain minimal intensity. The number of cycles of repetition that occur in one second is known as the "frequency" of sound, and this accounts for the pitch of a musical note. Low frequencies, with slow rates of repetition, produce a low note; high frequencies, with high rates of repetition, produce a high note.

The *pitch* of a sound depends upon the length and diameter of the tube in which it is produced. The shorter and narrower the tube, the higher the pitch. Since each succeeding branch of the tracheobronchial tree is shorter and narrower than its predecessor, the pitch of the sound produced within succeeding branches becomes higher and higher, finally reaching a peak in the terminal bronchioles.

The *intensity* of a sound, or its loudness, depends on both the energy with which it is transmitted and its frequency. Sound loses its intensity if it has to pass from one medium such as air into another medium such as water, because the sound waves are reflected and absorbed at the fluid-air interfaces.

The *timbre* of a sound is distinct from its pitch or intensity, in that timbre represents its character or quality. It depends on the relative proportion between the fundamental tone and the overtones. It is by means of the timbre that one is able to distinguish between sounds of the same pitch and intensity produced by different instruments.

VOCAL SOUNDS. Voice sounds are produced by the vibrations of the vocal cords in the larynx, which act like a reed instrument. The sound is then carried upwards into the oral cavity and the paranasal sinuses, thereby increasing its intensity and producing its particular tonal quality. The vocal sound is also carried downwards through the tracheobronchial tree as far as the chest wall, causing the thorax to vibrate in unison with the laryngeal sounds. It is thought that the major portion of the vibrations are conducted within the lumen of the bronchi, while the remainder are conducted down along the bronchial walls.

The sound produced within the trachea has been estimated to have vibrations of approximately 400 cycles per second, whereas that produced within a terminal bronchiole possesses vibrations of approximately 1700 cycles/sec. It is believed that the alveoli act as a "selective transmitter" of sound, in that they dampen the high frequency vibrations produced in the bronchial tree. In this way, those sounds with a frequency of 100 to 150 cycles per second are allowed to pass through the alveoli to the chest wall, while those of a higher frequency are not. It is

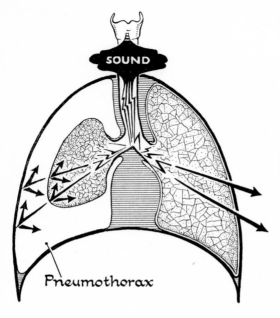

FIGURE 42. The reflection of sound waves at fluid-air interfaces in a pneumothorax.

Pneumothorax

presumed that the lung gradually loses its ability to act as a "selective transmitter" when it becomes diseased. Thus, as the number of normally functioning alveoli decrease, there is a progressive increase in the transmission of the higher frequency vibrations to the chest wall.

VOCAL FREMITUS. Vocal sounds produce vibrations over the chest wall which are called vocal fremitus. When the vibrations are felt by the palpating hand, they are known as tactile fremitus, and when they are heard by means of a stethoscope they are known as auditory fremitus.

The intensity of vocal fremitus is the same over both lungs except for an area over the apex of the right lung. The intensity of the fremitus is increased over the right upper lobe, because the larger bronchi are situated close to the chest wall. Vocal fremitus would appear to be less intense in women and children than in men, presumably because their voices are less resonant.

The vocal fremitus increases in intensity when the underlying lung parenchyma becomes more dense as a result of some disease process. When normal air-containing alveoli are no longer present, as in pulmonary consolidation, in which all the alveoli are filled with inflammatory exudate, the spoken vowels and consonants are clearly felt and heard on the overlying chest wall, provided the bronchus is patent. These sounds differ from those actually produced by the vocal cords, however, in that they have a decidedly nasal, bleating quality, like that of a goat; hence the name "egophony." Presumably the diseased lung parenchyma has lost its "selective transmitter" property and permits the higher frequency vibrations to pass through to the chest wall.

The vocal fremitus is decreased in intensity when either fluid or air is present in the pleural space (Fig. 42) because the sound waves from the underlying lung parenchyma are reflected and absorbed at the increased number of fluid-air interfaces. Most of the sound vibrations which manage to pass through the visceral surface of the fluid or air are reflected by the parietal surface, so that the vibrations are either diminished in intensity before they finally reach the chest wall or disappear completely. Vocal fremitus also becomes decreased if the chest wall is very muscular or obese, since the distance through which the sound must travel is increased.

Breath Sounds. Most of the breath sound which is produced within the tracheobronchial tree during inspiration and expiration is conducted within the lumen of the bronchi in a manner similar to that of the spoken voice. The passage of air into and out of the bronchial tree during respiration is illustrated in Figure 43. During inspiration eddies and turbulence are produced when the air current strikes the sharp borders of the bronchial bifurcations. As the air moves outwards during expiration, it mixes with air currents coming from other small airways and strikes against the wall of the parent bronchus, creating turbulence and small eddies, but presumably fewer than in inspiration because the out-going air does not encounter any sharp bifurcations.

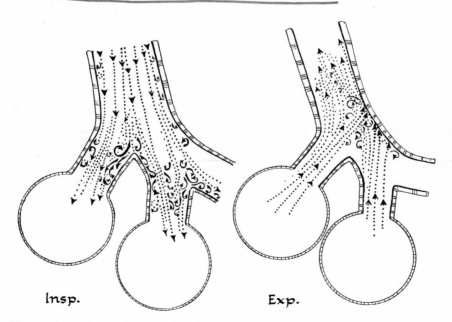

Insp.   Exp.

FIGURE 43. The production of turbulence in the airways during inspiration and expiration.

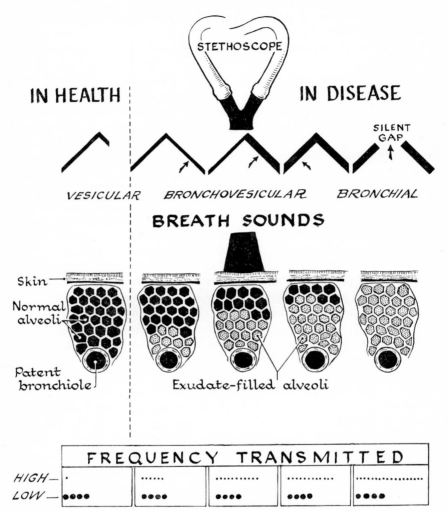

FIGURE 44.   The changes which breath sounds undergo as the alveoli become diseased.

The breath sounds heard over the chest wall during auscultation result from the turbulence produced by the movement of air within the tracheobronchial tree. The sounds heard over the chest with a stethoscope differ considerably both in quality and intensity, however, from those actually produced within the bronchial tree.

VESICULAR BREATH SOUND.   The sounds which are heard over normal lung parenchyma are called vesicular breath sounds. The inspiratory breath sound is easily heard over healthy lung tissue during auscultation, but the expiratory sound is fainter and is approximately one-third the length of the inspiratory note. These sounds can be detected over all areas of a normal lung except the apex of the right lung, where the breath sound is bronchovesicular in quality because the bronchi are closer to the chest wall and are covered by a smaller amount of lung tissue.

BRONCHOVESICULAR BREATH SOUND. The bronchovesicular breath sound is normally heard only over the apex of the right lung. In disease states, however, the "selective transmitter" properties of the pulmonary alveoli become altered so that some of the higher frequency vibrations pass through to the stethoscope on the chest wall.

Figure 44 demonstrates the successive changes in the breath sound heard during auscultation as the proportion of diseased alveoli to normal alveoli increases. At first, the short, faint, expiratory note of the vesicular breath sound becomes louder and higher in pitch. At the same time it progressively lengthens, finally reaching the length of the inspiratory sound. The inspiratory sound then becomes higher both in pitch and intensity until it equals that of the expiratory sound.

A bronchovesicular breath sound always implies that some of the alveoli in the diseased area of the lung are still functioning normally. In its more advanced stage, it may frequently be mistaken for a "bronchial" breath sound, which it closely resembles. The breath sound is bronchovesicular, however, as long as the end of the inspiratory sound blends with the beginning of the expiratory sound.

BRONCHIAL BREATH SOUND. When the disease process in the lung parenchyma has progressed to such an extent that all the alveoli are involved, true "bronchial breathing" becomes evident. This is the type of breath sound which is heard when an area of lung becomes consolidated, as long as it is in close apposition to a patent bronchus. The sound is produced because the lung has lost its "selective transmitter" property so that all the high frequency vibrations within the bronchial tree are now transmitted to the chest wall. Inspiration and expiration are equally affected with respect to pitch, intensity and duration. Characteristically, the bronchial breath sound is high-pitched and loud, being identical to that which is normally heard in auscultation over the trachea. It is distinguished from the bronchovesicular sound by the presence of a gap between the end of inspiration and the beginning of expiration. The explanation for this silent phase has never been clarified.

Adventitious Sounds. Vibrations produced by pathological processes within the lungs and the tracheobronchial tree are called adventitious sounds. These are never detected over healthy lung tissue; their presence always indicates that some type of pathological process has developed in the affected portion of the lung or pleura.

RHONCHI. A rhonchus, a term derived from the Greek word meaning wheezing, is a prolonged musical note, produced within the lumen of the tracheobronchial tree. Whenever a portion of the tracheo-

Dry sound ~~ **RHONCHI** Inflamed walls

Produced during forced, prolonged EXPIRATION.

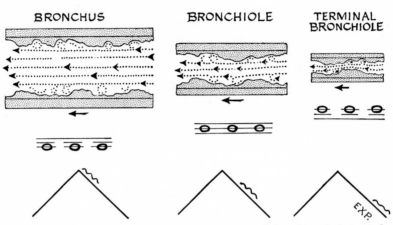

FIGURE 45.   The relationship between the origin of rhonchi and their pitch.

bronchial tree becomes narrowed, the resistance to air flow increases, producing turbulence and eddy formation. Since the bronchi normally shorten and narrow during expiration, the turbulent resistance increases more during this phase of respiration. Consequently, rhonchi are usually more pronounced during expiration, and especially during the expulsive phase of a cough. Occasionally minor degrees of bronchial obstruction may not produce rhonchi during normal respiration. Under such circumstances rhonchi may be elicited if the patient expires forcibly or coughs vigorously.

The pitch of a rhonchus depends on the diameter of the tube in which the sound is produced. A rhonchus originating in a large bronchus has a low-pitched quality and is known as a "sonorous" rhonchus; one originating in a terminal bronchiole has an extremely high-pitched quality and is called a "sibilant" rhonchus. Sibilant rhonchi are heard characteristically in chronic obstructive emphysema or during an attack of bronchial asthma. Narrowing of one of the intermediate bronchial branches produces rhonchi whose pitch varies accordingly; these are known as "medium-pitched" rhonchi. The different types of rhonchi are illustrated in Figure 45.

RALES.   A rale, a term derived from the French word meaning rattle, is a short, interrupted bubbling sound. It is believed that most rales are produced by the bursting of the surface film of bubbles of fluid within either bronchi or alveoli, although evidence to substantiate this has been difficult to obtain. Rales are more evident during inspiration, perhaps because the intrathoracic pressure is more negative during that phase of respiration so that the bubbles burst.

The pitch of a rale depends on the type of lesion and on the diameter of the chamber containing the bubbles of fluid (Fig. 46). If secretions are in the terminal bronchioles, the rales have a very high-pitched quality. If the secretions are in the smaller bronchi, the rales are lower in pitch. If the secretions are in the larger bronchi, the rales have a considerably lower pitch.

Rales have been classified clinically into three types, depending both on their pitch and on the predominant phase of inspiration in which they occur (Fig. 47). If there is exudate in the larger or medium-sized bronchi, as in a case of purulent bronchitis, low-pitched or coarse rales are produced predominantly during the initial part of inspiration. If the smaller bronchi are involved, as in bronchiectasis, medium-pitched rales are produced predominantly during the middle phase of inspiration. If the parenchyma alone is involved, however, high-pitched or fine rales are produced predominantly during the last part of inspiration. This phenomenon occurs when the alveoli are filled with either serous fluid, as in pulmonary congestion, or with inflammatory exudate, as in the early stages of pulmonary tuberculosis. It has, therefore, been suggested that the temporal position of the rales during inspiration may yield information regarding the anatomical location of the disease process. Unfortunately, it is difficult to obtain evidence to substantiate this obviously important hypothesis.

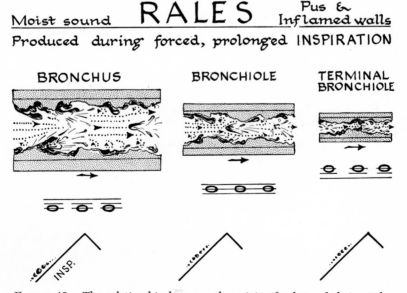

Moist sound   **RALES**   Pus &
Inflamed walls

Produced during forced, prolonged INSPIRATION

BRONCHUS   BRONCHIOLE   TERMINAL BRONCHIOLE

FIGURE 46.   The relationship between the origin of rales and their pitch.

RALES

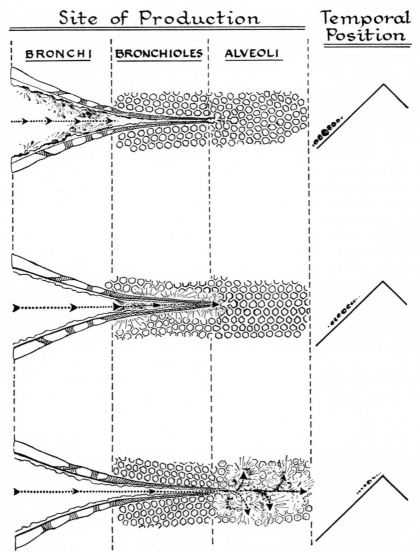

FIGURE 47.   The relationship between the origin of rales and their temporal position.

If there is only a minimal amount of disease in the alveoli, rales may not be elicited by an ordinary deep inspiration. On the other hand, they can often be detected during the beginning of the inspiration following a cough. These "post-tussic" rales (from the Latin word "tussis" meaning cough) are presumably produced by the separation of sticky alveolar walls which have become adherent during the compressive phase of the cough.

A creaky, interrupted, dry sound may occasionally be heard in patients who are suffering from fibrosis of either the lung parenchyma or the peribronchial tissues. As illustrated in Figure 48, this sound characteristically extends uniformly throughout the whole of inspiration and of expiration. It has been suggested that it is caused by the stretching and relaxing of the fibrous tissue during respiration.

PLEURAL RUBS. These dry, creaking, coarse, leathery sounds are diagnostic of pleural irritation. They are probably produced by the inflamed surfaces of the two pleural layers rubbing against one another during respiration. They therefore predominate during the latter part of inspiration and the early part of expiration. Since the greatest movement of the lungs, and therefore the greatest excursion of the pleural surfaces, occurs over the lower lobes, friction rubs are most frequently detected over the lower areas of the chest wall. Pleural rubs are only very occasionally heard over the upper areas of the chest wall because the movement of the upper lobes and the excursion of their pleural surfaces are comparatively small.

Signs Associated with Air or Fluid in the Pleural Cavity. THE COIN CLICK. When two coins are clicked together over the anterior chest wall, the sound which is heard over the posterior chest wall is muffled and faint as long as there is no air in the pleural space. When there is a large collection of air, especially if it is under tension, the sound has a clearly heard metallic quality, probably because the lung is almost completely collapsed, so that the number of interfaces at which the sound might be reflected is reduced.

SUCCUSSION SPLASH. When air and fluid are both present in the pleural cavity, a splashing sound may be produced when the thoracic cage is shaken. This sound, which is detected by the stethoscope, is called a succussion splash.

When a bronchopleural fistula is present, a gurgling sound may

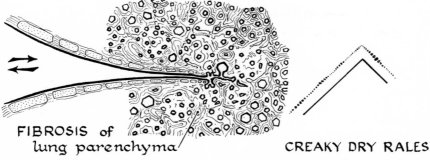

FIBROSIS of lung parenchyma   CREAKY DRY RALES

FIGURE 48.   The creaky dry rales produced by pulmonary fibrosis.

be detected during inspiration. This is probably caused by air entering the pleural fluid through the fistula.

THE PULMONARY VASCULAR RESISTANCE

As a result of alterations in the pulmonary vascular bed, the resistance within the vessels frequently becomes increased so that the pressure in the pulmonary artery rises. The level of pulmonary hypertension usually correlates well with the degree of oxygen unsaturation. The physical signs which indicate that the normal vascular hemodynamics have become altered are produced by the pulmonary hypertension. The lungs themselves give no indication of the presence of pulmonary hypertension, the only signs indicative of this abnormality being found during the examination of the heart.

The intensity of the second pulmonic heart sound yields a great deal of information about the possibility of pulmonary hypertension. The second heart sound is caused by the closure of the aortic and pulmonary valves. During inspiration the pulmonic second sound may be split into two parts, an earlier aortic component and a later pulmonary component. The aortic and pulmonary components are normally almost superimposed during expiration. This splitting is normally readily detected in most children and young adults, but it may also be present in many older persons. The splitting is the result of a delay in the closure of the pulmonic valve because of an increased right ventricular filling and a prolonged systole of the right ventricle during inspiration. On the other hand, when there is severe pulmonary hypertension or right ventricular failure due to pulmonary disease, the second sound may not split during inspiration. In addition, when pulmonary hypertension is present, the second pulmonic sound is very much louder than normal, and if severe, it may be transmitted to the apex. If the second pulmonic sound becomes so accentuated that it can be felt by the palpating hand, the pulmonary vascular resistance is exceedingly high.

When pulmonary hypertension from any cause is present, a high-pitched early systolic ejection click in the pulmonary artery may be heard. This is probably due to accentuated ejection vibrations. In addition, there is frequently a presystolic gallop rhythm.

An increased pulmonary vascular resistance imposes a very heavy burden on the right ventricle, so that it frequently hypertrophies. The position and character of the cardiac impulse, if visible or palpable, may be indicative of right ventricular hypertrophy. When the right ventricle is enlarged, a prominent pulsation may be visible along the left border of the sternum. This is usually associated with a conspicuous retraction further to the left over the left ventricle, so that the anterior chest has a rocking motion which is synchronous with the heart beat.

When right-sided heart failure develops, the condition is called cor pulmonale. There is no exact correlation between the height of the pulmonary arterial pressure and the development of cor pulmonale. In general, however, it has been said that a sustained mean pulmonary artery pressure above 40 mm. Hg is associated with both a significant alteration in the electrocardiographic tracing as well as a radiological enlargement in the size of the right ventricle.

SECTION

3

THE PATTERNS OF

RESPIRATORY DISEASE

BRONCHIAL DISEASE

PULMONARY PARENCHYMAL DISEASE

PULMONARY VASCULAR DISEASE

PLEURAL DISEASE

MEDIASTINAL DISEASE

DIAPHRAGMATIC DISEASE

DISEASES OF THE CHEST WALL
  AND THORACIC CAGE

CARDIORESPIRATORY INSUFFICIENCY

CHAPTER VII

Bronchial Disease

THE BRONCHI are involved in most pulmonary diseases. Some diseases involve the bronchi diffusely and others are limited to a single bronchus or one of its subdivisions. In the latter group of diseases it is essential to identify the involved bronchopulmonary segment during the physical examination. A knowledge of the pattern of the bronchial tree and the bronchopulmonary segments is therefore essential for the proper understanding of bronchopulmonary disease.

BRONCHOPULMONARY ANATOMY

The trachea extends anteriorly from the lower edge of the cricoid cartilage to the level of the second costal cartilage. This level corresponds posteriorly to the lower border of the body of the fourth thoracic vertebra. Here the trachea divides into the right and left major bronchi, which serve each lung.

The right major bronchus divides into three main branches, each serving an individual lobe of the right lung. From above downwards these consist of a bronchus to the upper lobe, one to the middle lobe and one to the lower lobe. The left major bronchus divides into only two branches, one to the upper lobe and one to the lower lobe. The lobar bronchi then divide into smaller branches, which are known as "segmental bronchi," each supplying a portion of a lobe called a "bronchopulmonary segment." These are illustrated in Figures 49 to 52. A given segment has not only its own bronchus, but in addition its own artery, vein and lymphatics. For this reason a segmental resection can be carried out with impunity, for removal of a lung segment does not compromise the blood supply of other parts of the lung.

THE RIGHT LUNG

The bronchus supplying the upper lobe of the right lung arises from the lateral aspect of the right major bronchus, about 2.5 cm. beyond

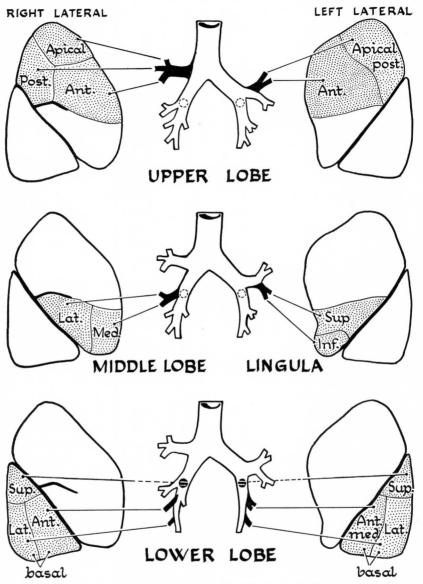

FIGURE 49.   The segmental bronchi and lateral view of the bronchopulmonary
segments.

the bifurcation of the trachea, and almost immediately divides into three
branches. The anterior branch supplies the anterior segment of the
right upper lobe, which is situated anteriorly between the levels of
the clavicle and the fourth rib. The apical bronchus supplies the apical

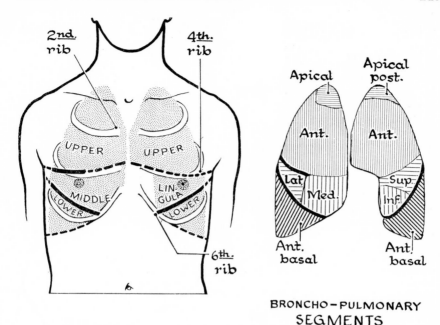

BRONCHO-PULMONARY
SEGMENTS

FIGURE 50. The bronchopulmonary segments (anterior aspect).

segment of the upper lobe, which lies in the area above the level of the clavicle. The third branch, or the posterior bronchus, supplies the posterior segment of the upper lobe, which lies posteriorly to the other segments of the upper lobe.

The middle lobe bronchus of the right lung arises from the anterior aspect of the right major bronchus, about 2 cm. below the opening of the upper lobe bronchus. It runs in a downward, forward and lateral direction, finally dividing into two branches which supply the medial and the lateral segments of the middle lobe.

After giving off its branch to the middle lobe, the right main bronchus gives off the superior or apical branch posteriorly and then continues its downward course and finally divides into four branches, each supplying a particular segment of the lower lobe. These are the anterior basal, the medial basal, the lateral basal and the posterior basal segments.

THE LEFT LUNG

The bronchus to the upper lobe of the left lung arises from the anterolateral aspect of the left major bronchus, about 5 cm. from the bifurcation of the trachea. Unlike the right major bronchus, it then splits into an upper and a lower division.

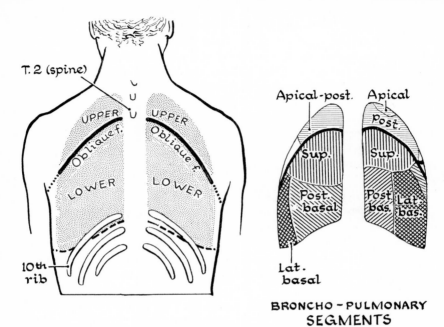

FIGURE 51.   The bronchopulmonary segments (posterior aspect).

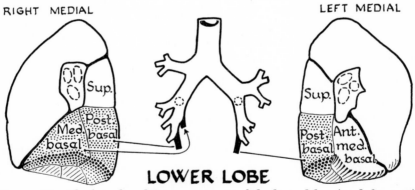

FIGURE 52.   The bronchopulmonary segments of the lower lobes (medial aspect).

The upper division of the left upper lobe bronchus divides into two branches, one supplying the anterior segment, and the other the apical-posterior segment of the upper lobe. The anterior segment corresponds to that of the right upper lobe, whereas the apical-posterior segment corresponds to both the apical and posterior segments of the right upper lobe. They therefore underlie the same areas of the rib cage as do their counterparts on the right side.

The lower division supplies the lingula. Although actually a part of the left upper lobe, the lingula corresponds morphologically to the middle lobe of the right lung. The bronchus to the lingula divides into two branches supplying the superior and the inferior segments of the lingula, which are situated one above the other.

The lower division of the left major bronchus continues its downward course, in a manner similar to that of the right major bronchus, to form the left lower lobe bronchus. This divides into four branches which supply the superior or apical segment, the anterior-medial basal segment (which corresponds to both the anterior basal and the medial basal segments of the right lung), the lateral basal segment and the posterior basal segment.

It should be noted that the upper lobe of the left lung, including its lingular portion, corresponds morphologically to both the upper and middle lobes of the right lung. Similarly, the segments of the left lower lobe correspond to those of the right lower lobe, with the exception of the anterior basal segment and the medial basal segment of the right lower lobe. These correspond to the anterior-medial basal segment of the left lower lobe.

All the larger bronchi are surrounded by plates of cartilage, but this is only occasionally true of the more peripheral bronchi. The bronchioles possess no supporting cartilage at all. When a portion of the lung collapses, the more proximal bronchi may remain patent because of their cartilaginous plates, whereas the peripherally situated bronchi behave like bronchioles and alveoli, in that they collapse with their walls lying in apposition with each other.

BRONCHIAL OBSTRUCTION

When a portion of lung parenchyma becomes diseased, the bronchus draining the area may be involved as well because of mucosal swelling or inflammatory exudate within its lumen. This narrows the lumen, thereby interfering with the normal movement of air into and out of the alveoli. Impaired drainage of secretions plays an important role in the progress of the pathological process within the lung tissue.

The term "bronchial obstruction" is a relative one. For instance, the severity of the obstruction of an affected bronchus varies inversely with the diameter of its lumen. Mucosal swelling does not produce the degree of obstruction in one of the larger bronchi that it does in one of the finer bronchi. Inflammatory swelling of even the larger bronchi may have serious obstructive effects in an infant, because of the smaller diameter of all its bronchi. A healthy person can, by coughing, easily expel thick bronchial secretions which are temporarily producing an obstruction. On the other hand, if the cough mechanism is inefficient,

these secretions may result in a sustained bronchial obstruction with
serious consequences.

PATHOGENESIS OF BRONCHIAL OBSTRUCTION

The three mechanisms by which a bronchial lumen may be narrowed are depicted in Figure 53. The cause may be extramural, in which case the narrowing of the bronchus is produced by external pressure, as with enlarged mediastinal lymph nodes occluding the right middle lobe bronchus. Bronchial obstruction may also be mural, the obstruction resulting from a pathological lesion within the confines of the bronchial wall, such as a bronchogenic carcinoma, which may increase in size and project into the lumen of the bronchus. Mucosal edema may lead to bronchial obstruction in a similar way. There are also intraluminal causes of bronchial obstruction, such as an inhaled foreign body or thick inflammatory secretions.

A bronchial obstruction may be either partial or complete. In a partial obstruction, the flow of air and drainage of bronchial secretions still take place although they are impaired. In a complete obstruction, both air flow and drainage of secretions no longer take place.

Partial Bronchial Obstruction. A partial bronchial obstruction always acts as either a by-pass valve or a check-valve, depending both on the degree of narrowing of the bronchial lumen and on the nature of the pathological process producing it.

BY-PASS BRONCHIAL OBSTRUCTION. The by-pass type of valvular obstruction is illustrated in Figure 54. In this type of obstruction, the lumen of the bronchus is only slightly narrowed, so that although the resistance is increased, air is still able to flow in and out past the site of obstruction. A partial bronchial obstruction occasionally produces distention of the lung parenchyma distal to the obstruction, because the resistance to air flow is particularly increased during expiration.

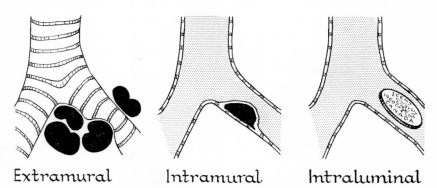

Extramural   Intramural   Intraluminal

FIGURE 53.   The causes of bronchial obstruction.

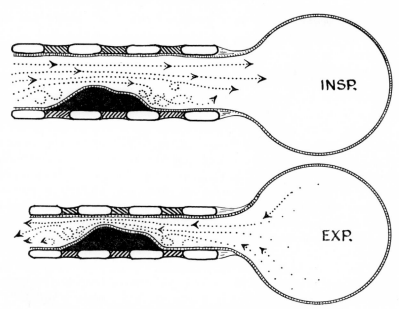

FIGURE 54.   The by-pass partial bronchial obstruction.

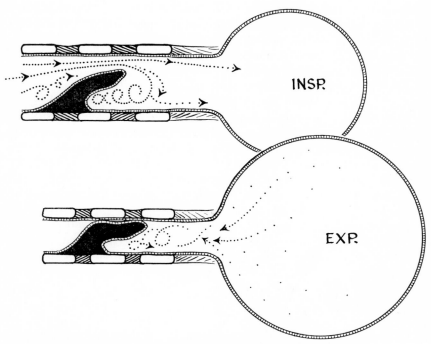

FIGURE 55.   The check-valve partial bronchial obstruction.

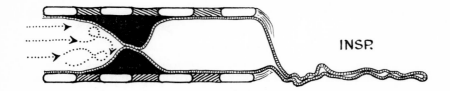

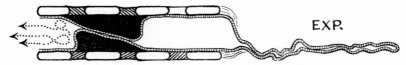

FIGURE 56.   The complete bronchial obstruction.

CHECK-VALVE BRONCHIAL OBSTRUCTION.   This type of bronchial obstruction differs from a by-pass valvular obstruction in that the bronchial lumen is completely occluded during expiration so that the egress of air is prevented. This is illustrated in Figure 55. An endobronchial tumor attached to the bronchial wall by means of a pedicle is an example of this type of obstruction. During inspiration, the bronchial lumen widens so that air passes over the tumor. During expiration, however, the lumen is completely occluded because of the expiratory narrowing of the bronchial lumen. As a result, air is trapped in the affected pulmonary segment, so that the alveoli become overdistended.

Complete Bronchial Obstruction.   In the complete or stop-valve type of obstruction, which is illustrated in Figure 56, the bronchus is completely occluded so that air cannot move in or out. The consequence of this type of obstruction is an atelectasis of the affected portion of lung which develops because the total pressure within the pulmonary capillaries is approximately 700 mm. Hg, while that within the alveoli corresponds to that of the atmosphere. Provided the blood flow to the affected lung segment is intact, the gases in the alveoli are gradually absorbed into the pulmonary capillaries. The elastic lung consequently retracts, so that the involved area of lung becomes airless and collapsed. The absorption of the alveolar air takes place slowly, so that the lung may not collapse immediately, even though the obstruction of the bronchus is sudden in onset.

CLINICAL MANIFESTATIONS

The clinical manifestations of airway obstruction depend on the type of obstruction and its location in the tracheobronchial tree. Complete obstruction of the trachea results in asphyxia and death. Partial tracheal obstruction produces distention of both lungs and an intense dyspnea which is largely inspiratory. Inspiration is forceful and prolonged, with visible indrawing over the sternal notch, the supraclavicular spaces, the intercostal spaces and the epigastrium. At the same time, a coarse, snoring, low-pitched rhonchus which is both inspiratory and expiratory in time can be heard over the trachea and at the open mouth.

If an inhaled foreign body is lodged at the tracheal bifurcation, the orifices of the two major bronchi may become obstructed in different ways. One major bronchus may be completely obstructed, whereas a by-pass or check-valve obstruction may develop in the opposite bronchial orifice.

If obstruction of a large bronchus should develop gradually there may be no symptoms aside from a cough. On the other hand, if the obstruction develops abruptly, intense dyspnea is always experienced. The extent of the symptoms which develop when the finer bronchi or bronchioles become obstructed depends on the number of bronchi involved. If the obstruction is localized to a few smaller bronchi, there may be no symptoms. If there is diffuse involvement of the smaller bronchi throughout both lungs, however, as in bronchial asthma, the patient experiences intense dyspnea.

Interference with bronchial drainage is a frequent consequence of bronchial obstruction, and because bacteria grow very easily in retained secretions, infection frequently develops in the affected area of the lung. Consequently, a cough is almost always associated with any type of bronchial obstruction. As the degree of obstruction increases, so does the cough. If the cough is ineffective the retained secretions often become infected and create a vicious cycle with the production of more secretions and more cough.

In a by-pass obstruction, eddies are produced in the air currents at the site of the obstruction, and the resultant vibrations produce a wheezing sound or rhonchus, particularly during expiration, when the bronchus shortens and narrows, and more particularly if the expiration is prolonged and forceful. Since the pitch of a rhonchus depends on the diameter of the lumen of the involved bronchus, a low-pitched, coarse, snoring sound is produced when there is a partial obstruction of the larger bronchi, and high-pitched whistling rhonchi are heard when the finer bronchi are involved. When bronchi with diameters between these two extremes are partially obstructed, medium-pitched rhonchi of various degrees are produced. The rhonchi are conducted through the parenchyma of the lung to the overlying area of the chest wall, as well as throughout the tracheobronchial tree, so that they may also be detected over the open mouth.

Rhonchi may be heard bilaterally over all areas of the chest cage or they may be confined to a single area. Generalized rhonchi indicate diffuse involvement of the tracheobronchial tree, a situation which occurs in bronchial asthma or chronic bronchitis. Rhonchi confined to a single area of the chest wall, on the other hand, indicate a localized partial bronchial obstruction. This finding, however, gives no indication of the type of pathological process producing the obstruction. An early form of bronchogenic carcinoma produces exactly the same type of rhonchus as does a localized collection of thick bronchial secretions. If the cause of the obstruction is immovable, the rhonchus persists despite vigorous coughing, but secretions usually become dislodged, so that the wheeze disappears.

There are characteristic clinical manifestations of a check-valve type of obstruction. First, a rhonchus may be heard during inspiration but not during expiration, because the air is unable to escape past the obstruction. Second, because air is trapped in it, the affected segment becomes overdistended, and if a large portion of lung is involved, the mediastinum shifts towards the normal side. The movement of the chest cage is diminished, the percussion note is hyper-resonant, and the intensity of the breath sounds is reduced over the affected lung.

When atelectasis develops in a complete bronchial obstruction, the size of the affected lung decreases and the density increases. Consequently, there is a shift of the mediastinum towards the affected side, while over the area of atelectasis, the movement of the chest cage is diminished and the percussion note is dull. Since the affected bronchus is completely occluded, there is no movement of air within the bronchus distal to the obstruction, so that the breath sounds are usually inaudible. Bronchial breathing may occasionally be heard, however, if the collapsed lung parenchyma overlies another large bronchus which is patent.

RADIOLOGICAL MANIFESTATIONS

The radiological changes brought about by bronchial obstruction are those produced by the complications which develop. If there is a localized check-valve type of obstruction, the affected portion of lung is hyperinflated. During fluoroscopy, both lungs may be seen to inflate equally during inspiration, but the affected area of lung does not deflate normally during expiration. In addition, the difference in intrapulmonary pressure on the two sides may cause the mediastinum to shift towards the unaffected side during expiration. The persistent inflation of the affected lung and the mediastinal shift may also be demonstrated on x-ray films taken during both inspiration and expiration. An x-ray taken during expiration in such a situation is shown in Figure 57. When there is diffuse partial obstruction of the smaller bronchi, there is frequently generalized hyperinflation of the lungs. When a complete

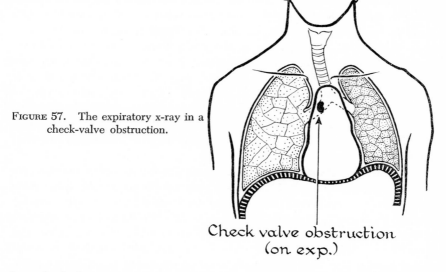

FIGURE 57. The expiratory x-ray in a check-valve obstruction.

Check valve obstruction
(on exp.)

bronchial obstruction is present, the manifestations of atelectasis, which are discussed later, are apparent on the roentgenogram.

FUNCTIONAL MANIFESTATIONS

The nature of the alterations in pulmonary function arising as a result of obstruction depend upon the type of obstruction present and on its location in the tracheobronchial tree. The commonest type of obstruction encountered clinically is the diffuse by-pass or check-valve type due to excessive secretions in the lumen of the bronchi or spasm of the bronchioles. The commonest clinical entities in which such obstructions are encountered are bronchitis, chronic obstructive emphysema, bronchiectasis and bronchial asthma. The functional manifestations of bronchial obstruction are therefore discussed under the appropriate sections, the first of which follows immediately.

BRONCHITIS

Bronchitis is a condition in which there is inflammation of the bronchial tree with the production of excessive mucus. It is possible that bronchitis is an allergic type of reaction, although specific antigens and antibodies have never been demonstrated. The acute variety of bronchitis is moderately common, and it usually leads to little disability. On the other hand, the chronic form is an important clinical entity, for it is inevitably associated with severe disturbances in respiratory function, is frequently followed by the development of chronic obstructive emphysema, and may ultimately lead to death from bronchopneumonia or acute respiratory insufficiency and right-sided heart failure.

In a healthy person, about 100 ml. of mucus, a viscid material containing various combinations of proteins and carbohydrates, is formed in the bronchial tree every day. This mucus is not expectorated, but is probably used to humidify and warm the inspired air. It is secreted from the goblet cells of the bronchial epithelium, which extend down as far as the terminal bronchioles, and from the mucous glands which are numerous in the walls of the trachea and the bronchi. The glands progressively decrease in number toward the periphery of the bronchial tree, so that only an occasional one is found at the bifurcations of the smaller bronchioles. The mucous glands are excited by vagal stimulation, but the goblet cells do not appear to be under nervous control, their hypersecretion apparently being stimulated directly by irritants such as atmospheric pollution, climatic changes and infection.

In acute bronchitis or in the earlier stages of the chronic form, there is hypersecretion of mucus by the bronchi due to either an increased number of secreting cells or an increased rate of mucus production, or both. In cases of moderately advanced chronic bronchitis, there is an apparent increase in the number of secreting cells, and the degree of hypersecretion varies. In a well-established case of chronic bronchitis, hypertrophy of the mucous glands and the goblet cells is evident. In the absence of an acute infection the cilia are usually intact, although if many goblet cells are discharging, the effective ciliary area may be reduced or the cilia may become inefficient so that drainage is impaired.

ACUTE BRONCHITIS

This condition may occur as a primary manifestation during the course of specific infectious diseases such as measles and typhoid fever, or as a concomitant of the acute bacterial pneumonias such as the lobular pneumonia of streptococcal origin. It develops most commonly as a consequence of a viral infection such as influenza, but generally this form becomes complicated by a secondary bacterial invasion. Sometimes, especially in patients with chronic bronchitis, acute symptoms appear to be precipitated by irritative rather than infective factors, the most frequent irritant being a high concentration of atmospheric pollutants.

Clinical Manifestations. The onset of acute bronchitis is heralded by a substernal burning discomfort, which is caused by the associated tracheitis. In addition, there is a harassing, rasping, painful cough, which may occur in exhausting, suffocating paroxysms. These paroxysmal attacks are precipitated by exposure to cold air as well as by the inhalation of irritants such as cigarette smoke. There is frequently an associated audible wheezing. Initially, there is characteristically only a scanty expectoration of mucus, but later it often becomes more abundant and mucopurulent. On recovery from the illness, little or no evidence of the disease usually remains, provided the offending irritant has been removed. For obvious reasons, little is known about the pathology of this condition.

Acute bronchiolitis is a very serious progression of this disease, especially in infants and children, not only because of the high resistance to air flow that is present, but also because of the lobular pneumonia which develops as a result of a lobular atelectasis and the consequent impaired drainage of secretions.

"RECURRENT" BRONCHITIS

As the term implies, there may be recurrent attacks of bronchitis, generally following in the wake of an upper respiratory infection. There is always an underlying chronic infection in some portion of the upper respiratory tract, such as chronic sinusitis or chronic rhinitis. A chronic purulent postnasal discharge can produce a chronic irritation of the mucosa of the trachea and bronchi, and an acute flare-up of sinusitis aggravates the condition.

Recurrent bronchitis is more liable to occur during seasonal changes. If the attacks are frequent enough or unduly prolonged, complete resolution of the inflammation may not take place, with the inevitable development of chronic bronchitis.

CHRONIC BRONCHITIS

Clinically, this condition is characterized by a chronic cough with expectoration which persists year in and year out. Pathologically, it is manifested by an excess secretion of bronchial mucus with edema and inflammatory changes in the bronchial wall. Functionally, it is associated with an increase in the resistance to air flow, particularly during expiration, as well as alterations of the ventilation-perfusion ratios.

Until recently, chronic bronchitis was considered to be a relatively rare condition on the North American continent, and was rarely felt to be a threat to life or even a common cause of prolonged disability. In the United Kingdom, however, chronic bronchitis outranks all other respiratory diseases as a crippler and a killer. It is responsible for an annual loss of nearly 27 million working man-days, and it is the cause of an annual death rate of 30,000. This is about 45 times greater than the number of deaths caused by chronic bronchitis in North America, and is twice the number caused by pulmonary tuberculosis. It may be possible that the disease is different in the two parts of the world, but it is likely that some of the "difference" is due to the criteria used in the diagnosis of chronic bronchitis. In fact, many of the cases labeled emphysema, intrinsic asthma or asthmatic bronchitis are probably cases of chronic bronchitis. It is therefore likely that the incidence of chronic bronchitis on the North American continent is much greater than has been assumed.

Pathogenesis. The factors involved in the etiology of chronic bronchitis have undergone considerable scrutiny, but the picture is still poorly understood. The frequency of deaths due to this disease increases with age, and there is a strong preponderance of males over females, the ratio being 4:1. Common to all cases of bronchitis are irritants in the tracheobronchial tree, one of the most important sources being the upper respiratory tract. Although it is often difficult to sort out which comes first, infection in the upper respiratory tract and postnasal discharge are common concomitants of bronchitis. Though the mouth and nasopharynx normally harbor many bacteria which are considered to be commensal organisms, the respiratory tract below the larynx is practically sterile. Many bacteria are probably inhaled during respiration, but normally these adhere to the layer of mucus in the bronchial tree and are removed by ciliary activity and coughing. In patients with chronic bronchitis, however, organisms can be isolated in variable proportions from the sputum. Many bacteriologists believe that the majority of these organisms are potential pathogens and that much importance should be assigned to them. Others consider that only a few organisms, namely, *Hemophilus influenzae* and pneumococcus, and occasionally *Staphylococcus aureus* and Friedländer's bacillus, have any pathogenic significance.

It is difficult to assess the role of the patient's occupation in the etiology of bronchitis, but the disease does occur more frequently in industrial areas. Bronchitis is prevalent among men who work in dusty occupations, especially coal miners, but there appears to be no close relationship with the duration of exposure to dust. It is interesting that there is a high incidence of bronchitis among the wives of these workers as well.

An environmental cause of chronic bronchitis is also often entertained. Pollution of the atmospheric air is strongly suspected of being a factor in the etiology and progression of chronic bronchitis. The fate and the physiological effect of these foreign particles in the respiratory tract depend on their size and chemical composition. Large particles of pollution, such as droplets in wet fog, are usually trapped in the nose and pharynx. Medium-sized particles are generally trapped in the upper bronchial tree, and particles smaller than 5 millimicrons in diameter may penetrate as far as the alveoli. They may be inert and innocuous, may act as irritants, may behave as fibrogenic agents, or may produce pneumonitis. By irritating the respiratory tract, they cause an excessive production of mucus and a diminution in the ciliary activity and possibly some bronchospasm, thereby promoting stagnation of bronchial secretions. It is of interest that as long ago as 1660 it was suggested that the pollution of air by coal dust might affect the lungs. The amount of air pollution caused by domestic chimneys is higher in Britain than in any other country. In the major English cities there is a significant correlation between the day-to-day condition of patients suffering from bronchitis and the average concentration of sulfur dioxide in the atmosphere. It should be pointed out, however, that although Copenhagen, the most industrialized city in Denmark, has approximately the same degree of air pollution as an English country town, its mortality rate due to bronchitis is about 20 times lower.

The role of smoking in the etiology of chronic bronchitis has not yet been fully determined. In a group of male medical practitioners over the age of 35, the mortality rate due to bronchitis was six times greater among heavy smokers than among non-smokers. The cigarette consumption in Denmark is approximately one-half that in Great Britain, and this has been suggested as the reason for the different incidence of chronic bronchitis in the two countries. It is postulated that nicotine acts directly on the bronchial mucosa, so that an excessive amount of mucus is secreted. However, not all cigarette smokers develop bronchitis, so that some individual or familial susceptibility must play an important part. The incidence of bronchitis is not high in pipe or cigar smokers.

Clinical Manifestations. The clinical course of chronic bronchitis is one of intermittent episodes of acute bronchitis, occurring chiefly in the winter months, from which recovery becomes progressively more difficult. The onset of the disease is usually insidious, although it may start acutely. Many patients trace their first symptoms to some acute infective episode such as pneumonia, measles, whooping cough or acute bronchitis. Others may attribute the chronic cough to smoking. Some patients develop a more severe form of recurrent bronchitis during the winter months with variable degrees of disability, but remain relatively well during the warmer months. The bronchitis may progress further to become a year-round affliction, with intercurrent acute exacerbations. This condition often leads to death from either bronchopneumonia or respiratory insufficiency and right-sided heart failure 20 to 35 years after its onset.

The clinical condition of patients suffering from chronic bronchitis may vary from day to day. The influence of weather is commonly recognized, the symptoms becoming aggravated during cold, damp or foggy weather, and recrudescence of infection is an important associated factor. The sputum is usually mucoid in appearance, but it frequently becomes copious and purulent during the acute episodes. The cough is frequently most productive on first awakening. Wheezing may be a prominent feature because of partial obstruction of the bronchi and bronchioles. Paroxysms of coughing and breathlessness may awaken the patient during the night, mimicking an attack of paroxysmal nocturnal dyspnea, but differing in that the attacks of dyspnea in chronic bronchitis are generally relieved as soon as sputum is raised.

As the bronchitis progresses, the lung parenchyma finally becomes involved, with the development of chronic obstructive emphysema. Shortness of breath is the prime symptom of this complication, the dyspnea progressively increasing in severity and becoming more and more disabling.

The physical signs depend on which portion of the tracheobronchial tree is involved and on the severity of the condition. Very few abnormal signs may be elicited during the examination of the chest unless special maneuvers are carried out. For example, rhonchi are frequently elicited if the patient expires forcibly for as long as possible while the examiner manually compresses the patient's chest. If only the trachea and major bronchi are affected, a few sonorous rhonchi may be detected bilaterally. Medium-pitched rhonchi are present if the medium-sized bronchi are involved, and high-pitched sibilant rhonchi are heard if the condition has progressed to involve the bronchioles.

Hyperinflation of the chest because of the bronchial obstruction is a common finding, so that the percussion note is hyper-resonant and breath sounds are faint. If there is superimposed atelectasis or pneumonia, it produces clinical signs indicative of an increase in density or change in lung size in the affected areas of the lung.

Radiological Manifestations. The abnormal radiological findings of bronchitis depend on the site and extent of the inflammatory process. If only the trachea and major bronchi are affected, no abnormal changes are present. If the more peripheral bronchi are involved the lungs may be hyperinflated.

Fluoroscopic examination may reveal evidence of a check-valve type of airway obstruction, such as poor aeration in some areas of the lungs during inspiration or failure to deflate during expiration. If the bronchial obstruction is severe, the diaphragm is often depressed and restricted in its movements.

Bronchograms frequently show small spike-like protrusions which project outwards from the main or segmental bronchi. These are probably caused by collections of radio-opaque media in the pit-like depressions formed by the abnormal openings of the ducts of the mucous glands. The caliber of the bronchi is often slightly narrowed, and irregularities of the bronchial lumen result from a mixture of stenosis and dilatation. Complete occlusions of the bronchi or bronchioles are frequently present. Occasionally a circular pool is seen at the abrupt ending of a long, narrow branch, giving it a beaded appearance; this probably represents a dilated bronchiole.

The presence of small, patchy, irregular opacities, usually confined to the bases of both lungs, is indicative of lobular pneumonia. A variety of other radiological changes are seen from time to time in association with chronic bronchitis. These include numerous thin-walled cysts, lace-like strands, changes related to the concomitant chronic obstructive emphysema and, occasionally, bronchiectasis.

Functional Manifestations. The main functional defect in bronchitis is ventilatory, the work of breathing being greater than normal. There is an increase in airflow resistance, but there is little alteration in lung distensibility, at least in the early stages. As a result, the vital capacity is usually normal in volume, but delayed in time, while the maximal mid-expiratory flow rate and the maximal breathing capacity are considerably reduced.

The distribution of gas is uneven, and the ventilation-perfusion ratios are altered throughout the lung, so that hypoxia is present. No retention of carbon dioxide occurs as long as the perfused areas of lung are capable of being hyperventilated. In the later stages of the disease, as obstructive emphysema develops, there is a fall in the diffusing capacity for oxygen due to obliteration and destruction of the pulmonary capillary bed. Still later, the alveolar ventilation may become so inadequate that carbon dioxide retention develops. Secondary polycythemia is a common complication. Pulmonary hypertension develops not only because of the reduction in the size of the pulmonary capillary bed, but also as a result of the effects of hypoxia, hypercapnia and possibly also polycythemia. The work of the right ventricle therefore increases and its wall may hypertrophy. Later, the right ventricle may fail and the full-blown picture of right ventricular failure may develop.

CHRONIC OBSTRUCTIVE EMPHYSEMA

Emphysema, derived from the Greek word meaning overinflation, implies a pathological process which consists of permanent overdistension of lung alveoli, with attenuation and loss of pulmonary septal tissues. Dyspnea is the cardinal symptom and is always present. The functional disturbances are those of air flow resistance, altered ventilation-perfusion ratios and reduced diffusing capacity. The clinical state of chronic obstructive emphysema would appear to be allied more closely to disturbances in pulmonary function than to the pathologic changes. For this reason, there is now a greater emphasis on the physiological definition of chronic obstructive emphysema.

Confirming the existence of this disease is probably the greatest diagnostic problem facing any physician concerned with respiratory diseases. Like "asthma," the term "emphysema" is often used very loosely; it may be a tag for a variety of conditions involving the tracheobronchial tree. In the classification which is most commonly used, there are four types of emphysema. These are chronic obstructive emphysema, senile or atrophic emphysema, acute vesicular emphysema and compensatory emphysema. Senile emphysema is a term used to denote senile degeneration of the alveolar septa. This is a natural result of aging and is rarely associated with any symptoms. Acute vesicular emphysema is a small localized overdistention of lung parenchyma due to a check-valve type of obstruction. This is usually reversible and therefore is not really a form of emphysema. Compensatory emphysema is an overdistention of lung parenchyma which develops in association with neighboring collapsed or fibrotic lung tissue. Any changes attributed to it are usually overshadowed by the underlying disease. The majority of patients suffering from symptoms due to emphysema therefore fit into the category of chronic obstructive emphysema.

PATHOGENESIS

Considerable controversy still exists about not only the etiology of chronic obstructive emphysema but also the mechanism of its development. The failure of the emphysematous lung to collapse when the chest is opened post mortem, the appearance of atrophied stroma and the fact that the pleural pressure fluctuates in the neighborhood of atmospheric pressure indicate that the elastic tissue of the lung is at fault. Some investigators have suggested that the elastic tissue becomes atrophic and broken, others that it is congenitally defective, and still others that it is merely stretched but not diminished. Laennec, a pioneer in the study of chronic obstructive emphysema, thought that the disease could be entirely explained by mechanical factors and claimed that it begins as a catarrh of the bronchi, which leads to partial bronchial obstruction during both inspiration and expiration. Current thinking has hardly improved on this concept. The disease probably develops as a result of bronchiolar obstruction due to infection, bronchial edema, secretions, bronchial muscular constriction or mucosal congestion, all of which lead to an increased resistance to air flow. Consequently, pulmonary overdistention may result. If this distention should persist over a long period of time, or if it is repeated over and over again, there may be destruction of alveolar walls so that there may be a loss of pulmonary elasticity and an irreversible emphysema may develop.

Defective defense mechanisms of the respiratory tract have been implicated in chronic obstructive emphysema because they are overloaded or because they are deficient. A check-valve type of obstruction and disruption of the normal collateral ventilation have also been blamed for the air trapping found in this condition. Inflammation results in the deformation and disruption of the bronchioli, with partial or complete occlusion of the lumen. In addition, the alveolar pores are involved so that they may not permit collateral ventilation. It has been shown that when bronchioli are obstructed, pressure gradients develop between collaterally ventilated and normally ventilated parts of the lung, particularly during the release phase of coughing. Air-trapping results because air enters alveoli but is unable to leave them, so that the alveolar walls are under stress. With repeated inflammatory episodes, there may be an increased number of obliterated bronchioles as well as greater air-trapping. More and more lung tissue becomes disrupted until, finally, the clinical picture of chronic obstructive emphysema becomes fully developed.

Recently it has been shown that obstruction of large numbers of pulmonary blood vessels, so that ischemia is produced, results in experimental emphysema in rabbits, the pathological picture being similar to that found in human chronic emphysema. It is possible that inflammatory obliteration of pulmonary capillaries and ischemia of alveolar walls may contribute to the development of chronic obstructive emphysema.

It should be pointed out that the relationship between alveolar distention and a loss of elasticity is not always simply a matter of cause and effect. It is likely that alveolar distention over a long period of time can hasten the loss of elasticity, but it is also true that a primary loss of elasticity may lead to alveolar distention. In other words, each may be the cause or the effect of the other, so that the loss of elasticity in chronic obstructive emphysema may be the basic defect or may be a secondary development.

The relationship between chronic obstructive emphysema and bronchial asthma is a controversial one. Evidence of emphysema is rarely found in the postmortem examination of the lungs of patients suffering from chronic bronchial asthma. On the other hand, episodes of dyspnea and wheezing precede the clinical picture of chronic obstructive emphysema in a number of patients. This finding is often difficult to interpret, but it is unnecessary to implicate asthma, for it is more likely that these episodes of dyspnea are due to acute bronchial obstruction as a result of infection. There appears to be no doubt, however, that there is a definite relationship between chronic bronchitis and chronic obstructive emphysema. In fact, many clinicians believe that chronic obstructive emphysema always occurs as a sequel to chronic bronchitis, although there is a definite group of patients in whom emphysema is not preceded by chronic cough, the disease being heralded by the onset of dyspnea. In these patients, it is possible that there is an inherent familial defect of the elastic tissue of the lung. Even in these patients, however, pathological evidence of bronchiolitis is frequently found at postmortem.

There also appears to be a relationship between bronchiectasis and chronic obstructive emphysema, particularly in cases of extensive bronchiectasis. In addition, there appears to be a high incidence of chronic obstructive emphysema complicating other chronic inflammatory diseases of the lung, particularly when both lungs are diffusely involved.

Two forms of emphysema are usually found on pathological examination of the lung, a centrilobular and a generalized form. Although evidence of bronchitis may be associated with both, it is much more predominant in the centrilobular form. Centrilobular emphysema commonly occurs as a minimal lesion. In this condition the periphery of the lobule appears normal, but there is considerable destruction of the air passages in its central portion. During the early stages, the dilated alveoli are located along the main bronchi and the superior surfaces of the interlobular septa. In more advanced stages, the respiratory and even the terminal bronchioles cannot be positively identified, and the periphery of the lobule becomes involved as well. Unlike bronchial asthma, the smooth muscle of the air passages as far as the alveolar ducts is often notably hypertrophied, a situation which is much more peripheral than that which is found in bronchial asthma.

CLINICAL MANIFESTATIONS

In spite of the difficulty in determining its pathogenesis, chronic obstructive emphysema has characteristic clinical features once it becomes established. In no other pulmonary condition is the radiological examination so singularly unrewarding. It can be diagnosed only from the history, the physical signs and an assessment of the pulmonary function.

The chief symptom of chronic obstructive emphysema is dyspnea. It usually begins slowly and characteristically is initially brought on by exertion. It is frequently present for a period of years before it begins to interfere with ordinary activity, so that patients may become habituated to it and are inclined to minimize it. It is aggravated by exposure to cold air and is, therefore, much more severe during the winter months. It is definitely expiratory, even if secondary bronchial spasm is not evident. The patient may have severe episodes of dyspnea associated with wheezing, which are usually precipitated by an upper respiratory infection and are often accompanied by an increased production of sputum. Conversely, a failure to expectorate sputum may in itself precipitate an attack of severe dyspnea because of the accumulation of secretions and the increased bronchiolar obstruction. In addition, nocturnal attacks of dyspnea and coughing may occur, probably as a result of bronchial obstruction by secretions. These attacks must be differentiated from attacks of paroxysmal nocturnal dyspnea which are due to left ventricular failure. The dyspnea usually progressively increases in severity, so that the patient is unable to accomplish his ordinary activities, and it may reach a stage at which he is unable to walk for even short distances without becoming tortured by dyspnea. When pulmonary congestion due to left ventricular failure supervenes in chronic obstructive emphysema, the dyspnea becomes extremely severe.

Coughing may be absent or inconspicuous during the early stages of the disease. Most patients suffer from chronic bronchitis, however, so that they may have been coughing for 15 to 25 years before the onset of dyspnea. The cough of chronic obstructive emphysema is quite characteristic and usually occurs in paroxysms in the morning on awakening or on exposure to cold air. The severity of the cough is frequently out of proportion to the amount of expectoration produced. Sooner or later, however, defective drainage is followed by infection and the production of mucoid or purulent sputum, so that ultimately, there may be profuse expectoration. At this stage the condition may resemble bronchiectasis, and indeed, bronchiectasis may finally supervene as a consequence of the frequent attacks of pneumonitis or lobular pneumonia and subsequent fibrosis.

Chest pain is occasionally felt in the parasternal regions or in the neighborhood of the rib margins. It is never very severe and is probably due to overinflation of the lungs and consequently increased pleural tension. On the other hand, pain resembling that caused by coronary insufficiency has also been described and has been attributed to pulmonary hypertension.

There is an increased incidence of peptic ulcers in patients suffering from chronic obstructive emphysema. The reason for this is uncertain, but it has been suggested that ulceration is due to the effect of hypoxia on the gastric and duodenal mucosa. There may be epigastric distress, especially after coughing, in severe cases. This becomes worse when right cardiac failure develops, probably because of liver engorgement.

The general nourishment is usually below normal in nearly all patients suffering from this disease, and weight loss increases with the severity of the disease. This is usually a slow process, but it occasionally may be so rapid as to suggest the presence of a neoplasm. Clubbing of the digits does not occur in a pure case of chronic obstructive emphysema; its presence usually indicates an associated or complicating septic condition or new growth.

The chest is in a position of hyperinflation because the elasticity of the chest wall is relatively unopposed when there is loss of lung elasticity, so that its resting position resembles that of a chest after a moderate inspiration. The diaphragm is gradually displaced downwards until it is so depressed that it can no longer function properly. Inspiratory indrawing may be noted over the chest wall, particularly in the areas overlying the insertions of the diaphragm. Since the chest is already expanded when inspiration begins, the accessory muscles of respiration are very frequently used to expand the chest still further. The pectoral muscles are particularly brought into play and cause the anterior part of the chest cage to rise in a "heaving" manner. As the chest expands, the diaphragm may paradoxically ascend rather than descend during inspiration. Since expiration must also be carried out by an active muscular effort, assistance from the accessory muscles is again required during this phase of respiration.

It should be pointed out that as a normal person becomes older, there is a decrease in the lung elasticity, although there is no alteration in the resistance to air flow. The chest may assume an inspiratory position and may have the clinical appearance of the "barrel-chest," which is manifested by an increase in the anteroposterior diameter and is associated with a hyper-resonant note on percussion. Such findings were formerly thought to be of great assistance in the diagnosis of chronic obstructive emphysema, but it is now appreciated that similar changes in the chest wall can occur in other obstructive diseases of the bronchi without being associated with emphysema, as well as in many healthy elderly people. Moreover, many patients with chronic obstructive emphysema may not exhibit the phenomenon of an increased anteroposterior diameter of the chest. It would appear that the development of a barrel-chest is related to changes in the thoracic vertebrae brought about by aging, although it is possible that it may tend to occur prematurely in patients who are suffering from chronic obstructive emphysema.

The movements of the chest cage are noticeably diminished but are equal bilaterally. Because of the hyperinflation of the lungs, the ratio of air-containing tissue to solid tissue is increased, so that fremitus, both tactile and auditory, is reduced and the percussion note is hyper-resonant. The breath sounds are characteristically distant, especially at the bases of the lungs, while in the late stages the lungs may become so silent as to suggest a pneumothorax. The expiratory phase is prolonged because there is an increased resistance to air flow requiring active muscular effort during expiration. Rhonchi are frequently present because of partial bronchial obstruction; they may not be detected during ordinary breathing, but extremely high-pitched sibilant rhonchi can frequently be elicited during the late phase of forced and prolonged expiration.

The heart sounds are often inaudible or may be heard very faintly at the apex, although they are usually easily detected in the epigastrium. If pulmonary hypertension has developed, the pulmonic second sound becomes accentuated, and it may not be split during inspiration.

The most serious threat to the life of the patient suffering from chronic obstructive emphysema is the sudden increase in hypoxia and hypercapnia which usually occurs during an acute infection. Acute right ventricular failure is a frequent result. As has been pointed out, symptoms and signs produced by severe hypoxia and hypercapnia are predominantly neurological and cardiovascular, the principal finding being disorientation and confusion. At such times the cough may be absent or ineffective, and secretions may accumulate in the trachea and bronchi.

Chronic right-sided heart failure is common in the late stages of the disease. This is manifested by cardiac enlargement, elevated venous pressure, hepatomegaly and edema. The severe hypoxia apparently causes an exacerbation of the previously existing increased pulmonary vascular resistance, leading to extreme pulmonary hypertension. This, together with the ill effects of hypoxia and hypercapnia on the myocardial function, appears to be responsible for the failure of the myocardium, and the hypercapnia, per se, may be responsible for further fluid retention.

RADIOLOGICAL MANIFESTATIONS

Roentgen films are not necessary to establish the diagnosis of chronic obstructive emphysema; indeed, they may often be misleading. The characteristic picture is that of increased translucency of the lungs, but this does not necessarily indicate the presence of emphysema. Nevertheless, certain findings in an x-ray film of the chest may corroborate the physical findings. The thoracic contour may be altered, the ribs running in a more horizontal direction, especially in the upper half of the chest. The lungs show an increased translucency which may be evenly spread throughout both lungs or may be limited to one or more lobes. The diaphragm is usually low and flat, commonly being adherent in the costal angles.

In advanced cases, a lateral view of the chest may present a striking picture. The kyphotic spine and the arched sternum frequently combine to produce a dome-shaped outline, the upper two-thirds of the thorax sometimes forming a true half circle. The anterior and posterior cardiac spaces may be increased in size and abnormally translucent.

The heart usually appears long and narrow, having been drawn downwards by the descending diaphragm. In the later stages, there may be evidence of hypertrophy of the right ventricle as well as an increase in size of the pulmonary artery shadow.

It must be stressed that, in the absence of heart failure, the radiological appearance of emphysema may be no different from that of overinflation due to diffuse bronchial obstruction, such as may occur in bronchial asthma. It has recently been suggested, however, that the two conditions can be differentiated by means of a full-chest tomogram, an x-ray film taken in a sagittal plane in approximately the central portion of the chest. Since chronic obstructive emphysema results in destruction of the alveolar walls and obliteration of the capillaries, the peripheral pulmonary vasculature is not seen in the full-chest tomogram of a patient suffering from this disease; in a patient without emphysema the vessels are usually prominent and can be followed out towards the periphery of the lung.

During fluoroscopy, the lungs are seen to be hyperinflated, characteristically failing to deflate during expiration. The diaphragm is low and relatively immobile, but it paradoxically may move upward during inspiration. In the later stages there may be an increase in the size of the pulmonary artery shadow and evidence of right ventricular hypertrophy.

FUNCTIONAL MANIFESTATIONS

Although the correlation between the severity of the clinical manifestations and the physiological disturbances is not perfect in chronic obstructive emphysema, the identification and understanding of the alterations in pulmonary function have led to considerable progress in the management of this disease. Since this condition is extremely serious and widespread, the physiological disturbances are dealt with here in some detail. They are presented under the headings of the mechanics of breathing, lung volumes, distribution of gas and blood in the lungs and gaseous exchange, regulation of respiration, and pulmonary circulation.

Mechanics of Breathing.   The resistance to air flow, both laminar and turbulent, is high in patients suffering from chronic obstructive emphysema, particularly during expiration. The resistance is increased further when there is a loss of lung elasticity, because the intrapleural pressure may rise above that of the airway pressure, thus compressing the airways. As a result, the resistance in the airways may rise to a point where there is no further increase in flow rate, despite all increasing efforts. The administration of nebulized bronchodilating agents reduces the nonelastic resistance in most patients, so that the work of breathing decreases.

Although the compliance of the lungs is greater than normal when inspiration is particularly slow, it is either normal or low during resting breathing when the respiratory rate is rapid. This suggests that, even though the over-all elastic properties of the lung may be diminished, the elastic resistance is increased during normal breathing, probably because the nonelastic resistance, which is also increased, is unevenly distributed. When inspiration is slow, air enters most areas of the lung, no matter whether the resistance is high or low, so a high value for the compliance of the lung is obtained. Conversely, when inspiration is rapid, air enters the areas of lung which offer little nonelastic resistance, so that they become overdistended and the calculated compliance is low. This principle has already been illustrated in Figure 11.

As the disease progresses, fibrosis and congestion in the presence of heart failure may occur. Under such circumstances, the compliance of the lungs is reduced even further as the lungs become more rigid. At the same time, the laminar and the turbulent components of the nonelastic resistance increase still further.

As is illustrated in Figure 58, the oxygen consumption of the respiratory muscles is greatly increased, apparently because the efficiency of the respiratory muscles is considerably reduced in these patients. The cause of the diminished efficiency has not been elucidated.

As a result of the altered physical properties of the lungs, the vital capacity is often normal in size, but there is considerable obstruction to air flow, so that the timed vital capacity, maximal mid-expiratory flow rate and maximal breathing capacity are reduced. As the disease

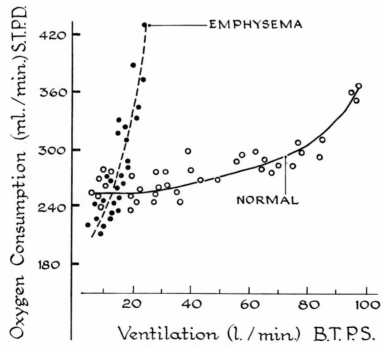

FIGURE 58. The changes in oxygen consumption with increasing ventilation in a normal subject and in a patient with chronic obstructive emphysema.

progresses, the vital capacity falls and the obstruction to air flow increases.

Lung Volumes.   As a result of the chronic hyperinflation of the lung, the total lung capacity is slightly larger than normal, the most striking features being increased residual volume and functional residual capacity. Although these findings are a reflection of the characteristic inability of the emphysematous lungs to empty, they are in no way diagnostic of this disease, for they may also be found in other diseases which are accompanied by diffuse bronchial obstruction. Furthermore, although the ratio of the residual volume to the total lung capacity is elevated in almost every case of chronic obstructive emphysema, the correlation between this ratio and the clinical severity of the disease is poor. Great variations in the functional residual capacity can occur in the same patient within a short period of time, especially when there have been exacerbations of bronchospasm or bronchitis. In addition, blebs, bullae and air cysts which communicate poorly or not at all with the tracheobronchial tree are inaccessible to physiologic measurement, so that in some cases the estimated total lung capacity is reduced despite an obviously hyperinflated chest.

Distribution of Air and Blood and Gaseous Exchange.   Because the loss of lung elasticity does not affect all parts of the lung equally, there is unequal expansion of the various parts of the lungs, leading to an exceedingly uneven and inefficient distribution of inspired air. In addition, injection studies of the pulmonary blood vessels and investigation of the hemodynamics of the pulmonary circulation during both rest and exercise suggest that the circulation of blood is also uneven in the emphysematous lung. An imbalance in ventilation-perfusion relationships is therefore a characteristic feature. Alveoli, which have a relatively small amount of blood flowing through them, are probably overventilated at the expense of others which are normally perfused. The physiological effect of this situation is similar to that of an increase in the dead space. The blood that perfuses the poorly vascularized, overventilated alveoli becomes fully oxygenated and probably excessively depleted of carbon dioxide. The quantity of blood flow is so small, however, that the total gas exchange in these alveoli is slight, and a greater than normal burden falls on the other alveoli. In such a situation, an adequate elimination of carbon dioxide can occur only when the normally perfused alveoli are hyperventilated.

The perfusion of poorly ventilated alveoli also results in arterial hypoxia and, in addition, a tendency towards carbon dioxide retention because not enough oxygen is added to, or carbon dioxide removed from, these alveoli. The physiological effect is similar to that of a true shunt from the venous to the arterial blood. Carbon dioxide retention may not occur if there is sufficient hyperventilation of the remaining well-ventilated, well-perfused alveoli, but the hypoxia cannot be corrected to any significant degree by this.

The ability of oxygen to diffuse across the alveolocapillary membrane is reduced in this condition, particularly in its later stages, probably because of the reduction in the size of the total pulmonary vascular bed. Many investigators, therefore, consider the findings of a reduced diffusing capacity in association with bronchial obstruction to be indicative of the presence of chronic obstructive emphysema.

Regulation of Respiration. Alveolar hypoventilation is a common occurrence in patients with this disease, so that the carbon dioxide tension of the arterial blood is frequently elevated, even at rest. Because of this, and because they do not increase their ventilation in a normal fashion when breathing carbon dioxide, it is thought that the sensitivity of the respiratory center is diminished. The situation is further complicated by the fact that the retention of carbon dioxide and the failure to respond normally to inhaled carbon dioxide are at least partially the result of the mechanical difficulty in ventilating the lungs.

The added insult of arterial hypoxia also plays an important role in these patients. When the medullary respiratory center loses its ability to respond to excessive levels of carbon dioxide, the hypoxia leads to stimulation of the peripheral chemoreceptors. Under such circumstances, these chemoreceptors may become the principal regulators of the respiratory drive, and hypoxia the prime stimulus, a factor which becomes extremely important when oxygen therapy is considered.

Pulmonary Circulation. Because the alveolar walls are destroyed, the pulmonary capillaries are obliterated. Because of the obliterative changes, the presence of hypoxia which constricts the pulmonary vasculature, and the secondary polycythemia, the pulmonary vascular resistance and the pulmonary artery pressure are both frequently elevated, even at rest, and they may rise considerably during exercise. The increased pulmonary vascular resistance imposes a heavy load on the right ventricle, so that it eventually hypertrophies and may even fail, producing the clinical picture of cor pulmonale.

BRONCHIECTASIS

The term "bronchiectasis" is derived from the Greek words "bronchia" and "ectasis," meaning extension. It is descriptive of a disease characterized by dilatation and distortion of either the bronchi or bronchioles, or both. The condition occurs when the bronchial walls become weakened by chronic inflammatory changes which not only involve the bronchial mucosa and submucosa but extend through the muscular coat into the surrounding lung parenchyma as well.

PATHOGENESIS

Many theories have been advanced to explain the pathogenesis of bronchiectasis, including congenital or developmental defects, distention of the bronchi by cough, destruction of the bronchial wall by necrotizing inflammation, obstructive mechanisms, atelectasis and fibrous retraction. It is now generally considered that bronchiectasis develops only in a portion of the lung, whether segmental or lobar, in which obstruction or atelectasis has been present. Since a greater than normal intrathoracic pressure is required to overcome the increased elastic resistance of the shrunken, airless lung, it tends to pull on the walls of the crowded bronchi within the atelectatic area, causing them to dilate. This may explain the cases of "reversible bronchiectasis" in which dilated bronchi, which are demonstrated after pneumonia, return to a normal size later. The degree of bronchial dilatation depends on the size of the bronchi affected. A large bronchus with its cartilaginous rings does not dilate as readily as the more muscular medium-sized and smaller bronchi. This is not necessarily so, however, because once infection has developed in their walls, bronchi of any size may become distorted.

If bronchial obstruction is relieved before infection has had a chance to develop, the dilated bronchi may recover their normal caliber when the atelectatic area re-expands. If bronchial obstruction has been prolonged, secondary infection inevitably supervenes, resulting in destruction of the bronchial walls and dilatation of the bronchi. The consequent reparative laying down of fibrous tissue further increases the traction on the bronchi, leading to still greater distortion. If the bronchial obstruction is caused by semifluid material such as a plug of viscid, purulent secretion or a blood clot, it may be sucked further in towards the periphery of the lung by the increased traction on the bronchial lumen. The material may be broken up and many obstruct the smaller bronchi or bronchioles, producing bronchiectasis in the new sites, even though the original bronchial obstruction has been removed.

Any lesion which narrows a bronchial lumen, be it extramural, intramural or intraluminal, may produce bronchiectasis distal to the obstruction. The condition may also develop when there is destruction of lung tissue, as in a lung abscess or tuberculosis. Certain pulmonary infections, particularly the pneumonias complicating measles, pertussis and influenza, are more liable to be followed by bronchiectasis. This applies especially to staphylococcal and streptococcal pneumonias, but only rarely to pneumococcal pneumonia.

Bronchiectasis is usually localized to a lobe or a segment, and the lower lobes, particularly that of the left lung, are most commonly involved. Fresh areas of bronchiectasis may subsequently develop in other parts of the same lung, but they are usually associated with a fresh bronchial obstruction. Bronchiectasis rarely occurs as a diffuse disease of the bronchial tree, although it has been described in a hereditary disease called mucoviscidosis, a disease of the exocrine organs in which there are abnormally thick, viscid secretions particularly involving the bronchial tree.

In many cases of bronchiectasis, the bronchial arteries tend to enlarge, often reaching the size of the pulmonary arteries at the same level. The bronchial and pulmonary systems frequently anastomose freely with each other. It has been postulated that the high bronchial artery pressure is transmitted to the pulmonary arterioles through the anastomoses and causes unoxygenated blood to be shunted away from diseased portions of lung to healthy areas, where there is a lower pressure in the pulmonary circulation.

CLINICAL MANIFESTATIONS

Cough is usually the predominant symptom in bronchiectasis, although the diseased, dilated bronchi may be insensitive so that purulent secretion may not always induce the cough reflex. In addition, the ciliary activity may be diminished or absent due to the inflammatory changes. In such cases, cough and expectoration of purulent material may be induced only after a change in posture, which may move purulent material into the larger bronchi, where the mucosa is normal. More frequently patients are asymptomatic except during periods of acute infection, when they develop a cough with expectoration of purulent sputum, and occasionally a fever. It is important to note that recurrent episodes frequently affect the same area of lung.

The amount of purulent secretions varies, depending on the size of the bronchiectatic cavities and the organisms involved. Poorly draining bronchiectatic cavities are often filled with stagnant, foul-smelling pus, particularly if the infection is caused by Vincent's organisms. The amount of sputum expectorated varies from a few ounces to several pints within 24 hours. Some patients may expectorate large quantities of purulent sputum, others small quantities of mucopurulent sputum, and still others, who are presumably suffering from a so-called "dry bronchiectasis," may have a nonproductive cough. Bronchiectasis affecting the upper lobes, which is usually secondary to arrested pulmonary tuberculosis, may be asymptomatic because the drainage from the upper lobe bronchus is very efficient in the erect position, as long as it is not obstructed.

The purulent secretion produced within a poorly draining bronchiectatic abscess is frequently very thick and viscid and, under ordinary circumstances, difficult to evacuate. The expectorated material, however, may be completely different from the pus in the bronchiectatic abscess. If the sputum is collected in a conical glass, it separates into three layers on standing: an upper, frothy, watery layer; a middle, turbid, muco-purulent layer; and a lower, opaque, purulent layer. The third or purulent layer may contain collections of small dirty-white or yellowish masses, known as Dittrich's plugs, or bits of elastic fibers if lung tissue has been destroyed.

A large proportion of patients with suppurative bronchiectasis also have chronic infection of the upper respiratory tract, particularly of the nasal sinuses. They are liable to acute exacerbations of sinusitis, which often may mask the lower respiratory tract symptoms. The causal relationship between infection in the upper and that in the lower respiratory tracts is debatable, but it is generally agreed that the sinuses very likely become secondarily infected by sprays of purulent sputum during paroxysms of coughing. On the other hand, chronic upper respiratory tract infection, with constant drainage of purulent secretion into the tracheobronchial tree, may lead to sepsis and even bronchial obstruction, with resulting abscess formation or bronchiectasis.

Although not a usual feature of bronchiectasis, dyspnea may become a distressing symptom if both lungs are extensively involved, and particularly when fibrosis develops. Secretions in the bronchi and distortion of the neighboring bronchial tree may increase the resistance to air flow and cause wheezing. In very chronic cases, however, dyspnea may not be experienced if the patients have become accustomed to the effort required for breathing.

Constitutional symptoms do not ordinarily occur in a patient with bronchiectasis, unless there is extensive chronic suppurative disease or an acute pneumonic infection. Under these circumstances, the patient may complain of undue fatigability, weight loss, profuse night sweats, anorexia and vague abdominal discomfort.

It is important to realize that the sufferer from bronchiectasis, particularly a young person, faces a serious psychological handicap. The recurrent bouts of pneumonitis result in long periods away from school or work. The patient may become retiring, introspective and asocial. He is unable to keep up with his schoolmates at games, because running or other forms of exercise usually induce a coughing paroxysm. In addition, he may be avoided by his associates because he is suspected of suffering from tuberculosis or because his breath or sputum is foul-smelling.

The physical signs depend on the degree of bronchiectasis, its location and the extent of pulmonary involvement. A solitary bronchiectatic segment may be detected by an astute clinical observer through the presence of rales. Some cases, however, may be discovered only by special radiological means. More extensive disease always produces physical signs.

Because of the basic atelectatic component of the disease and the progressive replacement of lung parenchyma by fibrous tissue, the physical findings are essentially similar to those found in atelectasis. If the left lower lobe is taken as an example, the trachea and apex beat of the heart are usually deviated to the left because of the decrease in the size of the left lung. Since the distensibility is decreased, the movement of the chest cage over the lower lobe is diminished. The diaphragm is higher on the affected side than on the opposite side and its respiratory excursion is reduced.

The density of the affected lung is increased so that the percussion note over it varies from dullness to flatness, depending on the extent of pulmonary consolidation and fibrosis. The vocal fremitus depends on the patency of the obstructed bronchus; if it is still occluded, vocal fremitus is absent, but if the offending bronchus is patent, vocal fremitus is often greater than normal. The audibility of the breath sounds also depends on the patency of the bronchus. If the bronchus is no longer obstructed, breath sounds varying in quality from the various gradations of the bronchovesicular to the frankly bronchial type may be heard, the type depending on the extent of the underlying pulmonary consolidation and fibrosis. The intensity of the breath sounds is diminished owing to the poor air-entry into the diseased dilated bronchi, which are filled with exudate. If the lung is consolidated, whispering pectoriloquy and egophony are both present.

It should be noted that all of these physical findings are dependent upon the extent of atelectasis, pulmonary consolidation or fibrosis, and that they bear no relationship to the extent or degree of bronchial involvement. The latter factor can be determined only from adventitious sounds. Rales are produced in the destroyed and exudate-filled smaller bronchi and alveoli. It has been suggested that the pitch and timing of the rales depends on the caliber and the anatomic location of the bronchiectatic dilatations. Coarse, low-pitched rales during the initial third of inspiration are thought to be produced by secretions in the larger bronchi, medium-pitched rales during the middle third of the inspiration by secretions in the smaller bronchi, and fine, high-pitched rales during the final third of inspiration by exudate within the airless, collapsed, surrounding alveoli. The rales during the initial and middle thirds of inspiration usually disappear if the patient makes a vigorous cough, but those in the final third usually persist. Expiratory rhonchi, whose pitch depends on the caliber of the bronchi involved, may be produced by an inflamed swollen mucosa, bronchospasm and secretions. Rhonchi detectable over both lungs, particularly during a forced expiration, are likely due to an associated bronchitis.

Constitutional manifestations occur more readily in patients suffering from extensive bronchiectasis. There may be a low-grade fever, a yellowish pallor, evident weight loss, generalized muscular wasting and other evidences of malnutrition. Clubbing of the digits may develop, particularly when there is extensive suppuration, and if this is severe enough, the clubbing may progress to the stage of hypertrophic pulmonary osteoarthropathy. The development of digital clubbing does not appear to be related to either the duration or the extent of the disease, however. Another complication in the patient with extensive suppurative bronchiectasis may be secondary amyloidosis.

RADIOLOGICAL MANIFESTATIONS

Dilated bronchi do not cast a radiological shadow; therefore, normal posteroanterior and lateral x-ray films of the chest do not exclude the diagnosis of bronchiectasis. It is only the complications of bronchiectasis that produce abnormal radiographic opacities. Peribronchial fibrosis may show up as irregular dense strands radiating downwards and outwards from the hilum. An atelectasis or a localized fibrosis causes a shift of the mediastinum to the affected side and elevation of the diaphragm. Occasionally, the dilated bronchi appear as thin-walled, translucent spaces, which may have a fluid level because they contain air as well as fluid.

These radiographic abnormalities are suggestive, but not diagnostic, of the presence of bronchiectasis. Special films called "bronchograms," in which the lumen of the tracheobronchial tree is outlined with a radio-opaque, iodine-containing medium, will establish the diagnosis. The radio-opaque contrast medium easily fills the dilated bronchi, provided they have been emptied previously by adequate drainage. In order to identify the affected bronchi, oblique views of the chest should be taken in addition to the standard ones. The bronchiectatic dilatations may occur in various forms. They may be "cylindrical," the bronchi showing a uniform generalized dilatation; "fusiform," the bronchi having the appearance of the fingers of a glove; or "saccular," with many small, rounded dilatations, resembling clusters of grapes.

FUNCTIONAL MANIFESTATIONS

The alterations in pulmonary function in bronchiectasis depend upon the number of bronchi involved as well as the associated parenchymal disease. With minimal bronchiectasis involving one bronchopulmonary segment, there is little effect on pulmonary function.

Usually the nonelastic resistance is mildly increased because of obstruction to air flow. Timed vital capacity, maximal mid-expiratory flow rate and maximal breathing capacity are reduced, and distribution of the inspired gas is impaired. These changes are probably due to excess secretions because of either the bronchiectasis or chronic bronchitis. The vital capacity may be little altered unless there is much pooling of secretions, or if there is atelectasis or fibrosis so that the elastic resistance is increased.

Even if the disease is mild, hypoxia may occur because of perfusion of poorly ventilated areas of lung, particularly if atelectasis or pneumonitis is also present. Hyperventilation of the uninvolved portions of the lung helps to maintain a normal or slightly lowered arterial carbon dioxide tension. When there is diffuse disease, the distribution of blood and gases is seriously altered because of accumulated secretions, and perhaps some associated bronchospasm as well. As a result, altered ventilation-perfusion ratios and alveolar hypoventilation may develop with consequent hypoxia and hypercapnia. The more diffuse the bronchiectasis or the associated bronchitis, the more severe the respiratory failure may be.

BRONCHIAL ASTHMA

"Asthma" literally means difficult breathing. Bronchial asthma is a condition in which there is an acquired hypersensitivity of the bronchi to a normally innocuous specific substance or substances. This produces spasmodic narrowing of the bronchial lumen and recurrent, paroxysmal attacks of wheezing. Because many physicians consider wheezing to be synonymous with bronchial asthma, this disease may be too frequently diagnosed. It is obvious from the discussion of bronchial obstruction, however, that although all patients suffering from bronchial asthma are subject to wheezing, patients who wheeze do not necessarily have bronchial asthma.

PATHOGENESIS

The clinical manifestations of bronchial asthma are presumably precipitated by the combination of an antigen with an antibody formed in response to a previous contact with the antigen.

An antigen is a foreign substance which stimulates the formation of an antibody within an animal or a man, and which is capable of reacting with that antibody. A specific antigen does not produce a specific clinical picture. The same antigen may produce bronchial asthma in one person, rhinitis in another, urticaria in a third, purpura in a fourth, and even different symptom complexes in the same person at different times.

An antibody is a protein, or at least it is inseparable from protein, which is presumably formed in response to an antigenic stimulus and is capable of combining specifically with the corresponding antigen. The site of antibody formation is not clearly established. Some workers consider that the lymphocyte is the primary site of antibody formation, but others have indicated that it may be the plasma cell.

Once sensitization is established, the antibodies may be widely distributed in the body. Nevertheless, certain "shock organs" apparently show a greater degree of reactivity to contact with an antigen, presumably indicating a greater concentration of antibodies in these areas. In bronchial asthma, sensitizing antibodies are presumably heavily concentrated in the bronchial mucosa so that the bronchial tree is considered to be the shock organ. Contact of an allergen with the sensitized bronchial mucosa elicits an antigen-antibody reaction which is believed to be associated with the release of histamine or a histamine-like substance, although serotonin and acetylcholine may also be implicated. The consequences are engorgement of the blood vessels, excessive production of mucus, development of edema and contraction of smooth muscle. The lumina of the smaller bronchi become greatly narrowed by swelling of the mucosa and spasm of the bronchial muscle, while the secretion of thick tenacious mucus by the bronchial glands further obstructs the bronchioli.

The allergens which cause bronchial asthma are many, the most important ones being inhaled organic dusts, such as pollens, mold spores, animal danders and feathers. The occurrence of bronchial asthma during the spring and summer months suggests that a pollen or one of the mold spores may be the offending allergen. Attacks in the spring are usually due to tree pollens; grass pollens are usually responsible for attacks in the early part of summer, and weed pollens for those occurring in the late summer. The occupational history may be important, for certain occupations involve exposure to particular allergens. Practically any food may occasionally be a cause of asthma, particularly in children, and drugs, such as morphine or aspirin, may precipitate attacks. In addition, it is exceedingly important to realize that in most patients, any irritant such as dust, smoke or drainage from an upper respiratory tract infection is capable of "triggering" an attack of bronchospasm in an already hyperirritable bronchial tree.

Heredity appears to play an important role in bronchial asthma. Although the hereditary background cannot be demonstrated in every case, allergic diseases tend to occur in certain families. The property that is inherited is probably not the specific allergy, but rather a tendency to develop a sensitivity to any of the antigens to which the individual may become exposed.

Psychic factors may precipitate attacks of bronchial asthma and also may influence the severity of symptoms, particularly in highly predisposed persons with an underlying bronchial hypersensitivity. It has been suggested that an emotional upset in a susceptible person induces hyperventilation, which in itself may precipitate an attack of bronchospasm. On the other hand, an attack may represent the reaction of an allergic "shock organ" to stimuli which in nonallergic people produce only the ordinary manifestations of emotion, such as weeping.

Since most allergic reactions involve blood vessels and smooth muscle, which are innervated by the autonomic nervous system, it is tempting to incriminate these nerves in the pathogenesis of asthma. The vagus nerves carry efferent fibers which innervate the bronchial smooth muscle and possibly also the mucous glands of the bronchial passages. In the experimental animal, stimulation of the distal end of a cut vagus nerve leads to bronchoconstriction and mucus production. The role of these efferent fibers in the human is unknown, although it is tempting to postulate that the bronchospasm and excess mucus seen in bronchial asthma are the result of overactivity of these fibers. Atropine, however, has no significant therapeutic value in the human subject suffering from bronchial asthma, whereas epinephrine and related sympathicomimetic drugs are particularly effective. Nerves from the stellate and adjacent thoracic sympathetic ganglia contain fibers which are capable of influencing the bronchi. However, various types of surgical procedures designed to resect the nerve supply to the bronchi have had little or no effect in patients with bronchial asthma, indicating that the nervous factor is rarely a predominant one.

Chronic bronchitis is frequently associated with bronchial asthma, for recurrent bronchial infection is a common manifestation. It is unlikely, though, that bronchial asthma ever leads to the development of chronic obstructive pulmonary emphysema.

CLINICAL MANIFESTATIONS

Bronchial asthma is characterized by recurrent, paroxysmal attacks of difficult breathing, which may be seasonal or may occur at any time of the year. The attacks often occur as a result of direct exposure to a specific allergen, an unusual exertion, a sudden change in temperature, some emotional stress, or infection of the upper or lower respiratory tract. There is usually difficulty in breathing, accompanied by wheezing due to excessive turbulent resistance to air flow in the tracheobronchial tree. The attack of dyspnea and wheezing may last for hours, and often ends spontaneously. On the other hand, some patients may remain in a state of continuous respiratory distress for days, a condition known as "status asthmaticus."

Paroxysmal attacks of coughing due to diffuse bronchial obstruction are a frequent manifestation of bronchial asthma. Thick gelatinous mucus, produced by the glands in the bronchial wall, is frequently present but exceedingly difficult to expectorate.

A patient with uncomplicated bronchial asthma often has no symptoms between the paroxysms of wheezing. In about one-quarter of the cases beginning in childhood, the attacks may cease spontaneously after adolescence. A considerable number of patients, however, remain in a chronic state of mild bronchial asthma, with symptoms particularly noticeable during periods of exertion or emotional excitement.

The physical signs are characteristically those of partial bronchiolar obstruction with a prolonged expiration and high-pitched rhonchi throughout both lungs. Since the lungs are frequently hyperinflated because of the airway obstruction, a hyper-resonant note is obtained on percussion, and the breath sounds are distant.

RADIOLOGICAL MANIFESTATIONS

There are no characteristic radiological changes in the lungs in bronchial asthma. The bronchial markings may be more prominent and the lungs hyperinflated, just as in other cases of diffuse bronchial obstruction. In contrast to the lack of peripheral vascularity noted in chronic obstructive emphysema on the "full-chest tomogram," the pulmonary vessels extend to the periphery of the lung in bronchial asthma.

FUNCTIONAL MANIFESTATIONS

During an acute attack of bronchial asthma the airway resistance is greatly increased so that the timed vital capacity, maximal mid-expiratory flow rate and maximal breathing capacity are all reduced. The volume of the vital capacity is also often considerably reduced, presumably because some bronchioles are completely obstructed. Since the bronchial obstruction is usually not uniform, the distribution of inspired gas is impaired. Hypoxia is frequently noted, but hypercapnia does not usually occur because there is compensatory hyperventilation of unobstructed alveoli.

Although a patient may appear to be clinically free of bronchial obstruction between attacks, there is often still some evidence of it when ventilatory function studies are performed. Its presence is manifested by an increased airway resistance and a nonuniform distribution of the inspired gas.

CHAPTER VIII

Pulmonary Parenchymal Disease

ATELECTASIS

THE TERM "atelectasis" is derived from the Greek "ateles," meaning imperfect, and "ectasis," meaning expansion. It is used synonymously with the term "pulmonary collapse," and it implies that the alveoli in the affected area of the lung have become airless and have collapsed. The condition may occur for several reasons, the most important of which is complete occlusion of the bronchus draining the affected area, with the subsequent absorption of air from the affected bronchopulmonary segment.

Several parts of the healthy lung barely expand during breathing and are therefore more susceptible to collapse than others. If the person is breathing shallowly, certain areas such as the apex of the lung, the upper part of the lower lobe and particularly the lung at the hilum expand very little. When the movement of a part of the chest cage becomes restricted because of distortion of the ribs or splinting due to chest pain, the underlying lung parenchyma does not inflate properly during inspiration and is, therefore, more susceptible to the development of atelectasis.

PATHOGENESIS

There are three main types of atelectasis: physiologic, compressive and obstructive.

Physiologic Atelectasis. The fetal lung is airless, the walls of its alveoli being almost in apposition, and a small quantity of amniotic fluid apparently moves in and out of the lungs. With the first inspiratory effort after birth, the thoracic cage is expanded so that a negative intrapleural pressure develops, and this pulls on the enclosed lungs. Since the lungs communicate with the atmosphere through the trachea, air is drawn into the lungs, thereby opening up the alveoli. Occasionally, these inspiratory efforts do not lead to complete inflation of the lungs and portions remain airless, probably because of an increased resistance to lung distention due to the surface tension between opposing bronchiolar and alveolar walls.

Compressive Atelectasis. This type of pulmonary collapse is caused by external pressure on the lung which hinders its expansion. This occurs when there is air or fluid in the pleural cavity or when there is a chest deformity such as kyphoscoliosis. The bronchi usually remain patent, so that the compressed lung is often capable of re-expansion when the external pressure is removed. If the compression has been maintained over too long a period of time, however, inflammatory changes followed by fibrosis may develop, so that the lung remains permanently smaller.

Obstructive Atelectasis. This type of atelectasis is a clinically significant condition which is always associated with a complete obstruction of the draining bronchus. The amount of collapsed lung tissue depends on the size of the obstructed bronchus. If a major bronchus is involved, the whole lung collapses. Similarly, a lobar bronchus affects a lobe, and a segmental bronchus, a segment. Because drainage is interfered with, infection is often superimposed in the atelectatic area.

Since bronchial obstruction may develop from many causes, so may atelectasis. An extramural obstruction of the bronchial lumen by direct pressure on its outer wall may result from either enlarged hilar lymph nodes due to such diseases as tuberculosis, sarcoidosis and malignancy, or an aneurysm of the aorta. A mural obstruction, such as a bronchogenic carcinoma or a bronchial adenoma, arising from within the bronchial wall is a common cause of complete obstruction of the lumen; ulceration and fibrosis due to tuberculosis can also result in stenosis of a bronchus. Finally, complete obstruction of a bronchus may develop from an intraluminal cause, such as a foreign body, or abnormal secretions that may be present in any chronic bronchial disease, whooping cough or lobular pneumonia.

THE DEVELOPMENT OF ATELECTASIS. If a bronchus remains obstructed for several hours, the air is completely absorbed from the affected portion of the lung. As a result, the lung shrinks in size and the pulmonary tissue may have the appearance and texture of the fetal lung. The alveolar gases are gradually absorbed into the pulmonary capillaries, and the lung tissue retracts because of its natural elasticity. Blood flow in the pulmonary capillaries is essential for atelectasis to develop; it does not take place if the pulmonary artery supplying the affected lobe is ligated before its bronchus is blocked.

The mechanism by which the alveolar gases are absorbed into the circulating blood can be best explained if a single alveolus is taken as an example. This alveolus is an elastic air-containing sac separated from the pulmonary circulation by the alveolocapillary membrane, through

TABLE 6

THE PARTIAL PRESSURES OF GASES IN ALVEOLAR AIR AND MIXED
VENOUS BLOOD

GAS	PARTIAL PRESSURE OF GAS (mm. Hg)	
	Alveolar Air	Mixed Venous Blood
Oxygen...................	110	40
Carbon dioxide..............	40	46
Nitrogen...................	563	563
H_2O.......................	47	47

which the gases diffuse. The extent of the diffusion depends on several factors, the most important being the partial pressures of the gases on either side of this membrane. Table 6 illustrates that the partial pressures of the individual gases in the alveolar air are different from those in the mixed venous blood because of the gaseous exchanges which take place in the tissues.

It is easier to describe the process of absorption of air from the alveoli as a sequence of exchanges of the individual gases, although all the gaseous exchanges actually occur simultaneously. Initially, because of the partial pressure gradients, oxygen moves from the alveolus into the pulmonary capillary, while carbon dioxide moves in the opposite direction. Because more oxygen is consumed than carbon dioxide is produced, more gas leaves the alveolus than enters it. The lung, by virtue of the elasticity of its alveolar walls, accommodates itself to this new volume and becomes smaller, so that the total pressure in the alveoli remains unchanged. The concentration and partial pressure of the nitrogen increase so that it also starts to diffuse out of the alveoli into the blood, and the lung again contracts to accommodate itself to its new volume. The concentration and partial pressures of the oxygen and the carbon dioxide in the alveoli now increase, so that they diffuse from the alveoli into the pulmonary capillary blood. This cycle continues until all the alveolar gases are absorbed and the alveoli are completely collapsed. The process whereby alveolar air is absorbed into the circulating blood takes place over a period of several hours, as there is little difference between the partial pressures of nitrogen in the alveolar air and that in the blood. On the other hand, if the alveoli should contain pure oxygen rather than nitrogen, complete atelectasis would occur in a matter of minutes. A sudden massive collapse of a lung or a lobe cannot be adequately explained on the basis of resorption of gas behind a blocked bronchus. It is possible that rapid collapse results from a ball-valve type of obstruction in which the air may be coughed past the obstruction during expiration but is not allowed to enter the bronchus during inspiration.

Atelectasis of a lobule may not take place if its bronchiole becomes obstructed because of the interconnections that exist between neighboring lobules through minute apertures in the interalveolar septa. Thus, even though the alveolar duct or the terminal bronchiole becomes blocked, an alveolus in a primary lobule or a secondary lobule may continue to contain air because it is supplied from the alveoli of neighboring lobules.

The atelectatic lung usually re-expands when the bronchial obstruction is corrected, provided it has not been collapsed for too long a time. The expansion of a collapsed area of lung takes place for the same reason as the initial expansion of a newborn baby's lung. As in the newborn, the resistance due to surface tension may be increased so that the initial intrapleural pressure which must be exerted to open the collapsed lung may have to be extremely great. Once the resistance is overcome, however, the collapsed portion of lung usually expands completely, and further respiratory excursions take place with the normal changes in intrapleural pressure.

CLINICAL MANIFESTATIONS

The alterations that take place within the thoracic cavity when a bronchus is completely obstructed vary with the size of the affected bronchus and the amount of lung tissue involved. Dyspnea and pain over the affected area of the chest are experienced if the atelectasis develops acutely. On the other hand, the patient may experience very little dyspnea, except perhaps on exertion, if the atelectasis has a gradual onset.

Atelectasis of segmental and smaller areas of lung produce such minimal abnormalities that it is usually impossible to detect them by physical examination, although they are generally demonstrable by radiologic means. When the atelectasis involves a greater portion of the lung, such as a lobe, certain characteristic clinical signs are easily recognizable by physical examination. These are the consequences of a decrease in size of the lung and an increase in density of the affected lung parenchyma.

The patient may show evident respiratory distress and cyanosis. The affected part of the chest wall may appear retracted, with the ribs closer together, and indrawing of the costal interspaces may occur during inspiration. The trachea and the apex beat of the heart are shifted to the affected side and there is diminished movement of the ribs over the affected lobe of the lung.

Because of the increased ratio of solid to air-containing tissue, the percussion note is dull, and the note over the hyperinflated part of the neighboring lung parenchyma may be hyper-resonant. The margins of the affected lobe can usually be determined by percussion, if one knows the surface markings of the oblique and transverse fissures. For example, the lower border of a collapsed right upper lobe is considerably higher than the normal position of the right transverse fissure, and the upper border of a collapsed right middle lobe is lower in position than the normal right transverse fissure. With an atelectatic right or left lower lobe, the lateral border is situated considerably more medially and closer to the thoracic spine than is the normal oblique fissure.

The vocal fremitus is reduced and the breath sounds are absent over the atelectatic area as long as the bronchus remains obstructed. If the obstructing material has subsequently been sucked down to the terminal bronchioles, the vocal fremitus may be increased and the breath sounds may become bronchial because, although the lobe is still airless, its bronchus is now patent. Bronchial breathing may also be heard over a collapsed right or left upper lobe because of the close apposition of the trachea. If the collapsed alveoli should contain retained secretions or inflammatory exudate, fine, high-pitched rales may be heard in the terminal phase of inspiration.

RADIOLOGICAL MANIFESTATIONS

Collapse of a lobe of a lung produces characteristic radiological signs. The airless lobe tends to assume a wedge-shaped form with concave borders. The apex of the wedge is situated at the mediastinum, and its base lies in apposition to the chest wall. The collapsed portion of a

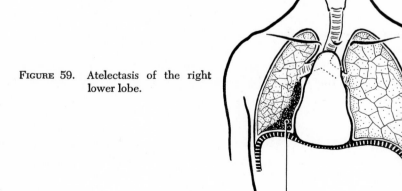

FIGURE 59. Atelectasis of the right lower lobe.

Atelectasis

lower lobe moves in a backward and medial direction, the anterior portion of the collapsed segment having a concave appearance. Figure 59 illustrates the radiological appearance of atelectasis of the right lower lobe.

A collapsed upper lobe shifts towards the apex of the lung, the hilus is displaced upward, and the trachea is deviated to the affected side. The wedge formed by the collapsed upper lobe moves in an upward and medial direction, the apex extending towards the superior aspect of the hilus. With collapse of either the right middle lobe or the left lingular segment, the base of the wedge moves medially towards the mediastinum. The apex of the wedge is directed laterally on the posteroanterior view and towards the hilus on the lateral projection.

FUNCTIONAL MANIFESTATIONS

The degree of functional impairment in atelectasis depends on the amount of collapsed lung parenchyma. The elastic resistance to distention increases so that the lung compliance is reduced. This is reflected by a reduced vital capacity. Although the elastic work is increased, the nonelastic work is usually unaltered in a pure uncomplicated atelectasis, because the unaffected airways in the bronchial tree remain patent and unobstructed. Usually, however, there is evidence of diffuse airway obstruction, and the timed vital capacity, the maximal mid-expiratory flow rate and the maximal breathing capacity are all lower than normal.

The distribution of inspired air is uneven if the bronchial obstruction is no longer complete or if there is evidence of partial bronchial obstruction elsewhere. Because of the increased resistance in the vessels perfusing the atelectatic alveoli, the blood is frequently shunted away from the poorly ventilated areas. Nevertheless, some blood still flows through their pulmonary capillaries, so that hypoxia develops because of the venous admixture-like perfusion. Carbon dioxide retention does not occur if the remaining alveoli are being hyperventilated.

Since the level of the diffusing capacity of the lungs is directly proportional to the size of the pulmonary capillary bed which is available for diffusion, there is no diffusion defect at rest unless a massive atelectasis is present. On the other hand, the alveolocapillary bed available for diffusion may be inadequate during exercise, so that hypoxia may develop.

PULMONARY CONSOLIDATION

The term "consolidation" implies that a portion of the lung parenchyma is firm or solid instead of soft and spongy. Consolidation of lung tissue is the result of a pathological process by which cellular material has completely replaced the air within the alveolar spaces. Destruction of the alveolar septa and the surrounding elastic structures is an infrequent occurrence, and although the alveoli are no longer able to function, their anatomical structure remains intact.

PATHOGENESIS

Consolidation results from either an inflammatory process or infiltration of the alveolar spaces with malignant cells. It may have a lobar, a segmental or a lobular distribution.

Inflammatory diseases of the lung parenchyma are commonly referred to as either "pneumonia" or "pneumonitis." These terms should not be used synonymously, however. "Pneumonia" usually refers to diseases with a self-limited course, in which the etiologic agent can be identified. In this group, the inflammatory process tends to heal without any significant damage to the tissues, there being little, if any, pathological involvement of the interstitial tissues. On the other hand, "pneumonitis" is an inflammatory condition of the lung in which the etiology is indeterminate. It may be acute, chronic or recurrent. Not only are the alveoli filled with an inflammatory exudate, but there is also an associated severe inflammatory involvement of the interstitial tissues and the bronchioles.

Pulmonary consolidation and pneumonia can be produced by a variety of specific or nonspecific agents.

Specific Pneumonias. The bacterial pneumonias are the most frequent types of pneumonia encountered in clinical practice. The commonest organism encountered by far is the pneumococcus. Infection by the hemolytic streptococcus, the staphylococcus, the Friedländer's bacillus and the tubercle bacillus may also lead to consolidation. These bacteria cause primary infections of the lung, and each tends to produce a characteristic clinical and pathological picture.

There is another group of acute pneumonias in which, despite exhaustive investigation, no evidence of a bacterial etiology can be ascertained. These pneumonias have certain characteristic features in common, presenting as an acute febrile infectious disease with clinical and radiological evidence of pulmonary consolidation which is lobular rather than lobar in distribution. In some cases, certain viruses have been established as the etiologic agents, but in the majority of these pneumonias, attempts at isolating a viral agent have been unsuccessful. Infection with the influenza viruses is the commonest condition encountered. Occasionally pneumonia may develop in a case of measles or as a result of infection with viruses of the psittacosis-ornithosis group, which causes a specific disease of birds.

Many pathogenic fungi are capable of producing pneumonia in man, either through direct inhalation or as part of a blood-borne dissemination from an extrapulmonary fungus infection. A mycotic pneumonia should be suspected if the patient has visited or resided in an area where certain fungus diseases such as histoplasmosis or coccidioidomycosis are known to be endemic. The ensuing pneumonia is generally characterized by necrosis and suppuration, although it is not definitely known how the pulmonary tissue becomes destroyed. Liberation of toxin by the fungi or the development of hypersensitivity on the part of the host to either the fungi or their breakdown products has been suggested.

Pneumonia is also an important feature of some rickettsial diseases such as Q fever, which is caused by *Coxiella burnetii,* and some parasitic diseases such as those due to *Endameba histolytica* and *Ascaris lumbricoides.*

Nonspecific Pneumonias.   PHYSICOCHEMICAL PNEUMONIAS.   There is a group of pneumonias which are basically nonspecific reactions of the lung parenchyma to a variety of different agents. There are many physical and chemical agents capable of inflaming the lung.

Aspiration pneumonia results from a breakdown of the defense mechanisms of the tracheobronchial tree, so that the organisms which normally inhabit the healthy upper respiratory tract are allowed to invade the pulmonary alveoli and set up an inflammatory reaction. During acute or chronic infections of the upper respiratory tract, thickened mucus or inflammatory exudate may be aspirated into the major bronchi. This eventually obstructs some of the smaller bronchi and bronchioles, with the production of various degrees of atelectasis. If the aspirated material is sterile and nonirritating, no inflammatory reaction takes place. On the other hand, if the material is infected or is an irritant, an inflammatory reaction is produced. A transient pneumonic infiltration of this kind is frequently seen in cases of chronic bronchitis or bronchial asthma, as well as in people in whom there is excess mucus production in the upper respiratory tract. The infected atelectatic areas in these pneumonias may have a lobular, a segmental or a lobar distribution. They are more liable to occur in debilitated persons, particularly in the aged and especially if they have been confined to bed for long periods. Patients who are in coma, deep narcosis or under anesthesia are also particularly liable to develop aspiration pneumonia.

Accidental aspiration of an irritating substance may also set up a severe inflammatory reaction in the lung parenchyma. Pneumonia may follow the aspiration of substances such as water or particulate matter in cases of drowning, vomitus by comatose or anesthetized patients, or regurgitated food in cases of esophageal obstruction. In addition, "lipid pneumonia" results from the aspiration of oil into the tracheobronchial tree; until their manufacture was discontinued, oily nose drops were a common cause of this condition. The administration of mineral oil for constipation, particularly if the oil is taken at bedtime while the person is in a reclining position, is another cause of lipid pneumonia. The oil tends to adhere to the posterior pharyngeal wall and is then easily aspirated into the lungs during sleep.

Large doses of irradiation to the thorax, as in the treatment of breast malignancy, can be injurious to the lung parenchyma. This usually causes an inflammatory edema, which is later followed by necrosis and fibrosis.

The lung may be injured by trauma even though there is no rib fracture or penetrating wound of the chest wall. The contused lung parenchyma becomes edematous and necrotic and is an ideal culture medium for the growth of bacteria, thus making the injured lung more susceptible to infection.

Finally, pneumonia often complicates a bronchial obstruction. Both bronchogenic carcinomas and bronchial adenomas originate in the bronchi and often cause bronchial obstruction, atelectasis, retained secretions and infection so that pneumonia is a common complication. Even though the bronchial obstruction is not complete, pulmonary infection may develop because of inefficient drainage of secretions. Recurrent pneumonia, pneumonia which runs an atypical course or pneumonia which recurs in the same area of lung, particularly in middle-aged or elderly patients, should always raise the question of malignancy in the examiner's mind.

CLINICAL MANIFESTATIONS

The symptoms of consolidation vary, depending on the specific type of pneumonia which is present. Each has its characteristic history and clinical course. Pneumococcal pneumonias are frequently preceded by an acute upper respiratory tract infection, the pneumonia often being heralded by violent chills, a rapidly mounting fever, and cough and sputum. Dyspnea and cyanosis may be severe. Similarly, Friedländer's pneumonia also may begin acutely with violent chills, rapidly mounting fever, cough and expectoration of copious amounts of sputum. Streptococcal and staphylococcal pneumonias often begin insidiously, with bronchitis a feature in the former, while the latter later develops into a critical illness with severe chills, dyspnea and cough. The viral pneumonias often begin as an upper respiratory infection with rhinitis, pharyngitis and tonsillitis, followed by symptoms of tracheitis and bronchitis. Often there are associated headache and generalized muscle aches and pains. The mycotic pneumonias are often more drawn out, with weakness, malaise, weight loss, night sweats, cough and expectoration.

The findings on physical examination depend upon the extent of the parenchymal tissue involved. Since the alveoli are full of exudate and offer an increased resistance to distention, the movement of the chest cage is restricted over the affected area of the lung. No displacement of either the trachea or the apex beat of the heart takes place because the alveoli are distended by the cellular material so that the size of the lung is unaltered and the end-expiratory intrapleural pressures are equal. The percussion note over the affected area is high-pitched or dull because the diseased alveoli are filled with cellular material, so that the ratio of solid tissue to air-containing tissue is increased. As the lung parenchyma has lost its "selective transmitter" property, the high frequency vibrations produced in the bronchial tree are transmitted to the chest wall and completely overshadow the low frequency vibrations; the breath sounds are therefore bronchial. The spoken voice is distinctly heard on the chest wall over the consolidated lung and has the bleating, nasal quality known as egophony. The whispered voice is also distinctly heard with a high-pitched, nasal quality—the "whispering pectoriloquy."

If the consolidation should have a lobular rather than a lobar distribution, the characteristic physical signs of consolidation may be difficult to detect. The affected areas are not only patchy and scattered, but are usually surrounded by normal lung tissue, so that the percussion note over them may still be resonant. Because the consolidated lobules are frequently bilateral, there may be no obvious diminution in movement. By careful auscultation, it may be possible to detect localized areas of bronchial or bronchovesicular breath sounds, but the most useful sign of all is that of whispering pectoriloquy, which can usually be detected over the patchy areas.

Rales can frequently be detected over a consolidated area of the lung. Since these are produced by the presence of cellular exudate within the alveolar spaces, they are generally fine and high-pitched in quality, occurring predominantly during the terminal phase of inspiration. When the secretions enter the bronchial tree, rhonchi may be present, and if the consolidation involves the visceral pleura, a pleural rub may be detected.

RADIOLOGICAL MANIFESTATIONS

Consolidated tissue shows up radiologically as a dense shadow in a part of the lung fields. It may be evident in one or two segments, a lobe or an entire lung. The mediastinum occupies its normal mid-line position. Figure 60 illustrates the radiological appearance of a consolidation of the right lower lobe.

In lobular consolidation, there may be scattered patchy opacities. Several of these may coalesce to involve several segments or even a whole lobe. These shadows are irregular in shape and are generally

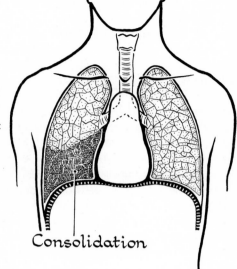

FIGURE 60.   Consolidation of the right lower lobe.

Consolidation

situated in the bases of both lungs. During resolution the shadow loses its homogeneity, becomes streaky and weblike, and finally disappears completely. Areas of translucency may develop in the radiological opacities. Although these may be mistaken for cavity formation, they actually represent re-aeration of the consolidated lung tissue in the process of healing. Occasionally, such appearances may be produced by ballooning of healthy alveoli in the neighborhood of the consolidated tissue, due to narrowing of the bronchial lumen by inflammatory swelling.

FUNCTIONAL MANIFESTATIONS

The amount of disturbance in pulmonary function depends upon the extent of the consolidation. In all cases, however, there is an increased elastic resistance to distention and therefore a reduced vital capacity. Unless secretions are present in the airway, there is no increase in nonelastic resistance, so that the timed vital capacity and the maximal mid-expiratory flow rate are essentially normal, while the maximal breathing capacity is only slightly reduced.

The distribution of gas is uneven because of the local alteration in elastic resistance. Hypoxia is frequent and is probably due to continued perfusion of the consolidated nonventilated lung, although it is possible that a diffusion defect may also be responsible. The carbon dioxide tension is frequently lower than normal because of the increased ventilation induced by hypoxia.

PULMONARY ABSCESS AND CAVITATION

A pulmonary abscess is a collection of pus within the substance of the lung resulting from a suppurative necrosis of pyogenic or fungal origin. It must be distinguished from other collections of pus, such as a bronchiectatic abscess.

When the necrotic material resulting from destruction of lung tissue in a suppurative pneumonia is expelled into the bronchial tree, the cavity that remains is known as an abscess cavity. Through long usage, a chronic tuberculous abscess is generally called a "cavity" while the term "abscess" is applied to a wide variety of suppurative diseases of the lung. It should be pointed out, however, that there is no difference between the lung excavation resulting from the discharge of tuberculous caseous material and that caused by the evacuation of the purulent material of a suppurative pneumonia. Although the latter is a much more acute process, they are both abscess cavities, the only difference being the etiologic agent.

PATHOGENESIS

A pulmonary abscess is not a distinct entity in itself, nor is it ever a primary condition. It is a pathological process which develops during the course of any number of inflammatory conditions of the lung, no matter what the cause, provided that there are associated suppuration and necrosis of the lung tissue. It usually develops because of the aspiration of infected or foreign material, but may also occur because of obstruction of the bronchial tree, a primary suppurative pneumonia or infected emboli. Rarer causes are infection of a pulmonary infarct, infection of a congenital cyst or emphysematous bulla, chest injury or an intra-abdominal infection that penetrates the diaphragm.

It has been well established that nasopharyngeal and oral secretions may be aspirated into the trachea during sleep. In the normal course of events, the bronchial defenses adequately deal with this noxious material, but to function effectively they depend on an intact nervous system and muscular apparatus. During such periods as surgical anesthesia, postoperative states, alcoholic stupor, traumatic shock or cerebral accidents with coma, the defenses are seriously impaired. In addition, if secretions are thick, tenacious and mucopurulent, or consist of clotted blood, even the ciliary activity becomes ineffective. Under such conditions, the aspirated secretions penetrate deeply into the bronchial tree and finally lodge in the finer bronchioles, where they produce a segmental atelectasis. This is even more likely to occur if solid material such as bits of tartar are aspirated during the scaling of teeth or pieces of tonsil or adenoid tissue are inhaled during their surgical excision.

Once an atelectasis develops, an inflammatory reaction inevitably follows. The severity of this reaction depends on the virulence of the infection and the resistance of the patient. The most common invading organisms are the saprophytic inhabitants of the mouth and nasopharynx, and these are usually followed by secondary invaders, such as the staphylococci, streptococci and Friedländer's bacilli, which produce suppurative pneumonia. Aspiration of a large quantity of irritant fluid, such as vomitus, usually results in a diffuse lobular pneumonia with multiple abscesses; solid matter, such as a piece of a tooth, usually causes a localized abscess. The site of aspiration abscess formation depends on the force of gravity as well as on the posture of the patient during aspiration. Aspirated material tends to lodge in the most dependent bronchus, so that if the patient is lying on his back at the moment of aspiration the bronchus to the superior segment of the lower lobe is probably the one involved. If he is lying on his side, the most likely site is the upper lobe, and if he is upright, such as during a dental extraction, the lower lobes are the ones most likely to be affected.

Bronchial occlusions produced by other intraluminal, mural or extramural lesions are less common causes of pulmonary abscesses. In conditions such as bronchogenic carcinoma, bronchial adenoma, an inhaled foreign body and stenosis of a bronchus due to external pressure on its wall there may be associated abscess formation in the atelectatic bronchopulmonary segment. An abscess cavity may occasionally develop within the substance of a pulmonary neoplasm, whether primary or secondary; it occurs most frequently in the squamous cell type of bronchogenic carcinoma. A cavity of this type may be caused by several factors. A deficient blood supply may produce an aseptic necrosis of the rapidly developing tumor tissue; obstruction of the communicating bronchus to the involved lung parenchyma may result in retention of secretions, which is followed by infection and suppuration; a hemorrhagic infarction following thrombosis of a pulmonary vessel in the region of the growth is another possibility. A malignant cavity characteristically has a thick wall and a shaggy, irregular appearance.

Primary pneumococcal and streptococcal pneumonias are rarely complicated by abscess formation, except in infancy or debility. Suppuration is a frequent occurrence, however, in pneumonias caused by the staphylococci, Friedländer's bacilli, tubercle bacilli and certain fungi such as *Actinomyces bovis, Coccidioides immitis* and *Histoplasma capsulatum.*

A pulmonary abscess due to *Endameba histolytica* may develop when an amebic abscess of the liver ruptures through the diaphragm into the lower lobe of the right lung. A traumatic hematoma of the lung, such as the laceration produced by a fractured rib or by shrapnel, is another rare cause of a pulmonary abscess; the extravasated blood acts as an ideal culture medium. Pulmonary abscesses may also develop by direct extension from septic foci in neighboring organs, such as the esophagus.

Lung abscesses have been produced experimentally in animals by introducing infected material, particularly infected blood clots, into the venous system. In the human, a sterile embolus from a peripheral phlebothrombosis may produce a pulmonary infarct, and very rarely the embolus becomes infected so that an abscess results. In some cases, a sterile pulmonary infarct subsequently becomes infected by means of aspirated material via the bronchial tree. Occasionally sterile necrosis and abscess formation may occur in a massive infarct, even in the absence of any primary or secondary infection.

A pulmonary abscess is caused by a combination of suppuration and necrosis of lung tissue. The necrosis may be produced by an associated septic thrombosis of the pulmonary vessels. The size of the slough varies from very small to so large that a whole segment of lung may be destroyed. The slough usually becomes separated from the surrounding lung tissue and lies free in the abscess cavity. The more chronic an abscess, the more thickened and putrid its contents become. The abscess gradually becomes distended by the accumulation of purulent material, and it finally ruptures into a bronchus, resulting in the evacuation of its contents and the entry of atmospheric air to form the abscess cavity. The extent to which a cavity is evacuated depends on the size of the lumen of the involved bronchus. If the bronchial lumen is small, a portion of the fluid may be retained in the cavity. If the bronchial lumen is large enough, there may be a complete evacuation of the contents, so that an abscess cavity remains.

Because of the unique structure of the lungs, a pulmonary cavity always contains air, either alone or in association with fluid, and it is generally spherical in shape. The presence of air within its confines is due to its communication with the outside atmosphere through a patent bronchus. The spherical shape is due to the elasticity of the surrounding healthy lung parenchyma. The principle may be illustrated by burning small, irregular holes in a thin elastic sheet of rubber; if the sheet is stretched taut, these irregularly shaped holes assume a perfectly round shape.

Occasionally a tension cavity may develop. In this case, the walls of the bronchus are involved and encroach on the bronchial lumen, producing a check-valve obstruction. Inspired air is trapped, so that the cavity enlarges and the intracavity pressure becomes considerably higher than that of the atmosphere. Tension cavities can develop fairly rapidly, over a period of weeks or even days. When the bronchial lumen becomes patent, they disappear almost as quickly with re-aeration of the compressed parenchyma surrounding the cavity.

When the bronchial outlets become completely occluded, the air within an abscess cavity is gradually absorbed by the blood in the pulmonary capillaries in a manner similar to that which takes place in an atelectasis. The rate of absorption depends on the permeability of the wall of the abscess as well as the amount of pulmonary blood flow in the surrounding parenchyma. If the wall is thin and the surrounding parenchyma little affected by disease, the absorption of air is rapid and complete so that the cavity collapses and resolves. On the other hand, if its wall is thick and fibrotic, with little blood-flow in its neighboring atelectatic and fibrotic parenchyma, little absorption of air takes place. A cavity whose wall has become calcified is obviously unable to collapse, since no absorption of air can take place.

CLINICAL MANIFESTATIONS

The symptoms and clinical course of a pulmonary abscess depend on the etiology and type of pre-existing pulmonary disease, the size and progression of the cavity and the presence of complications, such as empyema. Usually the clinical picture is dominated by the underlying pulmonary disease, the abscess frequently being discovered only by radiological means.

If a patient who has recently undergone a surgical procedure, particularly in the mouth, nose or throat, develops a febrile respiratory illness, the possibility of a pulmonary abscess should be suspected. This is also true of a patient who has been unconscious from any cause, or who has had a sudden choking spell while swallowing food.

The onset may be sudden, with a high fever, severe constitutional symptoms and an initially nonproductive cough. Any sputum produced by the inflamed bronchi in the neighborhood of the abscess is scanty, mucoid and odorless. An associated pleuritis may cause a localized pleuritic pain over the corresponding area of the chest.

Rupture of an abscess into a bronchus frequently occurs about 10 to 14 days after the onset of the illness and is indicated by the sudden expectoration of a large quantity of purulent sputum. There may be a fetid odor to the breath about 24 hours prior to the event. The sputum is green or brown, may be mixed with blood, and often has a very offensive odor. Large quantities of purulent sputum continue to be expectorated daily, especially in association with any sudden change in position. The patient's condition usually improves when the abscess ruptures. The temperature frequently returns to normal levels, the constitutional symptoms disappear and a sense of well-being returns. If the abscess should persist, however, the low-grade constitutional symptoms remain, and episodes of acute exacerbations alternate with periods of relatively good health.

The abnormal physical signs depend on the degree of the surrounding pneumonitis, the size of the abscess cavity and its distance from the chest wall. The usual findings are those related to the suppurative pneumonia with associated atelectasis and fibrosis: a shift of the mediastinum to the affected side, restricted movement of the chest wall over the affected area of the lung, an impaired note on percussion, bronchial breath sounds of diminished intensity and coarse rales during the second and third phases of inspiration.

An abscess cavity may occasionally produce distinctive signs of its own, but only if it is large, relatively empty of secretions and surrounded by a relatively narrow zone of consolidated parenchyma, and if its communicating bronchus is widely patent. Under such circumstances, a particularly loud, hollow-sounding form of bronchial breathing, known as "amphoric breath sounds," can be detected. It must be emphasized, however, that this type of breath sound is more frequently absent than present. The sounds may be diminished or absent either because the communicating bronchus is small and partially obstructed or because the cavity is situated some distance from the chest wall and is surrounded by parenchyma which has undergone compensatory overdistention.

Digital clubbing frequently occurs in the early stages of the disease and often progresses to the extent of hypertrophic pulmonary osteoarthropathy. This condition rapidly regresses when the abscess heals.

RADIOLOGICAL MANIFESTATIONS

An abscess cavity can be definitely diagnosed only by means of a radiological examination of the chest. Lateral and oblique views, as well as the standard posteroanterior one, are usually required to localize its position. An abscess can generally be recognized by the radio-translucent circular shadow it produces, the thickness of its border depending on the extent of involvement of the surrounding parenchyma. The most definite diagnostic feature of an abscess is the presence of a fluid level within the confines of its cavity. Owing to the presence of air, the fluid level is recognized by a straight horizontal upper border which moves if the patient changes his position during a fluoroscopic examination.

The radiological opacity produced by the surrounding pneumonitis may be so dense that it obscures the abscess cavity on the standard film. It may occasionally be demonstrated by the endobronchial instillation of a radio-opaque medium, provided that the material is able to flow into the cavity. Tomography is an even more convenient means of demonstrating the abscess cavity, particularly if the tomogram is done in the erect position.

FUNCTIONAL MANIFESTATIONS

Since an abscess cavity is essentially a localized process and a considerable amount of healthy lung tissue is still present, little disturbance in pulmonary function occurs. Nevertheless, if sufficient tissue is involved in the reparative process, the elastic resistance to distention may be increased so that the vital capacity is reduced and the distribution of inspired air is impaired. Alterations of ventilation-perfusion ratios occur so that minimal hypoxia may result.

CYSTS OF THE LUNG

In cystic disease of the lungs, whether congenital or acquired, the continuity of the lung parenchyma is interrupted by thin-walled, sharply defined open spaces containing either fluid or air, and often both. These may occur singly or there may be many in one or both lungs. They vary in size from a space so small as to be barely visible to the naked eye, to one that is so large that it occupies a whole lung. A solitary cyst may result from the coalescence of several smaller cysts. Multiple cysts may be confined to a segment, a lobe, or an entire lung, or both lungs may be riddled with small cysts, giving the involved tissue a honeycombed or spongy appearance.

The pathogenesis of cystic disease of the lungs has been a matter of debate for many years, and the etiology is still in doubt. Although the majority of investigators consider that there is strong evidence for a congenital origin, recent studies have shown that most cysts are acquired. For many years, it was considered that the presence of epithelialization of the cyst wall, particularly by stratified columnar epithelium, pointed conclusively to a congenital origin. It is now known that this type of epithelium can be present on the wall of an acquired cyst, however, and that the development of infection within a congenital cyst may destroy its epithelial lining. Thus, it is generally impossible to determine the origin of cystic disease of the lungs, unless it is found in the lung of a fetus or a newborn infant.

CONGENITAL CYSTS

It is now realized that congenital cystic disease is not as uncommon as it was formerly thought, since a large number of cases are being diagnosed by surgical excision. Both sexes are equally affected and there appears to be a familial tendency. Other congenital abnormalities are frequently associated. There is some difference of opinion as to the exact embryological fault leading to congenital cystic disease. It is generally agreed, however, that the cysts arise during the development of the lungs by separation of a fragment from the main bronchial buds or their derivatives, the forerunners of the bronchi. If only one bronchial bud is involved, a solitary cyst is formed; if many bronchial buds are affected, multiple cysts develop.

The walls of the cysts vary considerably in structure. They may contain tissues which resemble those of bronchi, bronchioles or alveoli. They may be lined with ciliated, columnar or cuboidal epithelium. They may contain muscle fibers, elastic tissue and cartilage. Pulmonary cysts may be filled with either air or fluid, the latter being less frequent. When the cysts contain fluid, it is usually clear and watery. On occasion, it may be viscid because of an increased content of mucus, or it may be foul-smelling and purulent if it is infected. After birth, a fluid-filled cyst may develop a communication with a bronchus and be transformed into an air-filled cyst. Since the lungs are normally sterile, cysts are rarely exposed to infection, but if they are, the infection is generally mild because of the resistance of their lining epithelium.

An air-filled cyst may enlarge if its bronchial communication becomes compressed by the cyst wall, so that a check-valve type of obstruction occurs. This is the usual manifestation in childhood. Such a ballooning cyst may crowd the mediastinum and compress the opposite lung. This may produce dyspnea on exertion, although symptoms are frequently completely absent until a complication such as a spontaneous pneumothorax or infection supervenes. Unless a routine x-ray film of the chest is carried out, the condition may remain undiagnosed unless a complication has occurred.

Another congenital lesion which may have the appearance of a cyst or cavity is a sequestrated lobe, which receives anomalous systemic vessels from the aorta or one of its branches.

Cystic Bronchiectasis.   There is little doubt that the majority of cases of bronchiectasis, even those which develop soon after birth, are acquired. There is, however, a rare form of proved congenital origin due to maldevelopment of the bronchi, which can simulate the acquired form of the disease, both clinically and radiologically. The origin of the congenital variety is similar to that of congenital cystic disease of the lungs, except that the bronchial sacculations probably develop from an outgrowth of bronchial tissue rather than from pinched-off bronchial buds. The saccules may attain several centimeters in diameter. Bronchography reveals large dilated bronchi entering the cysts. Bronchial cysts are generally found in the dependent areas of the lower lobes, and are prone to infection, thereby producing a clinical picture similar to that of acquired bronchiectasis.

ACQUIRED CYSTS

Blebs. Pulmonary blebs are collections of air which lie in the interlobular connective tissue just beneath the pleura. They are formed by ruptured alveoli, the escaped air tracking along the tissue planes of the lungs and finally becoming localized in the subpleural areas. Here, the air may be absorbed or it may rupture through the visceral pleura, producing a spontaneous pneumothorax. On rare occasions, the air may track medially and rupture into the mediastinum. The actual cause of the alveolar rupture is unknown, although it has been suggested that it is caused by a localized check-valve bronchiolar obstruction which produces distention of the alveoli.

Pneumatoceles. In contrast to a pulmonary bleb, a pneumatocele is a hyperinflated cavity deep within the substance of the lung parenchyma. A pneumatocele always contains air, but it may also contain inflammatory exudate. Its development is generally associated with a check-valve type of obstruction in the small bronchial branch draining a small segment of inflamed lung parenchyma. Because of the obstruction, the affected lung tissue becomes hyperinflated, so that the pressure increases within the alveoli, resulting in a rupture of the diseased interalveolar septa. The pneumatocele does not usually persist and it often subsides spontaneously.

Bullae. A bulla develops when several alveoli coalesce because of fragmentation of their interalveolar elastic tissue and subsequent rupture of their attenuated interalveolar septae. The condition is produced by a localized check-valve type of obstruction in the bronchioles. In chronic obstructive emphysema, there may be a single bulla or many, which may or may not communicate with each other. The walls, which are formed by the destroyed interalveolar septa, are roughened and poorly defined, possessing no true epithelial lining.

Honeycombing. Diffuse multiple cystic involvement of the lungs, also called "honeycomb lungs," is rare. In this condition the lung parenchyma is replaced by numerous thin-walled cysts, which may affect a portion of lung, an entire lung or both lungs diffusely.

The pathogenesis of this condition is not clear. It has been suggested that a defect in the embryological development of the terminal elements of the bronchial tree results in a failure of alveolar formation and that isolated segments of small bronchi and bronchioles then grow out in the form of cysts. Although honeycomb lungs are rarely found in either embryos or infants, the hypothesis is not disproved, for the bronchi continue to bud and form new alveoli for many years after birth. This kind of lesion is undoubtedly acquired as well, for many cases have been found in association with generalized systemic infiltrative diseases, such as the xanthomatoses, tuberous sclerosis, various pituitary diseases and collagen diseases.

No matter what the etiology, the gross appearance of the lung is identical in all cases. When the lung is sectioned, it has the appearance of a sponge or a honeycomb. The cysts, which are approximately 1 cm. in diameter, possess thin walls and contain air; a few may contain small amounts of fluid. There is minimal inflammatory reaction in the surrounding lung parenchyma and connective tissue.

CLINICAL MANIFESTATIONS

When single or multiple cysts are present in either lung or both lungs, the symptoms depend on the amount of lung tissue that is replaced and the degree of pulmonary compression which occurs when the cysts expand in size. The cysts usually produce no symptoms until some complication arises, so that they are frequently discovered during a routine radiological examination of the chest.

Cysts which contain fluid and are not in communication with the bronchial tree generally produce no symptoms. When such a cyst ruptures, the patient generally coughs up varying amounts of mucoid material. Air-filled cysts which are in communication with a bronchus are more liable to become infected, producing the symptoms of a suppurative lesion. If a tension cyst develops as a result of a tortuous, narrowed, check-valve type of bronchial communication, the cyst may enlarge to such a size that the mediastinum may be crowded over, compressing the opposite lung. This occurs more frequently in children than in adults. The loss of pulmonary reserve results in dyspnea, cough and cyanosis. If the pressure within the cyst becomes high enough, its wall may rupture, producing a pneumothorax.

In cystic bronchiectasis, hemoptysis is a relatively frequent occurrence, even in the absence of any superimposed infection. As the blood is derived from a dilated bronchial artery, the hemoptysis may be profuse.

In general, pulmonary cysts are difficult to detect by means of the physical examination unless there is a complication such as pneumothorax or suppuration. When these occur, the typical findings associated with these conditions are detected. A large tension cyst may produce signs which simulate those of a pneumothorax, so that it may not be possible to distinguish between these two conditions on clinical grounds.

RADIOLOGICAL MANIFESTATIONS

Cystic disease of the lungs is usually a radiological diagnosis. The number and the size of the cysts, as well as the nature of their contents, be it air or fluid, can be determined by means of the standard postero-

anterior and lateral films of the chest. A cyst which is filled with fluid
appears as a round or oval opacity with a sharply defined border. An
air-filled cyst is translucent, with a thin, sharply defined wall, and occasionally a fluid level. An infected cyst is generally surrounded by a
hazy opacity due to the associated pneumonitis, so that the outline of the
cyst may be obscured.

Unless there is some complication, the appearance and the size
of a cyst do not alter. An opaque cyst may become translucent, indicating that a bronchial communication has opened, or an air-filled cyst may
become opaque, indicating that it has filled with fluid, which is generally
of an inflammatory nature. The cyst may progressively increase in size,
indicating a check-valve type of obstruction. A tension cyst may become
so large that it is impossible to distinguish from a pneumothorax.

A pneumatocele superficially resembles a pulmonary abscess, but
it can be distinguished by its radiological appearance. The wall is thin
and the surrounding lung parenchyma is healthy. Another distinguishing
feature is its size, which may be seen to vary from day to day by serial
radiological examination.

If multiple small cysts are present over a large area, and particularly if both lungs are diffusely involved, the diagnosis of honeycomb
lung is relatively easy. If only a small area of lung is affected, particularly
the upper lobe, it may be obscured by the overlying healthy lung tissue.
It then has an irregular mottled appearance, so that it is frequently
mistaken for tuberculosis.

FUNCTIONAL MANIFESTATIONS

The disturbances in pulmonary function depend on the extent of
the disease. If the cyst is solitary and occupies little space, there may be
no alteration in function. If multiple cysts are present, the distensibility
is frequently reduced so that the vital capacity is diminished. No increase
in nonelastic resistance occurs unless the airways are compressed by an
elevated pressure within the cysts or there is an associated bronchitis.
Ventilation-perfusion ratios are usually altered so that hypoxia frequently
occurs. In some cases, the diffusing capacity is altered because of a
reduction in the size of the vascular bed, so that the hypoxia may be
severe. Carbon dioxide retention does not usually develop, except in the
later stages when alveolar hypoventilation and an increase in the work
of breathing occur.

PULMONARY FIBROSIS

The term "fibrosis" implies the presence of an excessive amount
of connective tissue in the whole or a part of an organ. It is a method of

tissue repair following any disease process causing inflammation or necrosis of the lung tissue.

PATHOGENESIS

The deposition of excess fibrous tissue in the lungs is not indicative of any one disease, but is usually a sequel to a variety of disease processes. The distribution of the fibrous tissue in the lungs varies in different disease processes, and the resulting scar tissue may be confined to either a small segment of lung parenchyma, a lobe or a lung, or may be found in both lungs diffusely.

A localized fibrotic area of the lung is the commonest type of pulmonary fibrosis clinically encountered. This is the usual consequence of a localized area of tissue necrosis, such as may follow suppurative pneumonitis, a pulmonary abscess or tuberculous caseation. The extent of the scar which develops depends on the size of pre-existing necrotic lesion.

A more extensive fibrosis, in which a lobe or a large portion of a lung is involved, usually follows those acute pulmonary diseases which produce large areas of tissue necrosis, such as atelectasis of a lobe in which suppuration has developed, acute tuberculous pneumonia or a large pulmonary abscess. A similar type of fibrosis may be produced by repeated irradiation of the lung. The aspiration of irritating substances may also result in an inflammatory reaction of the involved lung tissue, and this is usually followed by necrosis and fibrosis. The accidental aspiration of oily nose drops or liquid paraffin also produces an irritative chemical pneumonia which is followed by fibrosis.

The generalized form of pulmonary fibrosis, in which both lungs are diffusely involved, usually follows either some widespread pulmonary infection or the inhalation of irritating dusts or noxious fumes. Prolonged exposure to dusts containing minute particles of irritating inorganic chemicals such as silicon dioxide, silicates or asbestos frequently causes an extensive form of pulmonary fibrosis known as pneumoconiosis. Extensive fibrosis may also develop in certain types of noncavitating granulomatous diseases such as sarcoidosis or in the collagen diseases such as scleroderma. The accidental inhalation of high concentrations of irritant gases such as mustard gas or ammonia produces a diffuse, bilateral inflammatory reaction, which also generally heals by fibrosis.

The deposition of excess fibrous tissue and cicatrization of the lung may occur in the bronchiolar wall, within the alveoli and the interstitial spaces, in the pulmonary vessels or in the pleura.

Bronchiolar Fibrosis. The extent of cicatrization that occurs in the walls of affected bronchioles depends on the type of inflammatory process preceding it. If a superficial ulceration of the bronchiolar mucosa develops, as in mustard gas poisoning, granulation tissue fills the lumen of the bronchiole, and later fibrous tissue is deposited on the inner surface of the bronchiolar wall. If the walls of the bronchioles are destroyed by a suppurative process, fibrous tissue is laid down in the walls. The affected bronchioles may only narrow if the suppuration is mild and there is no actual destruction of the bronchiolar walls. This narrowing produces a check-valve type of obstruction and distends the alveoli. If the bronchiolar involvement is widespread, it may lead to chronic obstructive emphysema.

Parenchymal Fibrosis. This is the type of pulmonary fibrosis most frequently seen. It occurs as a result of an inflammatory process involving the lung parenchyma, so that its extent varies. Parenchymal fibosis is frequently associated with bronchiolar and interstitial fibrosis as well. It is the usual sequel to such conditions as suppurative pneumonia, tuberculosis and prolonged irradiation. The fibrosis not only obliterates the alveolar space but involves the interstitial tissue as well, so that the alveolocapillary membrane is thickened. The neighboring alveoli are frequently compensatorily hyperinflated, and this condition may occur in the opposite normal lung as well if the fibrosis is very extensive.

Pulmonary Vascular Fibrosis. Fibrosis of the wall of a pulmonary arteriole narrows or obliterates its lumen, increasing the resistance to blood flow, with the consequent development of pulmonary hypertension. The commonest cause of pulmonary vascular fibrosis is vascular obstruction by multiple emboli in the pulmonary arterioles. On the other hand, pulmonary hypertension, no matter what the etiology, may lead to sclerosis of the arterial walls and narrowing of the lumen.

Pleural Fibrosis. Involvement of the pleura by fibrous tissue, often to such an extent that symphysis of the two layers may take place, occurs after any form of fibrinous pleurisy, especially if it is associated with an effusion. It is particularly prone to develop after a pyogenic or tuberculous empyema or a traumatic hemothorax. The pleural fluid becomes organized and forms a thick fibrous layer which envelops the lung in a constricting vice, causing a compression atelectasis of the underlying pulmonary parenchyma. The respiratory movements of the affected lung are restricted and its pulmonary blood flow is diminished, while the opposite lung undergoes compensatory hyperinflation.

CLINICAL MANIFESTATIONS

The severity of the symptoms is related not so much to the extent of the fibrosis as to the pattern of the distribution of the scar tissue. The primary symptom associated with pulmonary fibrosis is dyspnea on exertion, its degree depending on the extent of the fibrosis. The dyspnea is usually masked by other symptoms due to the pulmonary conditions frequently associated with fibrosis, such as bronchiectasis, chronic obstructive emphysema and bronchopneumonia.

No symptoms may be present when there is gross shrinkage of a lung in a case of long-standing localized pulmonary fibrosis. When constitutional symptoms are present in such a case, they are usually due to an underlying suppurative process.

In peribronchial fibrosis the characteristic symptom is wheezing, which may be associated with cough and sputum. The characteristic sign is high-pitched sibilant rhonchi which may be produced only by a forceful and prolonged expiration.

The parenchymal type of fibrosis, when bilateral and diffuse, produces little in the way of abnormal physical signs unless there is a complication, such as chronic obstructive emphysema or pulmonary hypertension.

A localized parenchymal fibrosis such as the shrunken upper lobe of chronic tuberculosis reduces the size of the affected lung. The chest wall over the diseased area is retracted, its movement is restricted, and the trachea and the apex of the heart are shifted to that side. The percussion note is dull or flat, depending on the degree of parenchymal involvement. The breath sounds are usually bronchovesicular, although if a massive fibrosis involves the upper lobe of the right lung, the breath sounds may be loud and bronchial because the bronchus is elevated and is closer to the chest wall. Even in the absence of an underlying infective process, one can occasionally hear dry, interrupted, creaky sounds which extend throughout both the inspiratory and expiratory phases of respiration. These adventitious sounds, which are considered to be produced by the extension and retraction of the fibrous tissue, may be the only abnormal findings in an uncomplicated case of bilateral diffuse fibrosis of the parenchymal type.

Pleural fibrosis, which is also known as "fibrothorax," characteristically results in retraction of the affected hemithorax, with narrowing and indrawing of the interspaces and an elevated tied diaphragm. The movement of the affected side is restricted, and the mediastinum is shifted towards it. The percussion note is dull or flat, and the breath sounds are faint or absent. Adventitious sounds such as rales may be present if there is fibrosis or bronchiectasis in the underlying lung.

Clubbing of the digits may be present if there is extensive destruction of lung tissue or if the fibrosis is complicated by bronchiectasis or a lung abscess.

When pulmonary hypertension develops in perivascular fibrosis, there is an increase in the degree of dyspnea. Clinical examination of the heart demonstrates an accentuation of the pulmonic second sound and evidence of right ventricular hypertrophy. Later, with the development of cor pulmonale, the manifestations of right-sided heart failure become evident.

RADIOLOGICAL MANIFESTATIONS

The radiological appearance of the localized type of pulmonary fibrosis is usually that of an opacity which corresponds to the extent and distribution of the lesion. This is illustrated in Figure 61. Within the opacity there are hard linear strands of fibrous tissue, and the pulmonary vessels are crowded together. If the walls of the dilated bronchi are considerably thickened, they may become visible as narrow, hard lines. Denser areas caused by atelectatic segments and areas of increased translucency due to compensatory hyperinflation may be seen in the neighboring lung parenchyma. The pleura overlying the fibrotic area may be thickened. Because of the decrease in the size of the lobe, the fissure which forms its boundary is usually displaced. The mediastinal structures are shifted to the affected side, and the ribs over the fibrotic area are drawn closer together. The diaphragm is elevated and often irregular because of pleural adhesions.

The diffuse form of peribronchial or parenchymal fibrosis presents a somewhat different radiological picture. Because it is generalized and bilateral, coarse linear strands are visible throughout both lungs, and the mediastinum does not become displaced from its mid-line position. Multiple small, thin-walled cysts or honeycombing may be present throughout both lung fields.

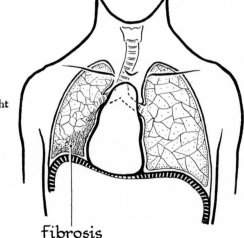

FIGURE 61. Fibrosis of the right lower lobe.

fibrosis

FUNCTIONAL MANIFESTATIONS

The disturbances in pulmonary function in pulmonary fibrosis depend upon the extent of the fibrosis as well as the pattern of its distribution. Whenever there is fibrosis of the lung parenchyma or the pleura, the distensibility of the lung is diminished, so the vital capacity is reduced, the extent of the reduction depending upon the amount of fibrosis. In bronchiolar fibrosis there is an increase in resistance to air flow, so that the timed vital capacity, the maximal mid-expiratory flow rate and the maximal breathing capacity are reduced. In the other types, however, there is little increase in nonelastic resistance, so that these ventilatory measurements are little altered.

If the distribution of the fibrosis is uneven, and particularly if it is peribronchial, the inspired air is distributed unevenly. In addition, there is frequently some associated perivascular fibrosis. As a result, there are alterations in ventilation-perfusion ratios so that hypoxia develops. Hypoxia is particularly evident in the parenchymal form of fibrosis in which there is a resistance to the diffusion of oxygen. On the other hand, carbon dioxide diffuses freely across the alveolocapillary membrane, and because of the increased ventilation induced by the hypoxia, the arterial carbon dioxide tension is frequently lower than normal. Whenever hypoxia is present, no matter what the form of fibrosis, and particularly when there is perivascular fibrosis as well, the pulmonary vascular resistance is increased, so that pulmonary hypertension eventually develops.

CHAPTER IX

Pulmonary Vascular Disease

THE CIRCULATION OF THE LUNG

THE LUNGS are one of two organs of the body with a double supply of blood, the other being the liver. One blood supply comes from the right ventricle through the pulmonary circulation, the other from the left ventricle through the bronchial circulation. The major portion of the circulation of the lung comes from the pulmonary arteries to the pulmonary veins, the bronchial arteries normally carrying only about one per cent of the blood. Although anastomoses have been demonstrated between the bronchial and pulmonary arteries, these have never been shown to function in normal lungs. In diseased lungs, however, these anastomoses dilate and the bronchial arteries may contribute a considerable part of the pulmonary circulation.

THE PULMONARY CIRCULATION

The pulmonary circulation constitutes a distensible reservoir which is situated between the right and left ventricles. Measurements of the pulmonary blood volume indicate that approximately 20 per cent of the total blood volume, or about 1.0 liter, is present in the pulmonary vessels at any given moment. Of this, 30 per cent is found in the arteries, and 65 per cent in the veins. The resting pulmonary capillary blood volume has been estimated to be about 6 per cent of the pulmonary blood volume, or 60 ml. Although this seems small, the surface area of the capillaries necessary to contain this volume of blood is 35 square meters. The pulmonary capillary blood volume is increased in congestive heart failure and it is reduced in pulmonary fibrosis.

The blood circulating through the lungs pulsates with a rhythm created by the heart beat. The perfusing blood pressure in the pulmonary blood vessels is less than 15 per cent of that in the peripheral circulation. The drop in the blood pressure from the main pulmonary artery to the left atrium is about 10 per cent of that between the aorta and the right atrium. In a normal person who is breathing quietly, the systolic and diastolic pressures in the pulmonary artery are approximately 23 and 8 mm. Hg, the mean pressure being about 13 mm. Hg. In the basal state, the pulmonary blood flow is very stable, averaging 3.0 liters per minute per square meter of body surface area.

The pulmonary circulation may be influenced by several different factors. The major portion of this vasculature is surrounded by a pressure which is less than that of the atmosphere. The pulmonary arteries and veins are exposed to the negative intrathoracic pressure, while the capillaries surrounding the alveoli are exposed to the more positive intrapulmonary pressure, which varies very slightly above and below that of the atmosphere. The blood flow, the blood pressure and the blood volume of the pulmonary circulation are therefore influenced by respiration, increasing during inspiration and decreasing during expiration. These changes are related chiefly to variations in the venous return to the right side of the heart, which in turn are associated with changes in the intrathoracic pressure.

When a normal subject exercises, the pulmonary arterial pressure does not rise appreciably until the blood flow increases three to four times. Thus, the pulmonary arteriolar resistance falls during exercise. The pulmonary capillary blood volume has been estimated to increase by 60 to 90 ml. during exercise, and the time spent by an erythrocyte in the pulmonary capillaries decreases from approximately 0.75 second to 0.33 second.

Hypoxia due to respiratory disease or a reduction in the oxygen tension of the inspired air raises both the pressure and the resistance in the pulmonary artery. The cause of this has not been established, but since sympathectomy affects this response, vasoconstriction has been considered. It has been suggested that the vasoconstricting stimulus is applied to the venous side of the capillaries, but it is not known whether this results from the direct effect of the hypoxic pulmonary venous blood or whether local nervous reflex mechanisms are involved. It has been suggested that this effect is particularly important because it causes the blood to be shunted away from the poorly ventilated areas of the lung towards better ventilated regions. No shunting of blood takes place if the hypoxia is very severe.

Mild increases in the concentration of carbon dioxide in the inspired air do not appear to affect the pulmonary circulation in normal subjects. In patients with chronic obstructive emphysema, on the other hand, mild increases result in an increase in both pulmonary blood flow and pressure but no increase in pulmonary vascular resistance. High concentrations of inspired carbon dioxide increase the pulmonary vascular resistance as well. Just as in hypoxia, this is presumably due to constriction of the pulmonary veins. The additive effects of hypoxia and hypercapnia have not been elucidated. Although hypercapnia has less effect than hypoxia on the resistance of the pulmonary vasculature, it is quite likely that the hypercapnia associated with pulmonary insufficiency further aggravates the already elevated pulmonary arterial pressure.

Certain pharmacological preparations affect the pulmonary circulation. Epinephrine produces a transient vasoconstriction of the pulmonary arterioles as well as a slight rise in the pulmonary artery pressure. Norepinephrine and serotonin appear to be potent pulmonary vasoconstrictors as well. On the other hand, injection of a small dose of acetylcholine into the pulmonary artery of a patient suffering from hypoxia and pulmonary hypertension causes a transient fall in the pulmonary artery pressure. The role of these substances in the development of pulmonary hypertension, however, is not clear.

THE BRONCHIAL CIRCULATION

In man, the bronchial arteries usually arise from either the proximal portion of the thoracic aorta or one of the first two intercostal arteries. Each lung possesses at least one bronchial artery. These vessels follow the course of the bronchial tree into the lung parenchyma, where they branch elaborately and rejoin to form plexuses around the bronchi and in the bronchial submucosa. The bronchial arteries supply the lower part of the trachea, the bronchi as far as the respiratory bronchioles, and the visceral pleura. By means of anastomoses with numerous other vessels, they also supply the vasa vasorum of the pulmonary artery and vein, the vagi and the mediastinal structures—particularly the pericardium—and the tracheobronchial lymph nodes.

In the normal person, blood brought to the lungs via the bronchial arteries may follow one of two courses during its return to the heart. In the proximal part of the major bronchi, some of this blood is carried via the bronchial veins into the azygos veins and then to the right atrium. More distally, the venous drainage enters into the pulmonary veins. The latter therefore normally carry small amounts of unoxygenated blood.

BRONCHOPULMONARY ANASTOMOSES

Extensive microscopic vascular connections at the capillary level and precapillary connections have been demonstrated between the pulmonary and the bronchial arterial systems in the normal lung. These shunts are located in the lobular subdivisions of the bronchopulmonary segments, as well as in the pleura.

When the vascular capillary bed is reduced by disease, the pulmonary artery may become thickened and even thrombosed. The lumina of the peripheral bronchial arteries frequently enlarge, often reaching the size of the pulmonary artery at the same level. The most striking changes are found in bronchiectasis, in which the bronchial arteries usually form a dense plexus of thick-walled, large-lumened channels. Their anastomoses with the pulmonary artery, which are situated distally in the walls of bronchiectatic sacs, may have a diameter as large as 2 mm. These plexuses of collateral arterial vessels may become very extensive, and conspicuous dilatation of the bronchial veins often takes place in such conditions as pulmonary embolism with infarction, abscess of the lung, tuberculosis, primary tumors of the lung and certain forms of congenital heart disease.

The burden of this collateral circulation must fall on the left side of the heart, for the blood is brought to the lung from the aorta and is then returned to the left atrium, principally by means of the pulmonary veins. In other words, there is a shunt between the aorta and the left atrium. The added work load on the left side of the heart may play a significant role in the development of left-sided heart failure, and it may also account for the left ventricular hypertrophy which is occasionally observed in cases of cor pulmonale. Conversely, blood shunted into the pulmonary arteries by way of these bronchial anastomotic channels tends to elevate the pressure within the lesser circulation, increasing the work of the right side of the heart and thereby predisposing to right-sided heart failure or cor pulmonale.

In patients with massive disease of one lung, there may be only slight desaturation of the systemic arterial blood. It has been postulated that the expanded bronchial arterial system, with its high pressure, prevents the flow of unoxygenated pulmonary arterial blood into the diseased portions of the lung and diverts it to normal areas. In this way, a fairly normal oxygen saturation is maintained in the efferent pulmonary veins. This high pressure collateral circulation probably also accounts for the pulmonary hemorrhages which may occur in bronchiectasis or other chronic pulmonary diseases. The large arterial vessels containing blood under systemic pressure are often situated superficially within the lamina propria of the bronchi, so that any ulceration may easily rupture them. The bleeding may be massive and may consist of obviously oxygenated, bright red blood.

PULMONARY HYPERTENSION

In a normal person who is breathing quietly, the systolic pressure in the pulmonary artery is approximately 23 mm. Hg, and the diastolic pressure is about 8 mm. There undoubtedly is a large pulmonary vascular reserve because the pulmonary artery pressure does not rise appreciably during exercise until there is a greater than threefold increase in pulmonary blood flow. The total pulmonary vascular resistance must therefore decrease because of either dilatation of existing channels or an opening up of new vessels, thereby increasing the size of the pulmonary vascular bed. Active vasodilatation has been suggested although there is no proof of this; it is more likely that new channels open up.

When there is a greater than threefold increase in pulmonary blood flow, the pulmonary artery pressure rises almost proportionately with the increase in blood flow. For practical purposes, it may be considered that when pulmonary hypertension develops in respiratory disease the resistance to blood flow is nearly always increased, except in left-to-right cardiac shunts, where the pressure in the pulmonary artery is elevated even though the resistance remains normal.

The pulmonary vascular resistance is determined from the formula:

$$\text{Resistance (R)} = \frac{\text{Pressure gradient}}{\text{Flow}}$$

$$\text{Thus, R} = \frac{\text{Pulmonary artery pressure} - \text{Left atrial pressure}}{\text{Pulmonary blood flow}}$$

This resistance is often expressed in units of force. Pressures, in mm. Hg, are converted to dynes per square meter; flows in liters per minute, are converted to milliliters per second. The normal gradient between the pulmonary artery and the left atrium is about 8 to 12 mm. Hg, and the pulmonary vascular resistance is about 80 to 160 dynes/sec./sq. cm.

As a result of alterations in the pulmonary vascular bed, the resistance within the pulmonary vessels frequently increases, causing an elevation of the pulmonary artery pressure. When the systolic pulmonary blood pressure is above 30 mm. Hg, and the diastolic pressure is above 15 mm. Hg, pulmonary hypertension exists. This may occur for a number of reasons, such as an appreciable elevation of the left atrial pressure, an increase in the pulmonary blood flow, obstruction or obliteration of the pulmonary vascular bed, or active pulmonary vasoconstriction.

ELEVATION OF LEFT ATRIAL PRESSURE

When the left atrial pressure is elevated, as in mitral valve disease or left ventricular failure, there is frequently pulmonary hypertension. In these conditions, both the pulmonary venous and the pulmonary capillary pressures are elevated, so that the pulmonary artery pressure is secondarily raised.

INCREASED PULMONARY BLOOD FLOW

When a large communication exists between the right and left ventricles, as in a ventricular septal defect, or between the aorta and the pulmonary artery, as in a patent ductus arteriosus, the pulmonary blood flow is increased. In the former situation, the left ventricular pressure, and in the latter the aortic systolic pressure, is transmitted to the pulmonary arterial system so that pulmonary hypertension develops.

OBSTRUCTION OF THE PULMONARY VASCULATURE

The pulmonary vascular resistance increases when the pulmonary blood flow is obstructed. Acute obstruction of one pulmonary artery by means of an inflatable balloon produces variable results, although usually it produces only a transient rise in the pulmonary artery pressure. This suggests that the vascular bed of the opposite lung, to which the blood has been diverted, is expansile. This procedure has been used as a prognostic test before a pneumonectomy is performed; if the pressure rises, the surgeon can anticipate a stormy postoperative course following pneumonectomy with both the pulmonary artery pressure and right ventricular pressure remaining persistently high.

In contrast to the experimental acute occlusion of a main pulmonary artery, acute occlusion of a pulmonary vessel by an embolus raises the pulmonary artery pressure. It has been suggested that this rise in pressure is caused by a reflex vasoconstriction which takes place when small pulmonary arteries are occluded but not when the main pulmonary arteries are obstructed. Another hypothesis is that the vasoconstriction is caused by the release of 5-hydroxy-tryptamine, or serotonin, from the blood clot.

OBLITERATION OF THE PULMONARY VASCULATURE

In such respiratory diseases as kyphoscoliosis, pulmonary fibrosis and chronic obstructive emphysema, the pulmonary capillaries may be obliterated or compressed so that the pulmonary vascular resistance is elevated. Hypoxia and hypercapnia, which are common to almost all of these disease states, are capable of producing pulmonary vasoconstriction and probably are also instrumental in raising the resistance and pulmonary artery pressure.

VASOCONSTRICTION OF THE PULMONARY VASCULATURE

Active vasoconstriction is probably associated with many of the forms of pulmonary hypertension which have been described. Most investigators believe that the pulmonary blood vessels possess tone and, therefore, that the tone can be altered. Hypoxia and hypercapnia appear to produce vasoconstriction and therefore elevate the pulmonary artery pressure. A number of observers have suggested that the pulmonary vasoconstriction is mediated through the sympathetic fibers and that the parasympathetic nerves initiate vasodilatation. The intense vasoconstriction which is seen after pulmonary embolism may be forestalled by elimination of the pulmonary sympathetic innervation by sympathectomy, anatomic block or the use of adrenergic-blocking and ganglion-blocking agents. When pulmonary hypertension is present, the infusion of acetylcholine into the pulmonary circulation may produce a fall in the pulmonary artery pressure suggesting active dilatation of the pulmonary vessels. On the other hand, elimination of the parasympathetic nerves in the experimental animal does not seem to affect the vasomotor events which follow pulmonary embolism.

PRIMARY PULMONARY HYPERTENSION

Primary pulmonary hypertension is a condition in which there is neither intrinsic cardiac or pulmonary disease nor any demonstrable mechanical obstruction in the vascular bed. An increase in vascular tone has therefore been implicated, although the possibility of multiple small pulmonary emboli has not been ruled out. The incidence of this condition appears to be slightly greater in females, and the majority of cases are found between the ages of 20 to 40 years.

Clinical Manifestations. The salient symptoms are those of exertional dyspnea and muscular weakness, both of which are probably related to a low cardiac output. Palpitation, exertional substernal and left-sided chest pain which is brought on by exertion, and syncopal attacks are present in about one-quarter of the cases. The syncope has been explained on the basis of acute elevations of the pulmonary vascular resistance so that the left ventricular output falls. Hemoptysis occasionally occurs, although the mechanism of its production is not clear. The terminal manifestations are characterized by the development of right-sided heart failure, and often there is a sudden demise.

The positive physical signs are usually limited to the heart and those organs which are affected by failure of the right side of the heart. There is evidence of right ventricular hypertrophy. The second pulmonic sound is accentuated and fails to split during inspiration. Distention of the neck veins, hepatomegaly and, later, peripheral edema develop.

Radiological Manifestations. An x-ray film of the chest demonstrates the right ventricular hypertrophy, a bulging pulmonary artery segment and prominent hilar vessels. These findings are associated with normal or decreased intrapulmonary vascular markings.

Functional Manifestations. The usual pulmonary function studies are all within normal limits. Hemodynamic studies during cardiac catheterization reveal an elevated pulmonary artery pressure in the presence of a normal systemic blood pressure and a low cardiac output. The arteriovenous oxygen difference is increased, but the arterial oxygen saturation is normal.

PULMONARY EMBOLISM AND INFARCTION

Pulmonary embolism and infarction are major circulatory emergencies. Unfortunately, they are often unsuspected clinically, frequently being discovered at the postmortem examination. Recently, however, it has become apparent that pulmonary embolism is one of the most important causes of morbidity and mortality, exceeding pneumonia in some centers.

PATHOGENESIS

Most pulmonary emboli originate as detached portions of venous thrombi located in the deep veins of the lower extremities. Occasionally, the thrombi may be in the right side of the heart or in the veins of the pelvic area or the upper extremities. Nonthrombotic materials, such as amniotic fluid, fat, air, bone spicules and fragments of organs, comprise a very small percentage of pulmonary emboli.

Venous thrombosis and pulmonary embolism occur predominantly in bedridden patients. Contrary to previously held views, most cases occur in nonsurgical patients, cardiac disease with congestive heart failure being the most important single condition predisposing to phlebothrombosis. The postoperative state is next in importance, especially that following abdominal or pelvic surgery in which there may be injury to the iliac veins. Pulmonary emboli are also common following operations of long duration or of such magnitude that there has been considerable injury to the tissues. Other factors which may predispose to phlebothrombosis are trauma to the lower extremities, pregnancy, varicose veins, carcinoma, obesity, polycythemia and other blood diseases, particularly when any of these conditions are associated with prolonged bed rest.

The mechanism responsible for the intravascular formation of blood clots is poorly understood. Pulmonary embolism is more prone to occur in many conditions which favor the formation of a blood clot in a vein. The factors which facilitate the production of intravascular clotting are retardation of the venous circulation, damage to the vessel walls and conditions favoring the coagulation of blood. Venous stasis is promoted by the combination of immobilization, shallow breathing and hypotension. Unlike the arm-to-carotid circulation time, which changes very little when a patient is immobilized after an operation, the foot-to-carotid circulation time gradually increases so that by the tenth day it is approximately 50 per cent greater than it was preoperatively. This increase in circulation time perhaps explains the frequency of thrombosis of the femoral veins and points out the danger of immobilization. Thrombi are also likely to develop in the cardiac chambers, particularly if there is either pooling of blood in the atrial appendage or any damage to the endocardium. This situation develops when there is cardiac dilatation due to heart failure, myocardial infarction, atrial fibrillation or endocarditis.

Venous thrombosis occurs frequently in polycythemia as well as in other hematologic abnormalities such as sickle-cell anemia and the sickle state. The increase in blood viscosity in these conditions, combined with the mechanical consequences of increased numbers of erythrocytes or the presence of sickled cells, predisposes to vascular stasis and thrombosis. Thrombosis in situ, due to a primary alteration in the clotting mechanism, has been produced experimentally in animals by the infusion of small quantities of certain serum factors, the only necessary adjuvant factor being venous stasis.

It has been thought that detachment of thrombi occurs more readily in phlebothrombosis than in a thrombophlebitis, but this concept has been criticized. There is no point in differentiating one from the other because any condition suggestive of venous clotting, with or without inflammation, is a potential source of an embolus. Once a clot fragment loses its anchorage in the vein, it is swept rapidly through the inferior vena cava and right heart into the pulmonary arteries. Similarly, a clot which originates in the right atrium may enter the pulmonary artery. Very large thrombi do not progress beyond the larger arteries, but smaller emboli pass into the narrower lobar arteries of the lungs. Emboli lodge in the vessels of the lower lobes, particularly the right lower lobe, more frequently than in the upper lobes. The posterior basal segments are most commonly involved, perhaps because these areas lie in the more direct axial stream of the pulmonary arteries.

Much has been learned from animal experimentation about the effects of pulmonary embolism. Embolization of the lungs with particulate matter invokes severe pulmonary hypertension, a fall in the systemic pressure, distention of the right cardiac chambers, engorgement of the peripheral veins and, often, death. It is probable that most of these effects are largely mechanical. Nevertheless, when the lungs of the animals are denervated at the height of the embolic reaction, the pulmonary hypertension gradually subsides, the left ventricular output increases and the animals survive. This finding suggests that the embolization produces a widespread pulmonary vascular constriction, which is mediated through sympathetic impulses. The vascular constriction might also result from either the local or reflex effects of 5-hydroxy-tryptamine or serotonin, which is known to provoke constriction of the pulmonary vasculature. It is postulated that the serotonin which is liberated from platelets in the process of blood clotting produces reflex pulmonary vasoconstriction, with a resultant increase in the right ventricular pressure, bradycardia, hypotension and apnea. The sensory receptors which are sensitive to serotonin appear to be located in the pulmonary circulation and in the ascending aorta; the afferent fibers run mainly in the vagus nerves.

Pulmonary Infarction.   It has been estimated that only about 25 per cent of pulmonary emboli result in infarction. A pulmonary infarct may develop if the embolus is large enough to obstruct either a lobar or a lobular branch of the pulmonary arteries. It is less likely to occur when the lungs are healthy. Infarction apparently develops only when embolic obstruction of a pulmonary artery is attended simultaneously by some additional factor which retards the blood flow through the lungs. Such factors are passive congestion due to congestive heart failure, previous pulmonary vascular obstruction and the hypostatic influences of posture. A pulmonary embolus is also more likely to lead to infarction of the lung if alveolar hypoventilation or an infection, such as pneumonia, should be present.

A pulmonary infarct is usually sterile, and secondary infection is an uncommon feature. Rarely, an abscess may develop from an infected embolus, necrosis or a secondary infection of a bland infarct. Since this type of abscess extends to the pleura, empyema may be an added complication.

CLINICAL MANIFESTATIONS

The diagnosis of pulmonary infarction is based chiefly on the symptoms and only partly on abnormal physical signs. Pulmonary embolism should be suspected in every elderly bedridden patient who develops a chest pain which is anginal or pleuritic in character and which is associated with acute dyspnea, unexplained vascular collapse, syncope, an unexplained fever, refractory congestive heart failure or edema of the lower extremities in the absence of sacral edema. A knowledge of the predisposing factors is of prime importance in leading to a suspicion of pulmonary embolism. In an average case, a slightly elevated temperature and a relatively rapid pulse rate for a few days prior to the event may be the only indications that a focus of phlebitis and venous thrombosis is developing.

Embolic occlusion of the main pulmonary arteries is usually rapidly fatal. The manifestations of smaller single or multiple thrombo-emboli or embolic episodes are exceedingly varied, and changing symptom patterns are frequent. Although most symptoms and signs of pulmonary embolism are manifest in the respiratory system, they may also be suggestive of a cardiac, neurological or intra-abdominal disease; in other instances, there may be no symptoms at all. When present, the symptoms may persist for weeks, months or even years.

Only a few cases demonstrate the classic syndrome of a pulmonary embolism, which consists of a sudden pleuritic type of chest pain, dyspnea, hemoptysis, fever, signs of consolidation, a pleural rub and evident venous thrombosis. In many subjects, pulmonary embolism is promptly followed by signs of circulatory collapse, a rapid and feeble pulse, and hypotension. Shock develops because so little blood passes the blockade in the pulmonary circulation that the left ventricle does not fill adequately and the cardiac output falls. This may result in manifestations of cerebral ischemia such as restlessness, apprehension, syncope and coma. Occasionally, a transient episode of unconsciousness and, in elderly patients, hemiplegia and convulsive phenomena, may be the chief signs of pulmonary embolism.

Pulmonary embolism most often presents itself with the sudden onset of chest pain, which may be of two types: one due to pleural reaction over the site of the infarction, and a severe retrosternal one indistinguishable from the pain of myocardial ischemia, which has been attributed to a fall in the coronary blood flow, although the substernal pain may also be due to distention of the pulmonary artery. As a general rule, the pain is pleuritic, being exaggerated by deep breathing. It is caused by pleuritis in the region of the infarct, the parietal pleura being highly sensitive to pain stimuli. There is usually an associated splinting of the chest movement as well as difficulty in breathing. Because most infarcts develop in the lower lobes of the lungs, the diaphragm may be involved in the pleuritis, so that the pain may be referred to the neck and shoulder.

On rare occasions, there may be severe upper abdominal pain and muscle guarding, so that intra-abdominal disease may be suspected. This is presumably a referred pain due to irritation of the lateral portion of the diaphragm. However, it may also be due to distention of the liver capsule if the pulmonary embolism has resulted in acute congestive heart failure.

An irritating cough may develop on the second or third day following the infarction. This is probably caused by irritation of the bronchial mucosa by secretions which have passed from the affected parenchyma into the normal bronchi. Hemoptysis is present in only a few cases and is probably the result of hemorrhage into the necrotic lung parenchyma as well as disruption of the bronchial vessels. The sputum produced during the early period of an infarction may be frankly bloody; it may contain dark blood during the healing process.

Dyspnea often begins suddenly and progresses rapidly to gasping respirations which may be out of proportion to the amount of lung tissue involved. On the other hand, it may be mild and hardly noticeable. The difficult breathing has been attributed to many factors, notably: bronchospasm; immobility or diminished excursion of the diaphragm; atelectasis; hypoxia; stimulation of receptors in the pulmonary artery, the right side of the heart and the superior vena cava; and possibly increased Hering-Breuer reflexes. The hyperpnea may be accentuated if fever is present, because this increases the rate of tissue oxidation. The height of the fever depends largely on the extent of the infarction and the development of a secondary pneumonitis, as well as on the presence or absence of phlebitis at the site of origin of the embolus.

The physical signs of pulmonary infarction are rarely distinctive, and the physical examination is entirely negative more often than not. Tenderness in the plantar veins of the foot or in the muscles of the calves is an early sign of venous thrombosis. Tenderness along the course of the great veins along the inner aspect of the thighs, swollen and tender inguinal lymph nodes and pitting edema are later developments. These signs are not necessarily found, however, and phlebothrombosis commonly exists without producing any signs or symptoms.

When respiratory signs are present, they are similar to those found in association with pneumonia or atelectasis. Diminished chest expansion on the side of the lesion, dullness to percussion, diminished breath sounds, bronchial breathing and rales are often present over the affected area, so that consolidation due to pneumonia may be suspected. A localized exquisitely tender area at the site of chest pain is a valuable diagnostic sign. It occurs most frequently in association with a small peripheral pulmonary infarction. Apparently it is produced by severe spasm of the intercostal muscles secondary to inflammation of the underlying pleura. Evidence of pleural irritation, shown by a friction rub, may develop on the second or third day. If a secondary pleural effusion should be present, both the breath sounds and the vocal fremitus may be diminished.

Tachycardia is observed in most patients. Arrhythmias are often present, and these may be responsible for the embolic episode in patients with heart failure. Paroxysmal cardiac arrhythmias, atrial fibrillation, atrial flutter and supraventricular tachycardia are possibly related to the stimulation of the autonomic nervous system, which occurs in conjunction with pre-existing myocardial disease or as the result of the hypoxia and cardiac strain engendered by the embolus.

Very minimal icterus may occasionally be noted. It is presumed that the hemolysis of erythrocytes in the hemorrhagic lung infarct is the source of the increased serum bilirubin, although it has also been suggested that the elevated serum bilirubin is related to hepatic dysfunction resulting from congestive heart failure.

Pulmonary hypertension and acute dilatation of the right ventricle are indicated by the presence of a prominent pulsation along the right border of the sternum, together with a loud pulmonic second sound, a pulmonic systolic murmur and a presystolic gallop rhythm. Because of the continued venous flow into the heart, acute right ventricular failure may occur and the peripheral veins become engorged. Obstruction of the distal branches of the pulmonary arteries by multiple pulmonary emboli may recur over a long period of time, so that right ventricular hypertrophy and cor pulmonale may develop very gradually. The minute emboli themselves appear to be innocuous, and it is not until there are numerous episodes of vascular obstruction that the function of the right ventricle deteriorates.

RADIOLOGICAL MANIFESTATIONS

The clinician relies too often on the presence of a radiological opacity for the diagnosis of pulmonary embolism, even though it appears in only a minority of cases. Nevertheless, the x-ray film may offer some valuable clues. For instance, there may be accentuation of the hilar shadows and elevation of the diaphragm on the side of the embolus. These findings are frequently misinterpreted as being caused by atelectasis. Occlusion of the larger branches of a pulmonary artery may occasionally be recognized by the abrupt termination and dilatation of a large pulmonary arterial shadow, and a wedge of increased radiotranslucency in a portion of lung field beyond it. This radiotranslucent area has been attributed to the avascularity of the parenchyma distal to the block.

The radiological appearance of a pulmonary infarction may at times suggest minimal or massive collapse of the lung. Although the pulmonary infarct frequently has a conical shape, with its apex in the direction of the hilum of the lung, it may appear as a round or oval opacity. Irregular shapes are common, simply because the long axis of the infarct is not opportunely situated to produce a triangular or round opacity. Often it presents as a hazy clouding or streaking at one base, which may change to a well-defined consolidation. When the infarct resolves it diminishes in size and takes on the appearance of a plate-like atelectasis.

Infarcts are commonly located at the costophrenic angles, and here they may produce a triangular shadow whose base is directed away from the hilum. This clouding may be observed within the first twenty-four hours and may be mistaken for a pleural effusion. On the other hand, a pleural effusion is not an uncommon complication and small amounts of fluid may accumulate in one or both pleural cavities. Occasionally pulmonary embolism and infarction may result in a massive hemorrhagic effusion.

FUNCTIONAL MANIFESTATIONS

As a result of occlusion of a branch of the pulmonary artery, alveolar spaces are no longer perfused by pulmonary capillary blood, although they are still ventilated. The air leaving the alveoli has the composition of inspired air, and therefore constitutes part of the physiologic dead-space. Because the end-tidal air is now composed of gas not only from well-ventilated and well-perfused alveoli but also from alveoli which are not perfused, the mean alveolar carbon dioxide tension is less than that of the arterial blood. This difference in the carbon dioxide tension between the alveolar air and the arterial blood has been used by some investigators as a diagnostic test for pulmonary embolism, the extent of the difference largely depending on the size of the artery which has been occluded. However, it must be pointed out that altered ventilation-perfusion ratios from any cause will produce this difference in carbon dioxide tension.

Arterial unsaturation occurs because of the alteration in ventilation-perfusion ratios, the extent of the hypoxia often being parallel with the degree of occlusion of the pulmonary vessels. On the other hand, a decrease in the diffusing capacity has also been observed and may account for some of the hypoxia. Rarely, carbon dioxide retention due to alveolar hypoventilation may occur, probably because of chest splinting.

In patients with multiple pulmonary emboli, the pulmonary vascular bed available for diffusion is reduced, so that the diffusing capacity for oxygen is very low. As a result of the increase in pulmonary vascular resistance, pulmonary hypertension with right ventricular hypertrophy and, eventually, right ventricular failure develop.

PULMONARY ARTERIOVENOUS ANEURYSM

Arteries and veins develop out of a common embryonic capillary plexus, so that opportunities are always present for persistent connections even after birth. There are normally small arteriovenous communications of the vascular systems of most tissues, including the lungs. These communications probably serve as a means of adjustment to changes in the external and the internal environments. For instance, it is believed that such anastomoses in the skin of the fingers and toes play an important part in heat regulation. Their function in the lung is not clear, although it has been suggested that they may act as safety valves to protect the lung capillaries from excessive increases in blood pressure and blood perfusion.

The existence of shunts between large blood vessels and between the chambers of the heart is normal only during fetal life. After birth, the major causes of abnormal vascular shunts are trauma, infection and malignant tumors. In adult life, multiple arteriovenous and other inter-vascular connections may develop in the lungs in association with chronic infection, such as bronchiectasis.

Normally, about 5 to 7 per cent of the total pulmonary blood flow does not become arterialized to the maximum extent, so that it acts like venous admixture. In certain pathological conditions, a large volume of blood may be shunted from the pulmonary artery to the pulmonary vein so that considerable hypoxia results. A pulmonary arteriovenous aneu-rysm provides an example of such a true venous admixture. This con-genital lesion is a pulmonary manifestation of a generalized systemic vascular disorder, hereditary hemorrhagic telangiectasis, which is char-acterized by localized dilatations of small vessels forming telangiectases or angiomata that have a tendency to bleed. These tiny ruby lesions are generally seen on the face, the nasopharyngeal and buccal mucous mem-branes, the lips, the skin of the body, and in the nail beds. Slight pressure on them causes blanching. The gastrointestinal, respiratory or genitouri-nary tracts, and even the brain or spinal cord may be affected.

PATHOGENESIS

Approximately one-half of the patients who have a pulmonary arteriovenous aneurysm have telangiectases of the skin or mucous mem-branes, and more than one-third of patients with telangiectasis have one or more similar lesions in the lungs. About 60 per cent have a family history of cutaneous telangiectasia. The cause of this inherited lesion remains unknown, but it is believed to be transmitted by a single domi-nant gene. Both sexes are affected and are able to transmit the disease, but females are more frequently involved. Occasionally, a generation may be skipped.

In most cases, the shunt takes place from a pulmonary artery to a pulmonary vein. The aneurysm frequently lies adjacent to the visceral pleura. One or more branches of the artery usually enter a loculated aneurysmal sac which is drained by a greatly enlarged and often tortuous vein. Veins from adjoining lobes may also drain the aneurysm, or it may be drained by completely anomalous veins.

It has been suggested that the vascular dilatation may be a mani-festation of a generalized weakening of the ground substance in the vessel wall due to a defect of the normal hyaluronidase-inhibiting mech-anism. Another suggestion is that the telangiectasis is produced by 5-hydroxy-tryptamine, which is normally detoxified in the lungs. Ac-cording to the latter hypothesis, the 5-hydroxy-tryptamine escapes de-toxification by by-passing the lungs via a pulmonary arteriovenous aneurysm. This postulate suggests, therefore, that the multiple telangiectases develop secondarily as a result of a primary pulmonary arterio-venous aneurysm, rather than vice versa.

CLINICAL MANIFESTATIONS

The pulmonary lesion is usually discovered during the third and fourth decades, although occasionally it has been found in children and even in the newborn. The disease may remain stationary for years, but frequently there is a definite tendency towards progression. There would appear to be two distinct clinical types: the type which is not associated with any clinical signs, and the type associated with the triad of cyanosis, polycythemia and clubbing of the fingers and toes.

When the shunt is small, there may be no noticeable clinical effects. When the shunt is large, the cardinal symptoms are due to the chronic hypoxia caused by shunting of unoxygenated blood through the aneurysm. The principal symptoms are dyspnea on exertion, which may be slight at first but later progressively increases in severity, weakness, palpitations and precordial pain. Neurologic complications are not uncommon; these may consist of headaches, vertigo, convulsions, syncope, paresthesias, diplopia, thick speech and paresis, as well as cerebrovascular accidents. The neurologic symptoms have been ascribed to a variety of causes, such as cerebral hypoxia and polycythemia, as well as telangiectasia in the brain with or without associated cerebral thrombosis.

Bleeding is a most important complication, the commonest type being epistaxis from telangiectatic lesions in the nasal mucous membranes. In addition, hemoptysis, hematuria, melena and cerebral hemorrhage may occur because of telangiectatic lesions in the tracheobronchial tree, genitourinary tract, gastrointestinal tract and central nervous system.

Cyanosis, clubbing and, occasionally, hypertrophic pulmonary osteoarthropathy are frequently found, although cyanosis may be absent.

If the lesion is large, a murmur is often heard on the chest wall over the site. The murmur is limited to a well-circumscribed area on the chest wall which may be quite small and thus may be easily missed. It is usually continuous, with a systolic accentuation, becoming more intense during deep inspiration and often fading out during expiration. A thrill may also be present. On the other hand, if multiple small aneurysms are present, there may be no abnormal signs at all.

RADIOLOGICAL MANIFESTATIONS

A large pulmonary arteriovenous aneurysm is often seen in a routine posteroanterior film of the chest. Its characteristic appearance is that of a lobulated or spheroid opacity with smooth discrete margins, which appears to be connected with the hilus by band-like linear or sinuous opacities. The afferent and efferent vessels may not be visible, however, in a conventional radiograph. In addition, the lesion itself may be so small as to be barely discernible. Any segment of either lung may be involved, although there appears to be a predilection for the lower lobes and the right middle lobe. In a few cases, the abnormal shadow may be hidden behind the heart. If multiple tiny lesions are present, no radiological abnormality may be evident.

Pulsations in the lobulated density, as well as in the hilus, may occasionally be seen on fluoroscopic examination. The vascular nature of the lesion may often be demonstrated by certain maneuvers, such as the Valsalva and Mueller tests. The use of tomography and angiocardiography is extremely valuable in the diagnosis of this condition. Although tomography can often give confirmative evidence, angiography is the most definitive and preferable procedure, for it not only provides information about the obvious radiological lesions but it also demonstrates the small lesions which are generally overlooked on a standard x-ray film.

FUNCTIONAL MANIFESTATIONS

A pulmonary arteriovenous aneurysm produces a true venous admixture. Some of the blood from the right ventricle returns to the left side of the heart without becoming oxygenated, so that hypoxia develops. Since the lungs themselves are normal and their ventilatory function is excellent, the hyperventilation induced by the hypoxia results in hypocapnia. The presence of true venous admixture is confirmed by the failure of the arterial blood to become fully saturated with oxygen when the patient inhales 100 per cent oxygen.

The cardiac output is nearly always normal, although it may be increased if the oxygen tension should become very low. Small shunts do not particularly affect the arterial oxygen saturation despite the drop in oxygen tension. With large shunts, however, the arterial oxygen tension falls considerably. This may stimulate erythropoiesis, so that both the red cell mass and total blood volume are increased. The amount of the shunt may be increased by the enlarged red cell mass because the increased viscosity of the blood may elevate the pulmonary vascular resistance. In some cases, the number of erythrocytes may be normal, but anemia, probably due to the chronic or repeated hemorrhages, may be present.

PULMONARY EDEMA

Pulmonary edema is an excessive accumulation of serous or serosanguineous fluid in the alveoli, bronchioles and bronchi. It is remarkable that fluid does not normally accumulate in the lungs since their structure offers little resistance to the passage of fluid from the capillaries. Ordinarily, in the systemic capillaries, the osmotic force of 30 mm. Hg exerted by the proteins in the capillaries is neatly balanced by the intracapillary hydrostatic pressure of about 25 mm. Hg. Even in the most dependent lung capillaries, however, the hydrostatic pressure is only about 10 mm. Hg, so any water or saline introduced into the alveoli is rapidly absorbed. The capillary hydrostatic pressure is even lower in the apices of the lung, indicating a considerable margin of safety for the alveoli.

PATHOGENESIS

When edema fluid accumulates in the lungs, the factors responsible are essentially the same as those concerned in the formation of edema fluid elsewhere. These can be any one or a combination of the following: an increase in the capillary hydrostatic blood pressure, a diminution in the colloid osmotic pressure of the blood, an increase in the permeability of the capillary walls, a reduction in the mechanical pressure in the tissues and an interference with the flow of lymph.

Increased Hydrostatic Pressure. When the resistance to the outflow of blood from the lungs is increased, as in mitral stenosis, the level of the capillary hydrostatic pressure may rise above that of the colloid osmotic pressure. A pulmonary arterial diastolic pressure of 40 mm. Hg or a mean "capillary" pressure of 35 mm. Hg is considered to be the upper limit of safety. If the pressures rise above this level, the blood pumped into the lung by the right ventricle tends to accumulate behind the obstruction. When this occurs, fluid passes through the capillary wall into the pulmonary interstitial tissues, particularly those of the dependent parts of the lungs.

The precipitation of pulmonary edema by the intravenous infusion of saline, plasma or blood suggests that pulmonary edema may also be elicited by a sudden increase in the venous return to the lungs, which increases the capillary hydrostatic pressure. Conversely, acute pulmonary edema is often relieved by factors which reduce the venous return, such as venesection, intermittent positive pressure breathing or the application of tourniquets to the extremities.

Pulmonary edema may also occur after a traumatic injury to the skull, cerebral hemorrhage or an attack of encephalitis. The pathways are not understood, but it has been proposed that stimulation of the central nervous system induces systemic vasoconstriction through the sympathetic nerves, increasing not only the resistance to the ejection of blood from the left ventricle but also the peripheral venous tone. These increases act to augment both the pulmonary blood volume and the pulmonary capillary pressure, so that the capillary hydrostatic pressure rises and produces pulmonary edema.

Diminished Osmotic Pressure.   The colloid osmotic pressure may be diminished by any condition which leads to a reduction in the plasma protein, particularly albumin. If the osmotic pressure is lowered, pulmonary edema may develop. A subacute form of pulmonary edema, which is possibly due to reduction in colloid osmotic pressure, is seen in uremia, acute nephritis and polyarteritis nodosa. It is possible that the rapid infusion of intravenous fluid may also reduce the concentration of the proteins and so cause acute pulmonary edema.

Increased Capillary Permeability.   Edema may develop as a result of changes in the permeability of the capillary walls because of chemical, bacterial, thermal or mechanical agents. In addition, it has been shown that capillary dilatation, per se, favors the outward movement of fluid. As protein escapes into the tissues, the osmotic gradient across the capillary wall is reduced, and further edema is favored. In this situation, the fluid has the characteristics of an exudate, possessing a high protein content.

Hypoxia has been implicated as the most important factor leading to increased capillary permeability in the lungs. Pulmonary edema and pneumonia are frequently found together at postmortem examination. In this case, pulmonary capillary damage is probably produced not only by inflammation but by a local interference with oxygenation as well. It is likely that the pneumonia not only increases the rate of fluid entry into the alveoli but also decreases the rate of fluid resorption by the lymphatics.

The lungs are irritated by acid gases such as chlorine and sulfur dioxide and by certain oxides of nitrogen such as ammonia and phosgene. The inhalation of water and nitric acid fumes or the ingestion of gasoline may also produce pulmonary irritation. The extent to which such irritants damage the lungs depends upon their solubility in water. A highly soluble gas is readily taken out of the inspired air by the first moist tissue it reaches. The upper respiratory tract may, therefore, bear the brunt of its action. On the other hand, a gas with a low solubility is slower in its irritating effect, and the most important damage usually occurs at the alveolar level. The effects of gas inhalation may vary, therefore, from slight tracheobronchitis to fatal pulmonary edema.

Reduced Mechanical Pressure.   Pulmonary edema may also occur in a patient with severe bronchial obstruction. During inspiration, the reduced intrapulmonary pressure may exert a suction effect on the capillaries so that serum exudes into the alveoli. In addition, the filling of the right side of the heart increases during inspiration, and the flow of blood from the left side of the heart is hindered. This may result in a progressive accumulation of blood in the lungs, with a consequent increase of the hydrostatic pressure in the capillaries. On the other hand, when obstruction to both expiration and inspiration is present, pulmonary edema does not develop, presumably because of the positive intra-alveolar pressure during expiration.

Interference with Lymphatic Flow.   Transuded protein and fluid from the pulmonary capillaries can either be removed by the numerous lymphatic collecting ducts or can move into the alveoli and bronchioli and then be expectorated. Pulmonary edema occurs when the fluid escapes into the lung tissue faster than it can be removed by the lymphatic system. Any factor which decreases the reabsorption of lymph in the lungs or obstructs the lymphatic channels favors the production of pulmonary edema. Since the lymphatic vessels empty into systemic veins, an elevated systemic venous pressure has an adverse effect on the reabsorption of transuded lymph from the lungs.

As long as the patient with congestive heart failure is in the erect position, the high intracapillary pressure in the areas of the body below the heart protects the lungs, so that edema fluid tends to accumulate in the dependent parts of the body. When he lies down at night, however, the edema fluid from the peripheral areas enters the blood stream and increases the venous return to the lungs. As a result, the pulmonary capillary pressure rises, and pulmonary edema develops. It is also possible that during sleep a considerable increase in the venous return to the heart may be produced by a sudden movement after a period of muscular relaxation. Additional factors which may be involved are an increased plasma volume and the increased capillary permeability which develops during sleep due to hypoxia. It is likely that, during the milder attacks of dyspnea, there is an acute edema of the interstitial tissues of the lung but that this fluid is removed by the lymphatics so that none escapes into the alveoli. If the transudation of fluid should persist, however, the lymphatics may be unable to cope with the excess fluid, so that it escapes into the alveoli and bronchioles, and pulmonary edema results.

CLINICAL MANIFESTATIONS

By far the commonest form of pulmonary edema encountered clinically is associated with cardiac disease. In patients with hypertensive and arteriosclerotic heart disease or aortic valvular disease, left ventricular failure and paroxysmal attacks of dyspnea frequently occur. The mildest form of dyspneic attack is paroxysmal nocturnal dyspnea, an attack of severe dyspnea and cough which suddenly awakens the patient. A more serious form is characterized by a persistent severe wheezing dyspnea which is associated with expiratory obstruction. The most severe form is due to the development of pulmonary edema.

Paroxysmal nocturnal dyspnea must be differentiated from the nocturnal attack which may develop in cases of chronic bronchitis, in which the patient awakens from his sleep gasping for air. The latter type of nocturnal dyspnea characteristically disappears after the expectoration of a plug of sputum. This is in contrast to the nocturnal dyspnea due to left ventricular failure which improves only after the patient gets up and walks around.

Acute pulmonary edema may begin with terrifying suddenness, or it may develop gradually, starting as a mild form of paroxysmal nocturnal dyspnea with wheezing, and then progressing to the full-blown clinical picture, which is characterized by an extreme respiratory distress. The breathing is noisy with audible wheezes or gurgling sounds. The patient not only must sit up to breathe but the distress is aggravated by a severe cough, with the expectoration of frothy, pink-stained sputum, which may be so profuse that it pours from the nose as well as from the mouth. He may suffer from an intense precordial oppression or actual pain, and he usually becomes panicky as the sense of impending suffocation grows more vivid.

He is cyanotic and the skin is often covered with a cold sweat. Moist bubbling rales are heard over extensive areas throughout both lungs. The blood pressure is usually elevated unless the patient is in shock, and tachycardia is a constant feature. Mild forms may subside spontaneously after a few minutes, but the attack may last for hours. It may end fatally during the first attack or during a subsequent episode. The chronic form of pulmonary edema may be insidious and often exists with such subtle clinical manifestations that it is easily misdiagnosed by the clinician as asthma or bronchitis.

RADIOLOGICAL MANIFESTATIONS

Pulmonary edema manifests itself as a dense, fluffy, radiological opacity which spreads outwards from the hilar areas into the central portions of the lungs. The peripheral portions remain clear, so that a butterfly shape is produced. Because the alveoli are filled with fluid, the bronchi which traverse this portion of the edematous lung are revealed as radiotranslucent linear arborizations. The pulmonary vessels are enlarged and hazy in outline and the heart shadow is usually increased in size. The central localization of the edema fluid in the lungs has been attributed both to the relatively greater excursion of the peripheral parts of the lung, so that the removal of lymph and fluid from the periphery is enhanced, and to accessory lymphatic drainage via the pleural lymphatics in these peripheral areas. Another possibility is that the x-rays are penetrating through more tissue centrally than peripherally.

FUNCTIONAL MANIFESTATIONS

Even a very large elevation in mean pulmonary vascular pressure does not greatly affect the distensibility of the lung. When pulmonary edema develops, however, the compliance of the lungs falls considerably and the vital capacity is therefore reduced. As the pulmonary congestion increases, the residual volume falls correspondingly, probably because bubbles of edema fluid at the mouths of alveoli render the measured residual volume to be less than that actually present. When frank pulmonary edema develops, the resistance to air flow increases by approximately three to four times. Edema of the airways and free fluid in the tracheobronchial tree might account for this, although the high resistance found in the early part of inspiration and the late part of expiration suggests that surface tension also plays a part. Because of the increase in nonelastic resistance, the maximal mid-expiratory flow rate and the maximal breathing capacity are reduced, and the work of breathing becomes exceptionally great.

In moderate degrees of pulmonary congestion and edema, the arterial oxygen tension is usually only slightly lower than normal, but in severe edema it may be very low, presumably because edema fluid in the alveolar spaces introduces a barrier to the diffusion of oxygen. On the other hand, when pulmonary edema is experimentally produced in animals, the diffusing capacity is not altered appreciably. Consequently, the drop in the arterial oxygen tension has been attributed to the continued perfusion of areas of lung whose alveoli are not ventilated because the bronchioles are blocked by edema fluid, which results in venous-admixture-like perfusion. The arterial carbon dioxide tension is usually lower than normal, presumably because of the easy diffusibility of carbon dioxide and the increased ventilation of well-perfused alveoli.

CHAPTER X

Pleural Disease

ANATOMY

THE PLEURAL cavity is normally only a potential space formed by the visceral pleura, which covers the lungs, and the parietal pleura, which invests the inner surface of the thoracic cage. The pleura consists of a serous membrane, lined on its free surface by a single layer of meso-thelium. This layer rests on a subserous, areolar layer which attaches the pleura to the underlying structures. The subserous layer is important, not only because of the considerable elastic tissue it contains, but also because of its rich network of blood vessels, lymphatics and nerve fibers.

The arterial blood supply of the visceral pleura is derived from the bronchial arteries; the venous return is via the pulmonary venous system. The arterial blood supply of the parietal pleura is derived prin-cipally from the intercostal and internal mammary arteries, and its venous return takes place through the corresponding veins. The lym-phatics of the pleura are closely connected with those of the lungs and the thoracic cage.

The nerve supply of the visceral pleura is derived from the au-tonomic pulmonary plexus. The parietal pleura is supplied by the inter-costal nerves. Both contain sympathetic and parasympathetic fibers and their efferent nerve endings lie near the surface of the pleura. Although both the visceral and parietal layers are richly supplied with nerves, the visceral layer is apparently completely devoid of any pain fibers. On the other hand, the parietal layer is richly endowed with pain fibers which are derived from the intercostal nerves. Irritation of the parietal pleura produces an exquisitely sharp pain which may be accurately localized to the site of irritation.

The outer rim of the parietal layer of the diaphragmatic pleura receives its sensory supply from the lower six thoracic intercostal nerves. Irritation of this area results in pain which is referred to the dermatomes of the lower thoracic intercostal nerves, so that it may be felt in the epigastric region or even in the lower abdomen. The painful area can be recognized as being confined to the thoracic dermatomes by the associated presence of hyperalgesia and hyperesthesia.

The central portion of the diaphragmatic parietal pleura receives its sensory supply from the phrenic nerves, which originate from the third, fourth and fifth cervical nerve roots. For this reason, irritation of the central portion of the diaphragm produces a pain which is referred to the neck and shoulder along the ridge of the trapezius muscle on the same side, the painful area again being associated with hyperesthesia and hyperalgesia.

The pressure within the pleural space is less than that of the atmosphere. In addition to initiating the flow of air into and out of the lungs, the negative intrapleural pressure produces a sucking effect on the superior and inferior venae cavae, thereby enhancing the venous return to the heart. The inspiratory descent of the diaphragm, by raising the intra-abdominal pressure, further assists the return of venous blood from the abdomen. Conversely, a lessening of negative pressure, such as occurs normally during a forced expiration, or in a disease such as chronic obstructive emphysema, impedes the venous return to the heart. The lymph flow is similarly assisted by the greater negative intrapleural pressure during inspiration and is sucked up from the abdominal cavity into the thoracic portion of the thoracic duct. Because of the presence of valves in the thoracic duct, backward flow is prevented and the lymph is squeezed into the subclavian vein during expiration.

PLEURAL EFFUSION

In healthy persons, the pleural cavity is virtually nonexistent, the layers being in close apposition to one another and separated only by a thin collection of serous fluid. This fluid acts as a lubricant, allowing the two layers to slide easily over one another during respiration, thus preventing any mechanical damage. The thin layer of lubricating serous fluid represents a balance between the outpouring of a transudate from the pleural capillaries and its reabsorption by the venules and lymphatics in both the visceral and parietal layers. Although this balance remains fairly constant, a larger amount of fluid can accumulate if the negative intrapleural pressure is increased as a result of some disease process. Although very rare, this situation may occasionally occur in atelectasis or in diseases associated with a widespread incomplete bronchial obstruction, such as bronchial asthma. A similar abnormal collection of fluid may take place if the venous pressure rises as a result of either cardiac decompensation or direct pressure on the venae cavae by an intrathoracic tumor. In addition, hypoproteinemia, by lowering the osmotic pressure of capillary blood, can lead to a pleural effusion. The latter situation is most commonly seen in chronic renal disease, hepatic cirrhosis and malnutrition.

In all of these situations, the fluid produced is a thin, clear transudate. Its protein content is usually less than 3 per cent, its specific gravity is less than 1.015, and only a few cells, chiefly lymphocytes, are seen microscopically. It does not clot on standing and no organisms are grown if the fluid is cultured.

In contrast to a transudate, an exudate is more viscous, less translucent and clots on standing. Its protein content is greater than 3 per cent, and its specific gravity is higher than 1.015. This type of pleural fluid usually collects as a result of a disease process which either has a damaging effect on the capillary walls, such as pneumonia or tuberculosis, or interferes with lymphatic drainage, such as a neoplasm. The cellular content of this type of effusion depends on the cause. Numerous cells are usually present. If the effusion is examined early, there are many polymorphonuclears, whereas, if the effusion has been present for some time lymphocytes predominate. If the primary lesion is malignant, tumor cells and red blood cells are frequently demonstrated. If it is bacterial in origin, the offending organism frequently can be identified.

A pleural effusion is usually secondary to some lesion outside the pleura, the only exception being a neoplasm of the pleura itself. The type of pleural effusion depends on the underlying disease process: inflammatory, noninflammatory, hemorrhagic, chylous or chyliform.

INFLAMMATORY PLEURAL EFFUSION

This type of effusion results from an inflammation of the pleura. It is always secondary to an inflammatory process involving the lung, the mediastinum, the esophagus or the subdiaphragmatic space. In its earlier stage, the inflammation produces a "dry" or fibrinous pleurisy, in which the inflamed pleural surfaces are covered with much fibrin and leukocytes, but there is little increase in pleural fluid. As the lesion progresses, an outpouring of pleural fluid occurs. This fluid is an exudate and possesses the characteristic features which have already been described. In the early stages of its formation, the pleural exudate is translucent, has a high fibrinogen content, and is usually described as "serous" or "serofibrinous." In the later stages the fluid may become frankly purulent, gradually becoming more opaque and thicker in consistency as the content of polymorphonuclear cells increases.

Empyema.   An empyema is a pleural effusion in which the fluid consists entirely of frank pus. It constitutes the final stage in the progression of an inflammatory exudate. It can be considered to be an abscess in that the pus is generally confined by adhesions to a localized area of the pleural cavity. Such an abscess usually contains thick, creamy, yellow-green fluid, although occasionally it has a thinner consistency. It is important that a purulent exudate be distinguished from an empyema. In the former condition, the purulent material is mixed with serous fluid and generally lies free within the pleural space. It is only when the material consists of pure pus with no serous fluid that an empyema, or pyothorax, is said to be present. The thick, shaggy, fibrinous exudate which is laid down on both the parietal and visceral pleural surfaces as a result of the suppuration tends to localize the collection of pus. The empyema is generally situated in the lowermost part of the pleural space, usually in the lateral or posterior aspects. It also very frequently tends to localize in one of the fissures between the lobes of the lung.

Aside from an infected traumatic hemothorax and an extremely rare infection of the pleura by a blood-borne septic embolus, all cases of empyema are secondary to a suppurative process in one of the structures adjacent to the pleura. Of these, the lungs are the most frequent offenders, and the mediastinum, the subdiaphragmatic space and the bony thoracic cage are less common sites of the infection. Empyema develops most commonly as a complication of the pneumonias, chiefly those caused by the pneumococcus, *Streptococcus pyogenes* and the staphylococcus. Among the less frequent causes are septic infarcts, tuberculosis, subdiaphragmatic abscess, amebic abscess of the liver and mycotic infections, particularly by *Actinomyces bovis.*

Empyema should be suspected if a case of pneumonia is not progressing satisfactorily and if there are persistent fever and constitutional symptoms. In general, the clinical picture is one of sepsis associated with a loculated pleural effusion. If a large empyema remains untreated, septicemia frequently develops. Spontaneous evacuation of the pus may occur by rupture through the lung into a bronchus or by extension through the thoracic wall (empyema necessitans). A small collection of pus may be gradually absorbed but it usually persists, leading in some cases to the development of amyloidosis of the kidneys, liver and spleen.

A neglected empyema may have disastrous effects on the thoracic cage and its contents. The extensive inflammatory exudate rapidly becomes organized, and thick fibrous adhesions form between the two pleural surfaces. The retracted lung and the displaced mediastinum are anchored, and the overlying thoracic cage is retracted and immobile. Penetration of the empyema through the chest wall may be indicated by a localized bulge, and a fistulous opening remains once it ruptures.

NONINFLAMMATORY PLEURAL EFFUSION

This type of fluid is a transudate, and its accumulation in the pleural space is referred to as a "hydrothorax." It is always associated with healthy pleura. It is a clear, pale, straw-colored serous fluid which does not clot on standing. It may occur in diseases associated with either a diminished osmotic pressure of the blood or retention of sodium. It is, therefore, most commonly found in patients suffering from generalized edema secondary to diseases affecting the heart, kidneys or liver. In cardiac decompensation, as well as in the nephrotic stage of chronic nephritis, effusions usually develop in both pleural cavities. On the other hand, for reasons not well understood, the hydrothorax may be unilateral, usually involving the right side in congestive heart failure. (It is usually predominant on the right side even though it is bilateral.) Effusions confined to the right hemithorax are also frequently found in cirrhosis of the liver. A unilateral transudate may also be produced by an obstruction of the large intrathoracic veins as a result of pressure by either a neoplasm or enlarged mediastinal lymph nodes.

HEMORRHAGIC PLEURAL EFFUSION

If the fluid in the pleural space is frank blood, the condition is referred to as a "hemothorax." Traumatic penetrating injuries of the chest wall with tearing of the intercostal arteries are a common cause. Hemothorax may also occur spontaneously when a bleb ruptures or when a pleural adhesion is torn. Rarely it occurs as a result of rupture of an intrathoracic blood vessel, such as an aortic aneurysm. The intrapleural bleeding may be slow, continuing over many hours. The blood usually clots very slowly because of the defibrinating effect caused by the movements of the lung and the heart. If infection should be introduced, however, clotting develops rapidly.

A pleural fluid consisting of a mixture of serous fluid and blood, so that its gross appearance is pink or red, is called "serosanguineous." This type of effusion is most commonly produced by a pulmonary infarction. Other less frequent causes of a hemorrhagic pleural effusion are a neoplasm—either primary in the pleura or metastatic from a primary site elsewhere—pulmonary tuberculosis, lymphomas and hemorrhagic disorders.

CHYLOUS PLEURAL EFFUSION

The presence of pure chyle in the pleural cavity is known as "chylothorax." This results from obstruction of either the thoracic duct and its tributaries or the left subclavian vein. It is most commonly caused by direct neoplastic invasion of the vessels or by metastatic involvement of the mediastinal lymph nodes, both of which obstruct the thoracic duct and interfere with the normal flow of chyle. Traumatic rupture of the thoracic duct may result from a penetrating or a nonpenetrating wound of the chest wall. Spontaneous rupture may occur in infants on rare occasions. Although chylothorax occurs more commonly on the left side, it may develop bilaterally. As the thoracic duct lies outside the pleural cavity, chyle tends to accumulate in the mediastinum before rupturing into the pleural space.

Chyle consists primarily of emulsified fats, being milky-white and opalescent. On standing, a creamy supernatant layer develops. The fat content may be as high as 4 per cent, the fat globules staining easily with Sudan III. Clotting does not usually occur, nor does the fluid putrefy. Its specific gravity is greater than 1.012, and it contains a variable quantity of protein. The cellular content is primarily lymphocytic, and it is sterile on culture.

CHYLIFORM PLEURAL EFFUSION

This type of fluid, which is also known as "pseudochyle," has the superficial appearance of chyle. No fat globules can be demonstrated, however, either microscopically or by staining with Sudan III. The milky appearance is due to the fatty degeneration of pus and endothelial cells which occurs in long-standing encysted purulent effusions.

FIBROTHORAX

A fibrothorax is an accumulation of nonelastic fibrous tissue within the pleural space, usually as a result of a prolonged pleural effusion of any kind, but more particularly a hemothorax or an empyema. Occasionally calcification may be associated with it.

The fibrosed pleurae inevitably contract and reduce the size of the lung so that the diaphragm becomes elevated and fixed in position. Because of the reduction in the size of the lung, the mediastinum is shifted to the affected side. The movement on the involved side becomes severely limited because of the thickened, fibrosed pleurae. As a result, only a small amount of air enters the underlying lung during breathing, and bronchial drainage is impaired so that chronic infection becomes a likely complication.

CLINICAL MANIFESTATIONS

The degree of disability produced by a pleural effusion depends not so much on the amount of fluid that is present but on the rapidity of its development. Provided the accumulation of fluid has been slow, very little distress may be experienced by some patients despite the presence of a very large effusion. On the other hand, a rapidly developing effusion, especially if bilateral, may produce extreme respiratory distress.

The degree of dyspnea that results from the compression of the underlying lung varies in different patients. It is a frequent symptom in fibrothorax.

If the pleural effusion is associated with or follows a "dry" or fibrinous pleurisy, chest pain is produced. This pain varies in severity, ranging from a dull, aching discomfort to an excruciatingly severe, sharp, stabbing pain, which tends to restrict the depth of breathing. The characteristic feature of pleural pain is that it becomes aggravated by a deep inspiration as well as by coughing. Since the pain is caused by movement of the inflamed pleural surfaces over each other, it tends to disappear when the two pleural layers are separated from each other by the accumulation of fluid. The pain is generally localized to that part of the chest wall overlying the area of pleural inflammation. If the lower part of the pleural space or the peripheral area of the diaphragmatic pleura is involved, however, the pain may be referred to the lumbar region or the abdominal wall. Irritation of the central portion of the diaphragmatic pleura results in pain along the same side of the neck.

Pleural inflammation frequently also causes a dry, useless, nonproductive cough. If a bronchopleural fistula is caused by an empyema, attacks of paroxysmal coughing with the expectoration of considerable amounts of purulent sputum may be noted, particularly with a change of posture.

Depending on the underlying cause, the temperature may be normal or considerably elevated in a patient suffering from a pleural effusion. If the course of events is favorable, this should subside in a matter of days. Empyema is the most serious form of pleural effusion and is usually responsible for a severe constitutional reaction. The fever associated with empyema may be continuous, remittent or intermittent. It may be accompanied by violent chills as well as night sweats. The patient usually feels miserable and ill and has severe anorexia, vague abdominal discomfort, fatigability and a progressive weight loss. The patient tends to favor the affected side, and usually prefers to lie on this side in order to diminish the intensity of pain.

Because a collection of fluid is, in effect, a space-occupying foreign body, it exerts certain mechanical effects. Because of its weight, the fluid tends to gravitate to the lowest recesses of the pleural space, unless it is hindered by adhesions. The presence of fluid in the pleural space compresses the underlying lung, so that its expansion is restricted during inspiration. Since the pressure in the opposite normal pleural space is now considerably more negative than that of the affected side, the mediastinum shifts away from the effusion. If the mediastinum is unable to move because of fibrous adhesions, however, the pressure in the affected pleural cavity rises even further, so that there is greater compression of the underlying lung.

Although the characteristic physical sign of a pleural effusion is the shift of the mediastinum, this may not occur if there is an underlying atelectasis, such as often occurs with a bronchogenic carcinoma. The mediastinum retains its central position even in the presence of a considerable collection of fluid, because the elevated pressure produced by the pleural effusion is counterbalanced by the lowered intrapleural pressure induced by the atelectasis.

The function of the diaphragm is also adversely affected by an overlying pleural effusion. The higher intrapleural pressure diminishes the extent of the expiratory ascent of the diaphragm, and the hydrostatic pressure of the fluid causes a flattening of its contour. Since it has lost its dome-shape, the diaphragm no longer elevates the lower ribs when it contracts during inspiration. Therefore, there is a decreased excursion of the costal margin on the affected side.

Depending on the amount of fluid present, vocal fremitus is either diminished or absent, and the percussion note varies from dullness to flatness. As the fluid increases in amount, the dullness is more evident in the axillary region and then in the lower part of the anterior area of the chest, the upper level of the fluid tending to be at a higher level in the axilla. When the patient is placed in a lateral decubitus position, free pleural fluid shifts to the most dependent part of the pleural space. No shift occurs if the collection of fluid is confined to a localized area by adhesions.

The breath sounds are usually reduced in intensity or are inaudible, depending on the amount of fluid present. Bronchial breath sounds and whispering pectoriloquy may be heard, however, if the layer of fluid is thin and overlies a compressed area of lung in the neighborhood of a patent bronchus. Bronchial breathing is a frequent finding at the upper level of a pleural effusion.

The slightly smaller hemithorax, retraction and narrowing of the interspaces and diminished movement are evident in a case of fibrothorax. The mediastinum is shifted towards the affected side. Vocal fremitus is diminished or absent. The percussion note is dull or flat depending on the degree of fibrothorax present, and the breath sounds are distant or absent. Rales or rhonchi may be heard if there is underlying bronchopulmonary infection.

RADIOLOGICAL MANIFESTATIONS

Both the x-ray film and fluoroscopy of the chest are invaluable in determining the site and the amount of the fluid. Unless the amount is very small, a pleural effusion is readily distinguishable by the characteristic shadow it produces. This is illustrated in Figure 62. The fluid casts a shadow which has the same density as that of the heart. It appears as a dense homogeneous mass occupying the lowest area of the chest, its upper border being hazy and gradually blending into the pulmonary area above it. The costophrenic angle is the first area to be obliterated. The upper border has a concave downward curve with the highest level in the axillary region. The presence of air above the fluid can be implied if the upper level of the fluid is a straight, abrupt, horizontal line. If the air has not been accidentally introduced during an attempted aspiration of the fluid, this finding indicates the presence of a bronchopleural fistula.

A shift of the mediastinum towards the normal side is usually evident, the degree depending on the amount of fluid present. No shift suggests that the mediastinum has become fixed by adhesions or that an atelectatic lobe is present in association with the fluid. If the pleural effusion is massive, the ribs may be spread and may have a more horizontal configuration than they have normally.

If the quantity of fluid is small, it tends to collect in the costophrenic space and produces a shadow which is often difficult to distinguish from adhesions between the diaphragmatic and parietal pleurae. The fluid occasionally accumulates between the lung and the diaphragm, where it is called an infrapulmonary effusion. This difficulty can be overcome if a film is taken in the lateral decubitus position.

In a fibrothorax the opacity produced by the thickened pleura may be as dense as that of a pleural effusion and may occasionally show areas of calcification. It is distinguished from a pleural effusion, however, in that the interspaces between the ribs are narrower, the mediastinal structures are shifted to the affected side, and the diaphragm is considerably elevated and fixed.

FIGURE 62.   Right-sided pleural effusion.

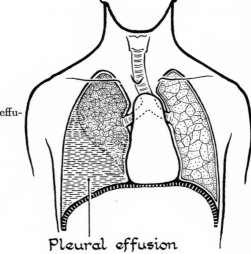

Pleural effusion

FUNCTIONAL MANIFESTATIONS

The degree of functional impairment depends on the size of the pleural effusion. As the fluid accumulates and the lung becomes more compressed, the elastic resistance to distention increases. This is reflected by a reduction in the vital capacity. Unless secretions accumulate in the tracheobronchial tree or kinking of the bronchi occurs, the nonelastic resistance is frequently unimpaired, so that the timed vital capacity and the maximal mid-expiratory flow rate may be normal. The maximal breathing capacity is usually slightly reduced, though not to the same extent as the vital capacity.

Because of compression, there may be local variations in the distensibility of the lung. The distribution of inspired air is therefore unequal. Venous-admixture-like perfusion may occur if the compressed lung is still being perfused, so that hypoxia develops, although there may be no carbon dioxide retention if the remainder of the alveoli are being hyperventilated.

Because of the increased resistance to distention of the affected lung, functional assessment of patients with fibrothorax reveals a reduced vital capacity and an altered distribution of gases. There is little increase in the resistance to air flow, unless kinking of the tracheobronchial tree or secretions are present. Since ventilation is reduced in the affected lung, the ventilation-perfusion ratios are considerably altered, so that hypoxia and possibly some hypercapnia may develop. An associated fibrosis of the lung may also develop as the fibrothorax progresses, resulting in a reduction in its vascular bed, so that the diffusing capacity for oxygen may fall.

ABSORPTION OF A PLEURAL EFFUSION

The absorption of a pleural effusion depends on the character and amount of the fluid present, as well as on the state of the pleurae. If the pleurae are healthy, as they usually are in the presence of a transudate, absorption is rapid once the initial cause of the effusion has been removed. Water, electrolytes and other diffusible substances are absorbed into the capillaries of the subserous areolar layer of the pleurae, while protein and other particulate matter are carried away by the lymphatic channels. Absorption becomes more complicated in the presence of an exudate, for it is considerably hindered by thickening and fibrosis of the pleurae. The fibrin in the fluid must first become liquefied and the obstructed lymphatics must again become patent before the fluid can be absorbed. If empyema is present, no absorption whatever may take place.

PNEUMOTHORAX

The presence of gas in the pleural space is referred to as pneumothorax; for practical purposes, this gas is always atmospheric air. Air can enter the pleural space through a bronchopleural fistula, through an opening of the thoracic wall due to a traumatic injury, or it may be deliberately introduced through a needle for therapeutic or diagnostic reasons. Rarely, anaerobic organisms may produce gas in the pleural space, as when a putrefactive pulmonary abscess ruptures through the visceral pleura.

OPEN PNEUMOTHORAX

In this type of pneumothorax, there is a persistent communication between the pleural space and the atmosphere, so that air can pass freely in and out of the pleural cavity. The most common cause is a traumatic injury of the chest wall which results in an external communication. An internal communication between the pleural space and the tracheobronchial tree, a bronchopleural fistula, also causes an open pneumothorax. Such a fistula may be produced by any condition which causes destruction of alveolar walls and visceral pleura. It can therefore occur in inflammatory disease of the lung, such as tuberculosis; malignant disease, such as a bronchogenic carcinoma; vascular disease, such as a pulmonary infarction; loss of lung elasticity, as in chronic obstructive emphysema; or rupture of a bronchial stump following operative removal of a lung or portion of a lung.

An open pneumothorax, particularly if caused by traumatic injury to the chest wall, presents a serious problem. Because of the free communication between the pleural cavity and the atmosphere, the intrapleural pressure on the affected side is equal to that of the atmosphere. As the elastic forces of both the chest wall and the lung are now unopposed, the chest cage enlarges while the affected lung collapses. If the mediastinum is mobile and not bound down by fibrous adhesions it moves to the unaffected side, where the intrapleural pressure is lower, and produces varying degrees of compression of the opposite lung. During inspiration, contraction of the respiratory muscles lowers the pleural pressure on the unaffected side. This may slightly lower the pressure on the affected side so that some air may enter through the opening in the chest wall and cause a further shift of the mediastinum towards the unaffected side. During expiration, the pressure in the pleural space on the affected side usually rises above that of the atmosphere, so that air escapes from the pleural space. The mediastinum then may move back towards its original position. This is illustrated in Figure 63, which also shows that some of the air expired from the normal lung may enter

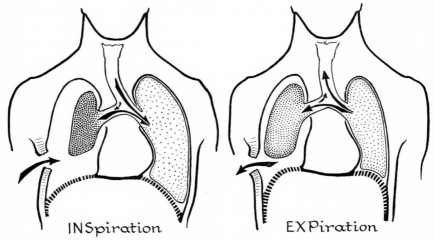

INSpiration   EXPiration

FIGURE 63.   The mediastinal shift and pendaluft in an open pneumothorax.

the collapsed lung, causing it to expand slightly. During the next inspiration, this "rebreathed air" may then again be inspired into the normal lung. This paradoxical movement of air, or "pendaluft," and the recurrent swing of the mediastinum, or "flutter," can be a serious menace to the patient's life.

CLOSED PNEUMOTHORAX

A closed pneumothorax implies that the air in the pleural cavity is no longer in communication with the atmosphere. This condition occurs after the rupture of a subpleural bleb, the tear in the visceral pleura being sealed off, or after the induction of an artificial pneumothorax. Once a pneumothorax becomes established, the gas usually is uniformly distributed, so that the intrapleural pressure is essentially the same throughout the pleural cavity. If the pleura is diseased, however, adhesions may prevent the uniform distribution of the gas so that it remains localized to one or several areas.

A closed pneumothorax may be spontaneous, traumatic, therapeutic or diagnostic.

Spontaneous Pneumothorax. A pneumothorax which develops suddenly in a person who has no obvious underlying pulmonary disease or in one who has bronchopulmonary disease is usually referred to as a "spontaneous pneumothorax."

The patient may have been free of respiratory symptoms and may have no apparent clinical or radiological evidence of an underlying pulmonary lesion. Spontaneous pneumothorax under these circumstances occurs predominantly in young people, particularly males, between fifteen and thirty-five years of age. Although the right lung is most commonly affected, it is not unusual for recurrent attacks to affect either one or both lungs. Since the healthy pleura is impervious to air, it is obvious that these apparently idiopathic cases of pneumothorax can only be secondary to a rent in the pleura and that they must be produced by some pathological process. Rupture of a subpleural bleb or bulla causes spontaneous pneumothorax in approximately 85 per cent of the cases. The remaining 15 per cent are most frequently produced by rupture of a tuberculous or pyogenic subpleural abscess, a tear in the esophagus during esophagoscopy or erosion of the esophageal wall by a malignant process.

Subpleural blebs may be congenital in origin, but more frequently they are found in association with scar formation due to some inflammatory disease. In such cases, no symptoms are evident until rupture of the bleb takes place. On the other hand, subpleural blebs are also found in association with an underlying pulmonary disease, such as bronchial asthma, bronchiectasis, chronic obstructive emphysema and the pneumoconioses. Under these circumstances, the symptoms preceding the event are those of the particular disease. It has been suggested that a bleb may rupture because of a sudden increase in the intrathoracic pressure, such as that resulting from an unusual exertion, coughing or sneezing. It is more likely that the rupture results from the repeated deep inspirations which precede these acts, particularly if, as is usually the case, the bleb has been caused by a check-valve obstruction.

A bulla is an air vesicle within the substance of the lung and is caused by a breakdown of alveolar septa. Alveoli may rupture if they are greatly overdistended as a result of a check-valve obstruction. The air escaping from the ruptured alveoli then tracks along the sheaths of the perivascular structures. The bubbles of air may travel either peripherally towards the pleural surface or medially towards the mediastinum. In either case a pneumothorax may result because of the rupture of either the visceral or mediastinal pleura. This may explain the occasional delay between the time of the actual exertion and the development of pneumothorax.

Traumatic Pneumothorax. Mention has already been made of the type of pneumothorax associated with an open, sucking wound of the chest wall. Pneumothorax may also occur in a traumatic, nonpenetrating injury of the chest wall. The sharp edges of fractured ribs frequently lacerate the parietal and visceral pleura and the underlying lung parenchyma, thereby allowing air to escape into the pleural space. Such injuries frequently cause hemothorax as well.

Therapeutic Pneumothorax. Until recently, the deliberate introduction of air into the pleural space was considered to be one of the most effective methods of treatment of pulmonary tuberculosis. Relaxation of the underlying lung was made possible by regulating the amount of air instilled, and actual compression of the lung was avoided. It was surmised, without definite confirmatory evidence, that reducing the size of the lung and restricting its excursions reduced the flow of blood and lymph, so that hematogenous spread of the disease was prevented and the growth of the tubercle bacilli was inhibited by the decreased supply of oxygen. In addition, the retardation of lymphatic flow would favor the development of fibrous tissue. The recent advent of specific antituberculosis therapy and surgical excision of tuberculous lesions has obviated the need for therapeutic pneumothorax.

Diagnostic Pneumothorax. When there is radiological evidence of a peripheral intrathoracic opacity the origin of which is difficult to determine, an artificial pneumothorax may be induced for purely diagnostic purposes. If the lesion is intrapulmonary, an x-ray film taken after the induction of the pneumothorax shows the opacity in the collapsed lung. If the lesion is attached to a rib or the parietal pleura, the opacity projects into the pneumothorax. Tumors arising from the diaphragm or the intercostal nerves can also be distinguished by this procedure.

VALVULAR PNEUMOTHORAX

If a tear in the visceral pleura does not become sealed off, it may behave like a check-valve and air from the tracheobronchial tree may enter the pleural space during inspiration but may be unable to leave during expiration. Large quantities of air may therefore accumulate in the pleural cavity within a short time, rapidly increasing the intrapleural pressure, which may reach or surpass that of the atmosphere.

A pneumothorax in which the pressure is greater than that of the atmosphere is known as a "tension pneumothorax." This condition is dangerous, since in addition to complete collapse of the affected lung, there is also a decided shift of the mediastinum to the opposite side. This, in turn, compresses the opposite lung and kinks and obstructs the great veins. As a result, the venous return to the heart may be retarded so that the cardiac output falls.

CLINICAL MANIFESTATIONS

The severity of the symptoms produced by a pneumothorax depends on the amount of air that has collected in the pleural space and the degree of collapse of the underlying lung. A small pneumothorax may often be asymptomatic and may produce no abnormal physical findings.

The onset of a spontaneous pneumothorax is usually abrupt and dramatic. The picture of a young man, in apparently good physical health, who is suddenly overwhelmed by exquisite chest pain and respiratory distress for no obvious reason, is very striking. The pain, generally confined to the affected side of the chest, is presumed to be caused by the sudden abrupt increase in intrapleural pressure and tension on any adhesions that may be present. It is usually sharp and stabbing and is aggravated by breathing and coughing. On occasion, however, it may be only a dull, aching discomfort. If the pain is very severe, it may be associated with symptoms of shock, apprehension and a feeling of chilliness. An irritative cough, due to stimulation of nerve endings in the pleural space or in the walls of the collapsed bronchi, may also be present.

A patient with a large pneumothorax is frequently in great respiratory distress, breathing rapidly and shallowly, and may be cyanosed. If shock is present, the skin is cold and clammy, the pulse rapid and thready, and the blood pressure low. Under these circumstances, the possibility of bleeding should be considered as well.

The affected hemithorax moves poorly or not at all and may be larger than the normal side. This enlargement is due to the unopposed elastic recoil of the chest wall. If the case is traumatic in origin and there are numerous rib fractures, there may be paradoxical movement of the chest cage, the affected side collapsing during inspiration and enlarging during expiration. The movement of the costal margin is also impaired because the rise in intrapleural pressure restricts the expiratory ascent of the diaphragm and flattens its contour. The mediastinum is deviated towards the normal side of the chest. Because of the increased ratio of air to solid tissue, vocal fremitus is diminished or absent over the affected hemithorax, and the percussion note is hyper-resonant. When a right-sided tension pneumothorax develops, downward displacement of the liver may be demonstrated by percussion of the upper limit of its dullness. The breath sounds are usually faint or inaudible over the affected side. If a bronchopleural fistula is present, a bronchial quality of the breath sound may occasionally be detected. The "coin-click" test is often positive in the presence of a large pneumothorax, particularly when it is under tension. On the other hand, a negative "coin-click" test does not rule out the presence of a pneumothorax.

If a significant collection of fluid is present in conjunction with the pneumothorax, it settles to the bottom of the pleural cavity, and the percussion note over it is dull or flat. In this situation, the upper limit of the flat note is horizontal, so that the change from resonance to dullness is abrupt. Since both air and fluid are present, a "succussion splash" may be heard with a stethoscope when the chest is shaken.

RADIOLOGICAL MANIFESTATIONS

A pneumothorax, unless very small, presents a characteristic and easily recognizable radiological picture in the posteroanterior view. If the collection of air is small, it may not be demonstrable in the film taken at full inspiration, but it often becomes visible if the exposure is made at the end of a maximal expiration because the translucency of the air in the pleural space is more apparent when contrasted with the density of the expiring lung.

The deflated lung appears somewhat denser than the opposite normal lung, and its periphery is recognized as a thin, fine line running parallel to the lateral margin of the chest cage. The pneumothorax space has a uniform translucency which is characterized by the complete absence of lung markings, although linear strands caused by adhesions may occasionally be seen running from the periphery of the lung to the costal margins. The collection of air is usually predominant in the upper part of the pleural cavity if the film has been taken while the patient is upright. It may be localized by adhesions and confined to a portion of the pleural space. If it is complicated by an effusion, the fluid occupies the lowest part of the space, the upper border being straight and horizontal.

During fluoroscopy of a closed pneumothorax, it may be noted that, unlike the opposite normal lung, the partially deflated lung enlarges only slightly during inspiration, so that the mediastinum moves towards the pneumothorax side. The paradoxical movement of the mediastinum is presumably due to the considerably larger change in size of the normal lung during inspiration. This is in contrast to the mediastinal movement in an open pneumothorax, which is towards the normal side during inspiration.

FUNCTIONAL MANIFESTATIONS

The degree of functional impairment resulting from a pneumothorax depends upon its size. As the pressure in the pleural space rises towards that of the atmosphere, the lung collapses and the chest cage expands because of its elastic properties. The vital capacity decreases proportionately with the amount of air introduced into the pleural space.

If the pulmonary circulation in the collapsed lung persists, the physiological effects of venous admixture, hypoxia and hypercapnia are produced. It has been shown that this state persists for only a few hours, after which the level of oxygen saturation in the arterial blood returns to normal. Apparently the mixed venous blood in the collapsed lung becomes diverted to the opposite functioning lung, so that only well-oxygenated blood reaches the left side of the heart. The diffusing capacity of the lungs varies inversely with the amount of lung that is collapsed, so that hypoxia may develop during exertion, although carbon dioxide retention does not occur if the remaining normal alveoli are hyperventilated. If paradoxical movement of the chest occurs, air may be shunted back and forth between the normal and the collapsed lungs. Air which has already taken part in gaseous exchange is rebreathed, so that the dead space is increased, resulting in hypoxia and hypercapnia.

ABSORPTION OF A PNEUMOTHORAX

The air of a pneumothorax is usually absorbed gradually, provided there is no communication between the pleural cavity and the atmosphere. Absorption of the air takes place through the subpleural venous channels, and the speed of absorption depends primarily on the state of health of the pleural surfaces. It is most rapid when the pleurae are healthy and is retarded if they are thickened and fibrosed as a result of disease. If the pleurae are calcified, no absorption may occur at all.

The process of absorption of air from a pneumothorax is similar to that which takes place in atelectasis. The pleural surfaces act as wet membranes, allowing oxygen, carbon dioxide and nitrogen to diffuse through them. Since the partial pressures of the gases in the pneumothorax approximate those of the atmosphere, while those in the venous blood are substantially lower, the gases in the pleural space diffuse into the venous blood until the pneumothorax becomes completely absorbed. As the pneumothorax diminishes in size, the lung gradually expands and the chest cage becomes smaller, so that the total pressure within the space is maintained. Expansion of the lung can be prevented, however, if it has become fibrosed or if the visceral pleura has become thickened through the deposition of fibrin.

CHAPTER XI

Mediastinal Disease

THE MEDIASTINUM, a word derived from the Latin "medius" meaning middle, refers to the space between the two pleural cavities in the central part of the thorax. Covered on both sides by the mediastinal pleura, this space forms a partition between the two lungs, enabling them to be functionally independent of each other. The pressure within the mediastinal space, like the intrapleural pressure, is subatmospheric and fluctuates with respiration.

Although the normal mediastinum is a relatively mobile structure, it maintains its central position within the thorax because the pressures in the two pleural spaces are equal. The mediastinum lengthens and narrows during inspiration, and it shortens and widens during expiration or when the body is in the supine position. Lateral displacement of the mediastinum occurs normally only in the lateral decubitus position, the shift to the dependent side amounting to as much as 3 to 4 cm. The mobility of the mediastinum varies considerably among normal people, and as many as 50 per cent may have a rigid, immobile mediastinum. Age appears to be a determinant of its degree of mobility, for a child's mediastinum is considerably more mobile than that of an adult.

ANATOMY

The mediastinum contains immensely important respiratory, cardiovascular, gastrointestinal, lymphatic and nervous structures. Any of these structures may be affected if the mediastinum should become involved by disease. The heart, which is the most important organ in the mediastinum, acts as the central structure by which the mediastinum is divided into its various compartments. It is enclosed in a fibrous sac, the pericardium, which is fused into the central tendon of the diaphragm inferiorly and ends superiorly at the level of the manubrio-sternal joint. The pericardium, therefore, is situated behind the whole body of the

248

sternum anteriorly and between the levels of the fifth to the eighth thoracic vertebrae posteriorly.

SUPERIOR MEDIASTINUM

The small portion of the mediastinum which lies above the upper limit of the pericardium is known as the superior mediastinum. Its lower limit is, therefore, a horizontal plane which extends posteriorly from the manubrio-sternal joint to the disc between the fourth and fifth thoracic vertebrae, and its upper limit is formed by the thoracic outlet. Within the confines of the superior mediastinum are located the following vital structures: the transverse portion of the aortic arch; the innominate, left carotid and subclavian arteries; the superior vena cava; the innominate and the left superior intercostal veins; the vagus, cardiac, phrenic and recurrent laryngeal nerves; the trachea; the esophagus and the thoracic duct; the remains of the thymus gland; and lymphatics.

ANTERIOR MEDIASTINUM

Situated anteriorly between the pericardium and the posterior surface of the body of the sternum is a small area called the anterior mediastinum. There are no vital structures within the anterior mediastinum, as it contains only some areolar tissue, fat and a few lymph nodes.

POSTERIOR MEDIASTINUM

The space behind the pericardial sac is known as the posterior mediastinum. Its upper limit is the superior border of the pericardium, and it extends downwards to the diaphragm. Its anterior boundary is the pericardium, and its posterior boundary is formed by the lower eight thoracic vertebrae. Within the posterior mediastinum are found the following structures: the descending portion of the thoracic aorta, the greater and lesser azygos veins, the vagus and splanchnic nerves, the esophagus, the thoracic duct and some lymph nodes.

MIDDLE MEDIASTINUM

The middle mediastinum is formed by the pericardial sac and its contents. Within this fibrous sac are situated the heart, the ascending aorta, the superior and inferior venae cavae, the pulmonary arteries and veins, and the terminal portion of the azygos vein. Above it lie the bifurcation of the trachea, the two phrenic nerves and the pericardio-phrenic vessels running on its lateral aspect.

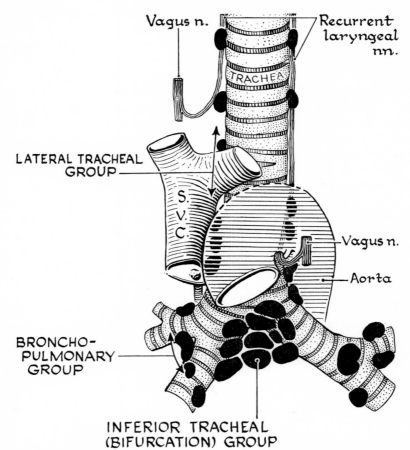

Figure 64.   The tracheobronchial group of mediastinal lymph nodes.

LYMPH NODES

The mediastinum plays a very important role in the lymphatic drainage of the body, for it receives lymph from the lungs, the esophagus, the pericardium, the neck, the abdominal cavity, the diaphragm and the anterior chest wall. The mediastinal lymph nodes are arranged into three major groups, the tracheobronchial, the anterior mediastinal and the posterior mediastinal groups.

Tracheobronchial Lymph Nodes. The most important of the three groups of mediastinal nodes are the tracheobronchial group, which are situated in three areas (Fig. 64). The lateral nodes lie alongside the trachea, with the main portion beneath the aortic arch and those on the left side in close relationship with the recurrent laryngeal nerves. Their afferents are derived from the bronchopulmonary, the anterior and the posterior mediastinal nodes, and their efferents drain into the bronchomediastinal lymph trunk and the inferior deep cervical lymph nodes. The inferior group of tracheobronchial nodes are situated beneath the bifurcation of the trachea and lie between the roots of the great vessels anteriorly and the esophagus and aorta posteriorly. They receive afferents from both the bronchopulmonary and the posterior mediastinal group of nodes. Their efferents empty into the lateral tracheobronchial nodes. The bronchopulmonary nodes lie in the hilum of the lung and receive lymph from the lungs and the pleurae, and then pass it onto the lateral and inferior tracheobronchial nodes.

Anterior Mediastinal Lymph Nodes. The anterior mediastinal lymph nodes are situated in the anterior mediastinum. They drain the

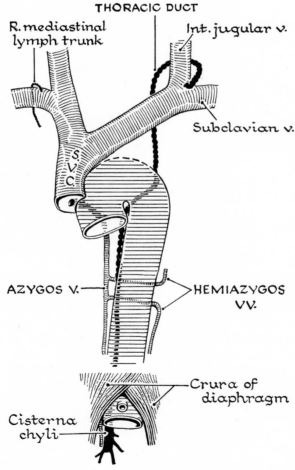

FIGURE 65. The course of the thoracic duct and the vena azygos system.

thyroid and the thymus glands, the pericardium, the heart and the diaphragm, as well as the upper surface of the liver. They receive afferents from the internal mammary lymph nodes, which drain the anterior chest wall, the breast and the abdominal wall. Their efferent lymphatics join with those of the tracheobronchial nodes to form the bronchomediastinal trunks.

Posterior Mediastinal Lymph Nodes. The posterior mediastinal lymph nodes are located in the posterior mediastinum, being chiefly situated along the aorta. Their afferent channels receive lymph from the esophagus, and their efferents terminate in the thoracic duct.

THE THORACIC DUCT

The thoracic duct, the course of which is illustrated in Figure 65, is the main channel for lymph in the thorax and also contains digested fat, or chyle. Beginning at the cysterna chyli within the abdomen, it receives afferents from the right and left lumbar lymph nodes, and then passes through the aortic hiatus of the diaphragm to enter into the posterior mediastinum of the thorax. Lying to the right of the thoracic aorta, it passes upwards towards the neck, crossing all the thoracic vertebrae. Just before reaching the level of the seventh cervical vertebra, it arches abruptly towards the left, and ends by entering into the angle formed by the left internal jugular and the subclavian veins.

OBSTRUCTION OF THE SUPERIOR VENA CAVA

When one considers the number of vitally important structures within the relatively narrow confines of the superior mediastinum, it is astonishing that space-occupying lesions or inflammatory processes in this area do not produce more serious effects. However, the anterior and posterior boundaries of the superior mediastinum are formed by rigid, unyielding bony structures, and its lateral boundaries are formed by soft, spongy, pliant lung tissue. When a space-occupying lesion develops within the superior mediastinum, therefore, it causes lateral expansion of this space.

Most of the organs in the superior mediastinum are resistant to compression. The cartilaginous rings of the trachea prevent its indentation by extrinsic pressure. The aorta and its main branches are able to withstand compression because their walls are strong, elastic structures, which are further strengthened by the high pressure of the blood within them. In addition, because they are relatively fixed structures, they are not displaced to any great extent. On the other hand, the trachea and esophagus are easily displaced from their central position. The trunks of the phrenic, vagus and recurrent laryngeal nerves are also mobile, so that they also are easily displaced.

Because of their thin walls and the low pressure of the fluid they contain, the large veins and the thoracic duct are the only structures incapable of withstanding any degree of pressure within the superior mediastinum. Of these, the thoracic duct is more strategically placed, because it lies posteriorly and is afforded protection as it courses behind the arch of the aorta and the left subclavian artery. The great mediastinal veins occupy a more anterior and unprotected position. The superior vena cava and its tributaries are therefore the first structures to be affected by any compressive force that may develop within the superior mediastinum.

THE COLLATERAL VENOUS SYSTEMS

The large superior mediastinal veins drain the head and neck, both upper extremities and the chest wall. If the venous return through these channels is prevented, the blood must travel through circuitous routes to the inferior vena cava in order to return to the heart. These routes, which consist of the azygos, internal mammary, vertebral and thoraco-epigastric venous systems, are interconnected with one another, and all take part in the collateral circulation. The predominant route utilized depends on whether the superior vena cava is obstructed above the entry of the vena azygos, at its orifice or below it.

The Azygos Venous System. The azygos vein, the course of which is shown in Figure 65, is the most important component of the azygos system. It arises from either the right lumbar or the right renal vein and enters the posterior mediastinum through the aortic hiatus of the diaphragm. It passes upwards to the right of the thoracic duct and the aorta and crosses the lower eight thoracic vertebrae. At the level of the fourth thoracic vertebra it abruptly arches across to the right to enter the superior vena cava, just before the latter structure pierces the pericardium. It drains all the intercostal veins except the right and left first intercostals, which empty into the vertebral veins.

The hemiazygos vein arises from the left lumbar or left renal vein and ascends into the posterior mediastinum by passing through the left crus of the diaphragm. It runs along the left side of the lower four thoracic vertebrae and then passes behind the aorta, the esophagus and the thoracic duct to the level of the eighth thoracic vertebra, where it arches to the right and enters the azygos vein. The azygos vein is also joined by the accessory hemiazygos vein, which descends from the superior mediastinum along the left side of the vertebral column to the level of the seventh thoracic vertebra. At this point it crosses over to the right to enter either the vena azygos or the hemiazygos vein.

By virtue of its connection with the common iliac veins through the lumbar, renal and other tributaries, the vena azygos system may have the important function of being a line of communication between the superior and inferior venae cavae. When the superior vena cava becomes occluded, venous blood from the head, neck and upper extremities returns to the heart by passing through the vena azygos system.

If the supeior vena cava is obstructed above the entry of the vena azygos, the blood flows in the normal direction from below upwards in the dilated vena azygos. If the obstruction of the superior vena cava is at the orifice of the vena azygos or below it, however, the blood flows downwards, towards the inferior vena cava.

The Internal Mammary Venous Route.   The vena azygos also communicates with a second important venous collateral system, the internal mammary route, which is composed principally of the internal, the superior and the inferior mammary veins, all of which empty into the left innominate vein. When the superior vena cava is obstructed, the venous blood is routed through the internal mammary system into the vena azygos, or when the azygos is not functioning normally, via the external iliac veins into the inferior vena cava.

The Vertebral Venous Route.   Both the azygos and the internal mammary routes communicate with a third important collateral system, called the vertebral route. This is composed of the vertebral and intervertebral veins and the internal and external vertebral plexuses, which drain into the intercostal, the lumbar and the lateral sacral veins.

The Thoraco-epigastric Route.   A fourth important collateral system is the thoraco-epigastric vein. This runs along the anterolateral aspect of the thorax and abdomen, connecting the lateral thoracic and the superficial epigastric veins with the great saphenous vein.

If the superior vena cava becomes obstructed above the entry of the vena azygos, the venous blood from the head, neck and upper extremities is carried by the internal mammary and vertebral systems to the azygos system, whence it passes into the inferior vena cava and then to the heart. If the obstruction is at or below the orifice of the vena azygos, all the venous blood is shunted to the superior vena cava via the azygos, internal mammary, vertebral and thoraco-epigastric systems.

PATHOGENESIS

The signs of the superior vena caval syndrome are produced by any lesion which interferes with the flow of blood through it, either by obstruction of the superior vena cava itself or indirectly by obstruction of both the right and left innominate veins. Occlusion of the superior vena cava can be produced by external compression of its wall by a lesion such as enlarged lymph nodes, invasion by a neoplastic process with secondary thrombus formation, or a primary thrombus within its lumen. The common causes of the superior vena caval syndrome are intrathoracic neoplasms, malignant lymphomas, chronic fibrous mediastinitis and an aneurysm of the ascending aorta. Most of these pathological processes develop slowly, so that the signs of vena caval obstruction are gradual in onset.

The lymph nodes primarily responsible for the development of superior vena caval obstruction are the right anteromediastinal and the right lateral group of tracheobronchial lymph nodes. The former group lies along the anterior surface of the superior vena cava and the latter along the posterior aspect of the superior vena cava and the superior surface of the vena azygos. A few of the inferior group of tracheobronchial lymph nodes also lie in contact with the lower portion of the superior vena cava.

The right lateral chain of tracheobronchial lymph nodes receives most of its lymph drainage from the right lung, the lower portion of the left lung, the lower part of the trachea and the major bronchi. The right anterior mediastinal chain drains some lymph from the right lung, the thymus gland, the pericardium, the heart, the diaphragm and the diaphragmatic and mediastinal pleurae. It is evident, therefore, that the right lateral tracheal and the right anterior mediastinal groups of lymph nodes drain most of the structures of the right thoracic cavity, the lower portion of the left thoracic cavity and the mediastinum. Therefore, any primary or metastatic neoplastic process or inflammatory lesion which involves any of these structures is a potential or actual threat to the patency of the superior vena cava.

The ascending aorta is situated anteromedially to the superior vena cava and lies along its side throughout its course. An aneurysm of the ascending aorta may therefore occlude the superior vena cava. In addition, the trachea and the right major bronchus lie on the posterior aspect of the superior vena cava, so that the wall of the vein can easily be infiltrated by a bronchogenic carcinoma.

CLINICAL MANIFESTATIONS

The syndrome of superior vena caval obstruction is characterized by an increased venous pressure in the areas drained by the superior vena cava, the production of collateral venous channels, and the presence of a pathological lesion which is responsible for the obstruction. It has been shown that the signs and symptoms of obstruction of the superior vena cava do not usually develop until the lumen of the vein has been narrowed to about three-fifths of its original diameter. The earliest manifestations of obstruction occur in both external jugular veins, which become distended and stand out as thick cords. Engorgement of the other veins in the neck and chest follows.

The symptoms are those produced by the increased venous pressure. They may be overshadowed, however, by the symptoms resulting from the primary lesion causing the obstruction, although a fibrotic process in the mediastinum or a primary thrombus within the lumen of the superior vena cava may produce no symptoms of its own.

The increased venous pressure causes a suffused, cyanotic swelling of the face and neck and dilated superficial veins. One of the earliest manifestations is an increasing difficulty in buttoning the shirt collar because of subcutaneous edema, which first involves the neck and then the face, the arms and the chest. The patient complains of a dull, throbbing, generalized headache and a giddy sensation when bending forward. Ophthalmoscopic examination of the fundi may frequently reveal the presence of dilated retinal veins and swelling of the optic discs. The veins in the neck and upper extremities are distended, even when the patient is in the upight position, and large dilated, tortuous veins are visible over the shoulders, the chest and perhaps the abdominal wall.

Dilatation of superficial veins on the patient's trunk helps to differentiate clinically the site of a superior vena caval obstruction. The veins are always dilated in the head, the neck, the upper extremities and the chest wall. When the vena azygos is obstructed, however, the superficial veins of the abdominal wall also become dilated, the blood flowing in a downward direction. The venous pressure in an antecubital vein is greatly increased, while the pressure in the femoral veins is normal. If the pressure in one antecubital vein is greater than in the other, some of the tributaries of the superior vena cava on that side have become obstructed as well. The dynamics of the venous pressure are frequently altered. The venous pressure normally falls slightly during inspiration and rises slightly during expiration. When there is superior vena caval obstruction either at or below the entry of the vena azygos, however, the effect of inspiration and expiration on the venous pressure is reversed. In addition, the arm-to-tongue circulation time is usually prolonged.

RADIOLOGICAL MANIFESTATIONS

No radiological abnormalities may be apparent if the superior vena caval syndrome is due to primary thrombosis of the great vein or to mediastinal fibrosis. If the syndrome is secondary to some pathological process in the lung or the mediastinum, the radiological manifestations are those produced by these lesions. The radiological manifestations are therefore discussed in the appropriate sections.

TUMORS OF THE MEDIASTINUM

Because of the complex variety of structures in the mediastinum, it is not surprising that a variety of mediastinal tumors may occur. Expanding mediastinal tumors may be either solid or cystic. They may arise from embryonic elements, such as bronchogenic cysts, dermoid cysts or teratomata; from the thymus gland, such as benign or malignant thymoma; from the thyroid gland, such as colloid goiter or adenoma; from lymphoid tissue, as in sarcoidosis, Hodgkin's disease, lymphosarcoma, leukemia, tuberculosis or metastatic carcinoma and sarcoma; from connective tissue, such as lipoma, fibroma or sarcoma; or from nerve tissue, such as neurofibroma or neuroblastoma. Finally, they may be metastatic from a primary malignant process in the bronchus, the esophagus or the breast.

CLINICAL MANIFESTATIONS

Mediastinal tumors usually grow slowly and are commonly asymptomatic in their early stages, generally being discovered accidentally on a chest x-ray. It is only when these growths begin to exert pressure on neighboring structures that symptoms become manifest, and some mediastinal tumors, especially those involving the lymphatic structures, may reach an astonishingly large size without producing symptoms. The symptoms depend on the location of the lesion and have no relation to the underlying pathological process. Once symptoms appear, they progress slowly, although on rare occasions they may be rapid and fulminating. The degree of displacement and distortion of the adjoining structures varies, so that different combinations of symptoms and signs may develop. To a large extent, these depend on the anatomical location of the tumor within the mediastinum.

The most striking symptoms and signs are produced by compression of the superior vena cava. The venous circulation particularly is compressed by lesions in the anterior mediastinum and the superior mediastinum. In the latter situation, other structures such as the trachea, the esophagus, the recurrent laryngeal nerves and the vagus nerves may also be involved. If the lesion is in the posterior mediastinum, the trachea and esophagus and the intercostal nerves may be involved. The aorta is seldom constricted, although pressure on its wall may very occasionally lead to necrosis and rupture.

Compression of the trachea or one of the bronchi produces a paroxysmal wheezing cough, frequently with associated stridor. The sputum is variable in amount and consists of mucus produced by irritation of the bronchial glands. If erosion of the bronchial or tracheal wall occurs, blood is present in the sputum in varying amounts. The sputum is purulent if secondary infection follows obstruction of a bronchus.

Dyspnea is frequently an early symptom, being produced by either tracheal or bronchial compression, so that the resistance to air flow is increased. Although initially only present during exertion, it gradually progresses in intensity until orthopnea develops. There is an associated sense of oppression in the chest, which later increases in intensity to the point of pain. This is usually situated substernally and varies in severity.

The esophagus is mobile and tends to be displaced, rather than compressed, by extrinsic pressure. If compression occurs, however, it causes dysphagia. As a result, swallowed solid food sticks in the esophagus and produces a localized substernal discomfort, which occasionally corresponds fairly accurately to the site of the obstruction.

Irritation of one of the vagus nerves may produce a severe paroxysmal cough, spasmodic closure of the glottis and bradycardia, as well as a generalized bronchospasm, simulating an attack of bronchial asthma. Paralysis of a vagus nerve results in tachycardia, vomiting and dyspepsia. Paralysis of one of the recurrent laryngeal nerves results in hoarseness due to an abduction paralysis of the corresponding vocal cord. The left recurrent laryngeal nerve is more liable to be affected owing to its longer course within the chest.

Irritation of the sympathetic nerves produces a tonic elevation of the eyelid, protrusion of the eyeball, dilatation of the pupil, hyperhidrosis and flushing of the face on the affected side. If the sympathetic nerves are paralyzed, Horner's syndrome results, with ptosis, enophthalmosis, constriction of the pupil and anhidrosis of the face on the affected side.

Irritation of the brachial plexus produces pain which radiates down the corresponding arm. Involvement of the intercostal nerves results in pain and paresthesias along the chest wall. Irritation of the phrenic nerve may lead to hiccoughs and pain in the shoulder, followed later by the development of a unilateral paralysis of the diaphragm.

If the thoracic duct becomes obstructed along its course in the posterior mediastinum, there may be rapid weight loss and cachexia, occasionally associated with chylothorax. It is most unusual for constitutional symptoms to develop in cases of benign mediastinal tumors unless such a complication is present.

The abnormal physical signs produced by a mediastinal tumor are very meager, except when the superior vena caval syndrome is present. If the tumor is very large and is situated in the anterior mediastinum, there may be a localized bulging of the anterior chest wall or a fullness in the intercostal spaces associated with edema and distended venules. The thyroid gland may be enlarged and adenomatous, extending below the suprasternal notch. A substernal thyroid may be palpable in the suprasternal notch as it rises during the act of swallowing. The trachea is often deviated to one side or the other, particularly if the mediastinal tumor is due to a substernal goiter.

If the tumor is in the superior mediastinum, the percussion note over the manubrium sterni is flat instead of resonant. Grossly enlarged mediastinal lymph nodes or a large tumor in the posterior mediastinum produces a dull percussion note over the upper thoracic vertebrae, an area which is also normally resonant. The dullness may be associated with whispering pectoriloquy and diminished breath sounds because of compression of the overlying lung. Any associated condition, such as atelectasis or pleural effusion, can be distinguished by its characteristic physical signs.

In order to exclude one of the lymphomatous diseases, a search should be made for enlarged peripheral lymph nodes as well as an enlarged liver or spleen. The presence of the stigmata of neurofibromatosis, such as areas of brown pigmentation and cutaneous fibromas, or signs of compression of the spinal cord point to the neurogenic character of a mediastinal tumor.

RADIOLOGICAL MANIFESTATIONS

The radiological examination of the chest enables the examiner to assess the correct site, the size and the outline of the growth. Unfortunately, a definitive pathological diagnosis cannot be made from the radiological appearance, although certain possibilities may be assumed.

An important feature of mediastinal tumors is their failure to pulsate. If the border of the opacity is sharp and clearly defined, the lesion is more likely to be benign, whereas if its outline is hazy, it is likely to be malignant.

The site of the growth is also very important. If the tumor is in the superior mediastinum and rises into the neck, it is very likely a substernal goiter. Tumors in the anterior mediastinum are more commonly due to thymomas and teratomas. Neurogenic tumors are most commonly found in the posterior mediastinum, but bronchogenic cysts, lipomas and fibromas may be found in any part of the mediastinum.

INFLAMMATION OF THE MEDIASTINUM

THE FASCIAL LAYERS OF THE MEDIASTINUM

The mediastinal fascial layers are a direct continuation of the deep fascia within the neck, which forms a sheath enclosing the trapezius muscle posteriorly and the sternomastoid muscle anteriorly, and blends with the fascia of the opposite side in the mid-line. Superiorly, it is attached to the superior nuchal line of the occipital bone, the inferior border of the body of the mandible and the hyoid bone. Inferiorly, it is attached to the subcutaneous portions of the clavicle, the acromion and the posterior part of the spine of the scapula. The fascia lining the posterior surface of the sternomastoid muscle extends into the mediastinum to form its fascial planes by dividing into several important layers.

The Pretracheal Fascia.   The most anterior of these layers, the pretracheal fascia, lies anterior to the full length of the trachea and ends at the level of its bifurcation by blending with the fibrous pericardial sac. It splits to enclose the thyroid gland and helps to form part of the carotid sheath. Laterally, it blends with the prevertebral layer of fascia and by so doing forms a compartment which encloses the trachea, the thyroid gland and the esophagus.

The Prevertebral Fascia.   The most posterior fascial layer, the prevertebral fascia, lines the anterior surface of the vertebral muscles and also helps to form part of the carotid sheath. Laterally, it blends with the pretracheal fascia to form the compartment which encloses the trachea, the thyroid gland and the esophagus.

The Carotid Sheath.   The third fascial extension is situated between the pretracheal and prevertebral layers and blends with them to form a fibrous envelope called the carotid sheath, which encloses the common and internal carotid arteries, the internal jugular veins and the vagus nerve. It is doubtful whether the carotid sheath can ever be distended enough to allow the passage of pus, but it may occasionally be a route for the spread of infection.

Postesophageal Fascia.   A very important potential space extending from the superior mediastinum to the diaphragm is situated between the esophagus and the prevertebral fascia. It is not a completely free space, for it is divided into upper and lower compartments by the blending of part of the prevertebral fascia with the pericardial sac at the level of the bifurcation of the trachea. This is the route most frequently taken by inflammatory processes within the mediastinum.

The mediastinal compartments formed by the layers of fascia are only potential spaces. They become real spaces when they are distended by the accumulation of fluid, whether serous, purulent or hemorrhagic, or by the presence of air.

ACUTE MEDIASTINITIS

The most frequent source of infection of the mediastinum is a suppurative process involving the fascial planes in the neck as a result of a peritonsillar or retropharyngeal abscess, tuberculous caries of the cervical spine or suppuration of a cervical lymph node. Postoperative mediastinitis may also follow a tracheotomy or thyroidectomy. Another source of infection is direct extension of an inflammatory process involving a mediastinal viscus or one of the neighboring structures. Of these, the esophagus is the most important. Perforation of its wall may occur during esophagoscopy or may result from the accidental swallowing of a foreign body, such as a chicken bone. Other intrathoracic causes of mediastinitis are such inflammatory processes as pulmonary abscess, empyema, suppuration of a tracheobronchial lymph node, and tuberculous caries of a rib. In addition, rupture of a subdiaphragmatic abscess through the diaphragm may involve the mediastinal tissues.

Mediastinal inflammatory reactions vary from so mild that they are overlooked to acute fulmination. The mild variety is usually produced by a mild inflammatory process, but infection by virulent organisms may result in a diffuse cellulitis, which may lead to death from toxemia before pus has had a chance to develop. If suppuration occurs, it may be generalized or localized in the form of an abscess. The pus may rupture into the esophagus or the trachea, or it may find an outlet through one of the intercostal spaces.

CLINICAL MANIFESTATIONS

The symptoms and signs produced by acute mediastinitis may be overshadowed by those of the disease which is primarily responsible for the mediastinal inflammation. The milder variety may produce so few symptoms and such a slight constitutional reaction that its presence may be overlooked. In the more severe forms of the disease, especially those with an associated purulent collection of fluid, the symptoms and signs are primarily related to the effects of pressure, just as in a mediastinal tumor. The constitutional reaction is correspondingly more intense and varies with the severity of the infection, but in the presence of pus, there is a high fever as well as other evidence of severe toxemia.

Thoracic pain is an important feature in acute mediastinitis. It is caused by the inflammatory swelling or distention of the fascial spaces, as well as by the spread of the infection to neighboring structures, such as the pericardium and the pleura. It is a throbbing pain and it is usually situated over the sternum. Characteristically, it is aggravated by movement of the trunk, particularly on changing from the sitting to the lying position. If the esophagus has been ruptured just above the diaphragm, the pain may be situated in the epigastrium, and there may be associated muscular rigidity. Generalized thoracic pain due to involvement of the intercostal nerves may be produced by pus in the posterior mediastinum.

Other prominent symptoms are cough, dyspnea and pain on swallowing. Expectoration of pus indicates rupture of the abscess into a bronchus.

The physical findings may be very meager. If there is a collection of pus in the anterior mediastinum, there may be tenderness over the sternum and dullness to percussion in this area. An abscess in the posterior mediastinum usually produces no abnormal physical signs, except for occasional tenderness over the spinous processes of the thoracic vertebrae. If the superior vena cava is involved in an inflammatory process of the superior mediastinum, dilated tortuous veins may be present over the chest wall.

RADIOLOGICAL MANIFESTATIONS

An x-ray of the chest is often of considerable assistance in the diagnosis of acute mediastinitis, particularly if a localized abscess is present. In the early stages of an acute inflammatory process there may be few abnormal findings, aside from a thickening of the mediastinal pleura and distention of the pulmonary lymphatics. If an abscess develops in the superior mediastinum, the superior mediastinal shadow is broadened. The abscess is evident as a localized bulging to one side or the other above the hilum of the lung, with a less clear-cut border than that of a tumor. An abscess in the posterior mediastinum is indicated by a hazy opacity in the normally translucent space between the esophagus and the vertebral column. In the anterior mediastinum, an abscess distorts the cardiac shadow to one side or the other. If the abscess has been caused by a perforation of the esophagus, it may contain air and may demonstrate a fluid level. A similar radiological picture is seen if gas-forming organisms are present or if rupture has taken place into the trachea or bronchus.

CHRONIC FIBROUS MEDIASTINITIS

A mild form of fibrosis of the mediastinum may develop after recovery from an attack of acute mediastinitis. There is also a severe kind of chronic, diffuse cicatrization of the mediastinum which is unrelated to the acute disease. The etiology is obscure, although a number of specific infections such as rheumatic fever, tuberculosis and syphilis have been incriminated.

In chronic mediastinitis, there is a relentless progressive increase in the amount of the connective tissue of the mediastinum which causes adhesion and matting together of all the mediastinal structures, including the pericardium. It may be a diffuse process or it may involve only a localized portion of the mediastinum. If the superior and anterior parts of the mediastinum are principally involved, the lumen of the superior vena cava may become constricted and eventually obstructed. The trachea and bronchi may become stenosed, and the left recurrent laryngeal nerve may be paralyzed by the compression. In the posterior mediastinum, the esophagus may become involved, either by stenosis or by the development of an esophageal diverticulum. The parietal layer of the pericardium may be involved in the sclerotic process, becoming markedly thickened and adherent to the surrounding mediastinal structures. In contrast to constrictive pericarditis, in which the pericardial space is obliterated by the symphysis of the two pericardial layers, however, the pericardial space is preserved in chronic fibrous mediastinitis.

CLINICAL MANIFESTATIONS

The symptoms and physical signs produced by chronic fibrous mediastinitis depend on the site in which the fibrosis is predominant, as well as on the particular mediastinal structures affected by the cicatrizing process. The clinical manifestations are therefore similar to those produced by other lesions of the mediastinum. There may be a dull note to percussion over the sternum or the interscapular area. If the parietal layer of the pericardium is involved, the thickened pericardial sac interferes with the systolic contraction of the heart and is immobilized by its adherence to the surrounding structures. As a consequence, the left lower anterior chest wall may retract during each systolic contraction. A similar systolic retraction in the lower posterior aspect of the left chest wall, known as Broadbent's sign, is produced by adhesions between the pericardium and the posterior chest wall. Because of the inadequate systolic filling of the heart, the cardiac output may be low and the neck veins distended.

RADIOLOGICAL MANIFESTATIONS

There may be few abnormal changes in the x-ray of the chest in chronic fibrous mediastinitis. The mediastinal pleura may be thickened and the superior mediastinal shadow widened. Fibrous bands in the posterior mediastinum may show up as a linear mottling in the translucent space between the esophagus and the vertebral column. The cardiac shadow may be widened and may have hazy borders, and on fluoroscopy it may show decreased systolic contractions. When a radioopaque mixture is swallowed, the esophagus may be shown to be distorted, displaced or stenosed or to possess a traction diverticulum.

MEDIASTINAL AIR

PATHOGENESIS

The accumulation of air in the tissues of the mediastinum can be produced by a variety of conditions. It usually develops as a result of traumatic rupture of the trachea or a bronchus or of perforation of the esophagus following, for example, the accidental swallowing of a sharp object, such as a chicken bone. Trauma to the chest cage, with laceration of lung alveoli, also releases air which tracks along the sheaths of the pulmonary vessels towards the hilum and finally ruptures into the mediastinum. Accumulation of air may occasionally follow thyroidectomy or tracheotomy, the negative pressure of the mediastinum sucking air into its tissues along its fascial planes; or it may follow a pneumoperitoneum, when the increased intra-abdominal pressure forces the air through the esophageal hiatus of the diaphragm.

Mediastinal air occasionally occurs spontaneously in apparently healthy persons. Once again, there is a rupture of alveoli, the released air dissecting along the pulmonary vasculature into the mediastinum. The reason for the rupture of the alveolar walls is not clear. A check-valve bronchiolar obstruction has been implicated, and a congenital inadequacy in the development of the alveolar wall has also been suggested as a cause of attenuation and weakening of the wall. There is rarely any precipitating increase in the intrabronchial pressure, the accident usually occurring while the patient is at rest.

The fate of the air in the mediastinum depends on the amount that is released and on the pressure which develops in the mediastinal tissues. It either remains within the confines of the mediastinum and is gradually reabsorbed, or it escapes upwards into the tissues of the neck. A subcutaneous collection of air therefore develops, involving the face, neck and trunk, and eventually even the external genitalia. Occasionally, the air may rupture through the mediastinal pleura to produce a pneumothorax.

CLINICAL MANIFESTATIONS

The symptoms and clinical course depend largely on the cause of the condition. A spontaneous mediastinal collection of air usually runs a benign course and produces a fairly characteristic clinical picture. There is a sudden onset of substernal pain of varying severity, which may radiate straight through to the back or into the neck and shoulders. Occasionally the pain may simulate that of coronary ischemia, by radiating down the left arm. A characteristic feature of the pain is its aggravation by any change in position, a jarring motion, swallowing or twisting of the neck. There is often only minimal evidence of peripheral vascular collapse, and the temperature, pulse rate and respirations are normal.

If air continues to accumulate, the blood flow to the heart may become impeded by being dammed back into the veins of the head, neck, lungs and liver. The cardiac output may therefore fall, so that severe hypotension and shock may develop.

The detection of subcutaneous air in the tissues of the head, neck and thorax is of diagnostic importance. Percussion over the precordium may produce a hyper-resonant note. A distinctive physical finding is the presence of a peculiar crackling, crunching sound over the precordium, which is synchronous with the contractions of the heart; occasionally it may resemble a pericardial friction rub. This sound is produced by the thrust of the heart against the blebs of air in the anterior mediastinum. The intensity of the sound may be altered by respiration and change of position, and it may be heard only when the patient is in the left lateral position. The intensity of the sound bears no relationship to the amount of air, often being very pronounced even though the patient has little or no discomfort.

RADIOLOGICAL MANIFESTATIONS

Because the air-containing lungs surround the mediastinum, me-diastinal air is difficult to visualize unless it is localized or large in amount. If it can be demonstrated, it is visible in the anteroposterior view as a translucent area projecting from the lateral border of the mediastinum. Demonstration may be complicated by the presence of a pneumothorax.

HERNIATION OF THE MEDIASTINUM

There are two relatively weak areas in the mediastinum, the two sites where the mediastinal pleurae are in contact with each other. One is located anteriorly behind the upper part of the sternum at the level of the second to the fourth costal cartilages, and the other lies posteriorly in the inferior retrocardiac region between the esophagus and the aorta. These areas may give way if the intrapleural pressure rises sharply in one or other hemithorax in association with a relatively rigid medi-astinum. A bulge, or herniation, of lung takes place into the other side. This frequently occurs through the area which lies anterior to the su-perior mediastinum. The most common cause is a tension pneumothorax, but it may also take place if there is a large area of localized overdisten-tion due to a check-valve obstruction of a bronchus, or if there is a large, expanding pulmonary cyst.

CHAPTER XII

Diaphragmatic Disease

ANATOMY

THE DIAPHRAGM occupies the floor of the thoracic cavity and acts as a partition between the contents of the thoracic cage and those of the abdominal cavity. It is formed by two thin, dome-shaped sheets of striated muscle, each of which arises from the inner surface of the xiphoid process, the ipsilateral costal margin and the bodies of the upper lumbar vertebrae. Each hemidiaphragm is inserted medially into the central tendon, a firm tendinous aponeurosis which is adherent to the overlying pericardial sac. It is therefore in close apposition to the serous membranes of the pleural spaces, the pericardium and the peritoneum. The major component of each hemidiaphragm is formed by its costal or lateral portion, the fibers of which pass upwards in a vertical direction in close apposition to the inner side of the chest wall and then turn medially to form the dome prior to being inserted into the central tendon.

The normal diaphragm, as viewed from its peritoneal surface, is illustrated in Figure 66. On its posterior aspect, the peripheral part of each hemidiaphragm develops into three thick muscular bundles, known as crura. Each crus crosses the mid-line before being inserted into the anterior aspect of the bodies of the third and fourth lumbar vertebrae. In this way they form three archways. The inner archway, which is developed by the decussation of the two inner crura, lies posteriorly at the level of the twelfth dorsal vertebra. It serves as an opening, or hiatus, for the passage of the thoracic aorta into the abdomen. A second decussation at the level of the tenth dorsal vertebra forms an opening which is situated anterior and slightly to the left of the aortic openings. This permits the passage of the esophagus, its vessels and the two vagus nerves. The middle crura are responsible for apertures which allow the passage of the splanchnic nerves and the hemi-azygos vein on the left side.

In the embryo, the diaphragm originates in the cervical region and then gradually descends into the thoracic cavity. The fully formed diaphragm maintains a permanent connection with its original site in the neck through the phrenic nerves, which are the sole motor nerves of the diaphragm. In addition, these nerves carry sensory fibers and receive sympathetic fibers from the inferior cervical ganglion and occasionally from the medial cervical and first thoracic ganglia. The phrenic nerve supplies the sensory innervation to the anterior and central portions of the pleural surface of the diaphragm and the central portions of its abdominal surface by means of afferent fibers which originate in the dorsal root ganglia of the third, fourth and fifth cervical roots. Any irritative lesion in these areas evokes a pain sensation which is perceived along the ridge of the trapezius muscle in the ipsilateral shoulder. A similar pain is felt when the phrenic nerve is irritated by a lesion in any part of its course along the lateral aspect of the mediastinum. It has been suggested that the nuclei of the phrenic nerves in the spinal cord are connected with one another across the mid-line. This would explain why both leaves of the diaphragm may still function normally when there is a destructive lesion of one-half of the spinal cord above the level of the second cervical segment.

The diaphragm is the principal organ of respiration. Although

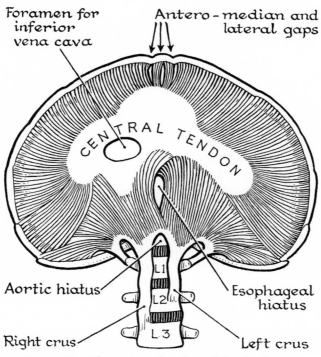

FIGURE 66. The peritoneal surface of the diaphragm.

its primary function is to enlarge the chest cage vertically during inspiration, it also plays a part in its transverse enlargement by elevating the lower ribs and the costal margin. At the end of a normal expiration, the upper limit of the dome of the right hemidiaphragm is at the level of the fifth rib, while that of the left hemidiaphragm is at the level of the fifth interspace. In a healthy person, a change from the erect to the supine position results in a rise in the resting level of the diaphragm which may be as much as 6 cm. A similar effect takes place when a healthy person assumes the lateral decubitus position. In this position, the lower hemidiaphragm rises, particularly if the subject lies on his right side.

Both leaves of the diaphragm move approximately equally, going through a range of about 2 cm. during quiet breathing. The central tendon is considerably less mobile, because it adheres to the overlying pericardial sac, which, in turn, is relatively fixed by its fusion with the fascia which extends up into the neck and by the great vessels and the hila of the lungs. The ascent of the diaphragm during expiration is a purely passive phenomenon, being produced by the elastic recoil of the inflated lungs and the tone of the abdominal muscles. The diaphragm begins its expiratory rise, even though the ribs are still in the inspiratory position. As soon as the ribs begin to descend, however, the diaphragmatic movement slows down.

The diaphragm also plays a very important part in the cough reflex. Its only active role occurs during the inspiratory phase prior to the closure of the glottis. During the compressive phase of the cough, the diaphragm remains in a state of tonic contraction. During the expulsive phase, however, the diaphragm is moved in an upward direction by the pressure of the abdominal organs. The diaphragm takes an active part in the acts of vomiting, defecation and parturition as well. In such circumstances, it acts synergistically with the contracted abdominal muscles to elevate the intra-abdominal pressure.

HERNIATION OF ABDOMINAL VISCERA

CONGENITAL HERNIATION OF THE DIAPHRAGM

All diaphragmatic hernias, with the exception of the traumatic, are related to a failure in the development, or a lack of fusion, of one of the various multiple structures which take part in the formation of the embryonic diaphragm. In the first month of intra-uterine life, the embryonic coelomic space, which is originally a continuous tube, subdivides into the pericardial cavity, the pleural space and the peritoneal cavity by the development of a membranous partition which is called the septum transversum. This septum remains restricted to the anterior half of the embryo, so that communication persists in the posterior part of the coelomic space, connecting the pleural space and peritoneal cavity. The two pleuroperitoneal canals are separated from each other by the dorsal mesentery, which is situated in the median plane and contains the growing esophagus.

During the second month of intra-uterine life, the pleuroperitoneal canals become closed by an ingrowth of the structures which form their walls, as well as by the proliferation of the dorsal mesentery and the urogenital ridge. Because the pleura and peritoneum have now developed, no communication exists any longer between them. The diaphragm is still a purely membranous structure at this stage. It is during the third month of embryonic development that the phrenic nerve begins its descent into the thoracic cage from its origin in the cervical area. As it descends, it is preceded by a premuscle mass which is derived from the cervical myotomes. These premuscle fibers enter the membranous diaphragm at the sites where it is pierced by the phrenic nerves and then develop into muscle fibers, which spread outwards throughout the membranous structures to transform them into the muscular diaphragm, the posterior part being the last portion to be affected. The central portion, which eventually forms the central tendon, is not involved in this process.

The anteromedial part of the fully developed diaphragm is formed from the septum transversum, its posteromedial portion from the primitive dorsal mesentery, and the lateral portion from the body wall. The gaps between the posteromedial and lateral portions eventually become fused with the dorsal mesentery. All these components of the diaphragm are of mesodermal origin. A failure in either the proper development or the fusion of any of these components results in an area of weakness or a loss of continuity in that portion of the fully developed diaphragm. The sites in which these defects occur are illustrated in Figure 67.

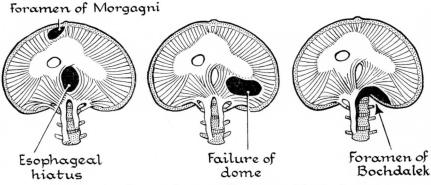

FIGURE 67.   The sites of congenital herniation of the diaphragm.

The Foramen of Bochdalek.   A failure in the closure of the pleuroperitoneal canal leads to an absence of the crura and crural attachments. This results in a triangular-shaped opening in the diaphragm which is situated in its posterolateral portion with its base facing the thoracic wall. This gap, the foramen of Bochdalek, forms a direct communication between the thorax and the abdomen. Because of its position, and since the opening may be large, the intestine is the organ which most commonly herniates through it, usually early in infancy or childhood. A bilateral defect may produce an opening so large that the posterior half of the diaphragm may be absent.

The Foramen of Morgagni.   A second type of congenital diaphragmatic hernia occurs anteriorly behind the sternum, on either side of the xiphoid process. Normally, there are small gaps in the retrosternal attachment of the diaphragm which allow the passage of the superior epigastric vessels. Failure in the development of the retrosternal attachment of the diaphragm results in a large opening, more commonly situated on the right side, known as the foramen of Morgagni. Such an area is deficient in muscle fibers, the gap being filled with areolar tissue and being covered only by the pericardium and the peritoneum. The organs which may protrude into the thorax through this gap are the colon and omentum.

The Esophageal Hiatus.   A third site of maldevelopment of the diaphragm is the esophageal hiatus. Herniation through this hiatus is the commonest type of nontraumatic hernia encountered. Here again, there is a failure of fusion of the various structures which form the hiatus, but this is complicated by the fact that the stomach has to descend to its normal intra-abdominal position before the esophageal hiatus can be fully developed. The embryonic stomach is originally formed in the cervical region and, as the esophagus elongates, it migrates downwards through the posterior mediastinum until it finally reaches its normal position below the diaphragm. There may be a delay in the descent of the stomach, or it may not descend completely. Incomplete descent of the stomach results in a shortened esophagus, with a portion of the stomach protruding into the thorax. If the esophagus is of normal length, the stomach protrudes into the posterior mediastinum by sliding through the abnormally enlarged esophageal opening along the side of the esophagus.

If the esophagus fails to elongate properly, the stomach becomes arrested in the lower portion of the posterior mediastinum, so that its fundus remains within the thorax, while the pyloric portion lies below the diaphragm. This situation is further aggravated by the negative intrathoracic pressure which tends to suck the stomach into the chest, and, in addition, any act which increases the intra-abdominal pressure tends to push it upwards. In time, the whole stomach may herniate through the dilated hiatus.

Another type of maldevelopment of the diaphragm occurs as a result of failure in the closure of the dome of the diaphragm. This produces a gap in the substance of the muscular diaphragm, while its posterior part is normally developed.

Although all these structural defects of the diaphragm are of congenital origin, herniation of abdominal contents need not necessarily appear in infancy unless the defect is already large. With a small defect, symptoms may become manifest only in adult life, especially if the patient becomes obese or pregnant. These conditions, by increasing the abdominal pressure, may enlarge the defect.

TRAUMATIC HERNIATION OF THE DIAPHRAGM

Herniation of abdominal contents into the thoracic cage can also occur as a result of a traumatic rupture of the diaphragm—for example, by a penetrating wound through the chest cage or the abdominal wall. In automobile accidents, a blunt traumatic impact to the thorax or abdomen can result in rupture of the diaphragm. Under these circumstances, the relatively weak diaphragm gives way under the impact of the solid abdominal viscera which pushes it against the more pliant thoracic contents.

Rupture of the diaphragm may also occur as a result of traumatic compression of the chest. As shown in Figure 68, the type of rupture depends on the site of compression. Compression of the anterior part of the chest towards the spine may result in a lateral tear of a leaf of the diaphragm. In contrast, compression of the side of the chest may result in a tear which runs in an anteroposterior direction. Traumatic rupture of the left hemidiaphragm occurs twenty times as frequently as that of

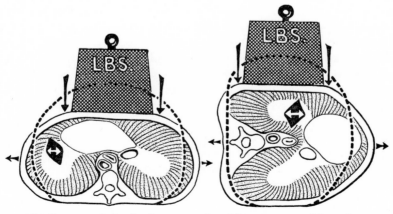

FIGURE 68.   Rupture of the diaphragm produced by anterior and lateral compression of the chest. The arrows indicate the direction of the tear.

the right, the right hemidiaphragm presumably being protected by the liver, which acts as a buffer. A traumatic tear of the left hemidiaphragm may result in a herniation of the stomach, colon and even the spleen into the thorax. On the right side, herniation may involve the liver and colon.

If there is a large defect in the diaphragm with massive herniation of abdominal viscera into the thorax, torsion and displacement of the mediastinum may occur. In such a case, the severity of the symptoms, particularly dyspnea and vomiting, is extreme. If the herniation is small, however, and there is very little effect on the intrathoracic structures, the symptoms may be mild.

DISEASES AFFECTING THE POSITION OF THE DIAPHRAGM

A disease process involving the diaphragm may result in either its elevation or its depression. Both conditions are associated with a decrease in its mobility.

PARALYSIS OF THE DIAPHRAGM

Interruption of the phrenic nerve results in paralysis of the ipsilateral hemidiaphragm. This paralysis is permanent if the nerve is cut or avulsed, whereas a return of its motor activity usually takes place within a period of approximately six months if it is crushed. Before the advent of chemotherapy and excisional surgery, crushing of the phrenic nerve was one of the methods used to induce relaxation of the lung in the treatment of pulmonary tuberculosis.

The phrenic nerves may become paralyzed by disease processes which involve them either centrally or peripherally. Centrally, the anterior horn cells may be affected by poliomyelitis, the spinal cord may suffer traumatic injury, or the nerve roots may be involved by meningitis or tuberculous caries of the spine. Peripherally, the nerves may be affected by diphtheria, lead poisoning, alcoholic neuritis or beriberi. An aneurysm of the aortic arch may press on the left phrenic nerve, or the nerve may be involved by a malignant intrathoracic tumor which has spread to the hilum.

An interruption of the nerve impulses to a hemidiaphragm leads to its paralysis. Provided that there are no adhesions, it then rises from 3 to 10 cm. higher than the hemidiaphragm on the nonparalyzed side. Interruption of the motor impulses to the diaphragm results in atrophy of the muscle, and gradual replacement of the muscle fibers by fibrous tissue. As the muscle fibers disappear, the diaphragm gradually rises higher, assuming its maximal elevated position in approximately six months.

EVENTRATION OF THE DIAPHRAGM

The term "eventration" is actually a misnomer, for there is no protrusion of abdominal viscera through an opening in the diaphragm, as the name would imply. This term is commonly accepted, however, as it was applied to the condition when it was first described in 1790. In this condition, the diaphragm is a thin, atrophic sheet of fibrous tissue with a complete absence of muscle fibers. Because of this lack, it assumes an abnormally elevated position, though still arching smoothly from its costal attachments.

The acquired form of eventration is commonly seen as the end-result of a lesion which causes paralysis of the phrenic nerve. In an infant it may develop as a result of a birth injury affecting the brachial plexus. A congenital origin has been postulated for a small percentage of the cases of eventration because of their occurrence in the newborn. In addition, the congenital hypothesis is enhanced by the occasional association of hypoplasia and other congenital abnormalities of the corresponding lung, as well as congenital abnormalities elsewhere.

FIBROTHORAX

Fibrous pleurisy, the end-result of an improperly treated empyema or hemothorax, is characterized by gross thickening of the pleura and involvement of the chest wall and underlying lung. The diaphragmatic pleura is always involved in this cicatrizing process. The diaphragm becomes elevated and its movements are severely restricted by both the adhesive pleuritis and the shrunken intrathoracic structures.

INTRA-ABDOMINAL CONDITIONS

Any condition which produces an increase in the intra-abdominal pressure may elevate the level of both leaves of the diaphragm, thereby restricting their movements. Bilateral elevation of the diaphragm may be caused by pregnancy, an artificial pneumoperitoneum, ascites, distention of any part of the gastrointestinal tract or obesity. In addition, an operative incision through the abdominal muscles, particularly in the upper part of the abdomen, is frequently associated with elevation and fixation of a hemidiaphragm. This occurs because the peripheral costal portion of each hemidiaphragm interdigitates with the transverse abdominus muscle, which receives the same nerve supply from the lower thoracic nerves.

INFLAMMATORY DISEASES OF THE DIAPHRAGM

Although primary myositis of the diaphragm does occur, it is considerably less common than that which arises secondarily. The difference in incidence is easily understood if one remembers the intimate relationship between the diaphragm and the pleural, pericardial and peritoneal membranes. Because of its position in the thoracic cage, the diaphragm can become secondarily involved by even the smallest collection of inflammatory exudate in the pleural space. The situation is somewhat different on the peritoneal side of the diaphragm, for inflammatory exudate in the peritoneal cavity tends to gravitate towards the pelvis. If the infective process involves the subdiaphragmatic space, however, the diaphragm always becomes secondarily involved.

SUBDIAPHRAGMATIC ABSCESS

The exceedingly rich plexus of lymphatics which traverse the diaphragm forms communications between the pleural and peritoneal spaces and thus permits the spread of infection from one space to the other. In pleural or pulmonary suppuration, secondary involvement of the subdiaphragmatic space is exceedingly rare. On the other hand, a subdiaphragmatic abscess very commonly spreads to involve the pleurae and lung parenchyma. It has been suggested that this occurs because of the sucking effect on the lymphatics produced by the negative pressure within the pleural space.

A localized collection of purulent exudate or pus in the subdiaphragmatic space is an extremely serious complication which may follow any form of intra-abdominal suppuration. It most commonly occurs as a result of peritonitis following perforation of a portion of the gastrointestinal tract by acute appendicitis, a peptic ulcer or a neoplasm. The right subdiaphragmatic space is most commonly affected, being involved five times more frequently than the left. Thoracic extension of the infection is a frequent occurrence, so that a serous pleural effusion, empyema, pyopneumothorax and pulmonary suppuration may develop. Although thoracic extension is usually due to lymphatic spread, it may also follow perforation of a necrotic portion of the diaphragm. Even a perinephritic abscess has occasionally been associated with a pleural effusion or empyema.

The most common causal organisms are the *Bacillus coli,* the staphylococci and gas-forming bacilli. The gas produced by the latter organisms collects within the abscess cavity under the diaphragm and produces a characteristic radiological appearance which is suggestive of a pneumoperitoneum.

PRIMARY INFLAMMATION OF THE DIAPHRAGM

This extremely rare condition is an acute myositis, probably of viral etiology, which develops without any associated involvement of the pleurae, lung parenchyma or peritoneum. It is a self-limited process, usually clearing spontaneously within a few weeks; although it has a tendency to recur, the subsequent attacks being considerably milder.

SPASMODIC CONDITIONS AFFECTING THE DIAPHRAGM

Hiccup is an irregular, clonic spasm of the diaphragm involving either one or both leaves. It is associated with an abrupt closure of the glottis during the act of inspiration. It is a common disorder in healthy people, often being caused by some trivial condition, such as a mild form of dyspepsia. On the other hand, it may be associated with diseases affecting the stomach, gallbladder or peritoneum. Hiccup may also be a serious manifestation of a toxemic state such as uremia, a central nervous system disease such as meningitis, or involvement of the phrenic nerve by a malignant process. If it persists over a lengthy period of time, it can contribute to a patient's physical exhaustion.

Tonic spasms of the diaphragm may occur in association with rabies, tetanus, tetany and strychnine poisoning. They may also occur in the early stages of an epileptic convulsion.

Diaphragmatic flutter is an extremely rare condition which differs from tonic and clonic spasms in that the attacks consist of a series of very rapid, rhythmical contractions which may reach as many as 100 to 300 per minute. It may develop in such conditions as encephalitis lethargica and tetany.

MANIFESTATIONS OF DIAPHRAGMATIC DISEASE

CLINICAL MANIFESTATIONS

Irritation and inflammation of the diaphragmatic pleura, the diaphragmatic peritoneum, the diaphragmatic muscle or the phrenic nerve produce similar painful stimuli. As these structures have the same nerve supply, it is not possible to distinguish which is affected. Irritation of the central portion of the diaphragm produces a pain which is referred to the neck and shoulder on the same side, principally to the ridge of the trapezius muscle. If the peripheral rim or the posterior third of the diaphragm is involved, the pain is referred to the lower posterolateral part of the chest and the upper abdominal wall on the same side. Both types of referred pain may be present at the same time if a larger area of the diaphragm is affected. Referred diaphragmatic pain is usually induced or aggravated by deep breathing, coughing, sneezing or straining. It is always associated with hyperesthesia of the skin at the site of the pain. The pain is aggravated by lying on the affected side because the range of the costal movement is decreased and diaphragmatic movement is increased. The findings on physical examination are similar in all cases of diaphragmatic irritation, whether primary or secondary. The lower part of the affected side of the chest including the costal margin shows restricted movement. The diaphragm is elevated and is also restricted in its movement.

The symptoms produced by paralysis of the diaphragm depend not only on the presence of associated pulmonary disease, but also on the development of paradoxical movement. Although dyspnea may be produced, it may be only transient if the lungs are healthy. If the pulmonary reserve is already low, however, the additional hazard of diaphragmatic paralysis may jeopardize the life of the patient. If the phrenic nerve interruption has been produced by invasion or compression of the nerve by an intrathoracic lesion, the symptoms produced by the primary disease may overshadow those caused by the paralyzed diaphragm. On physical examination the diaphragm is found to be high and the chest movement on the affected side diminished.

When a herniation of abdominal contents is present, mechanical pressure on the mediastinum or lungs by the displaced abdominal viscera may produce symptoms. The respiratory symptoms consist of dyspnea, cough and wheezing. Torsion of the mediastinum may cause palpitation, tachycardia and anginal pain due to coronary insufficiency. Displacement of the abdominal viscera, particularly on the left side, may also produce abdominal discomfort and anorexia, regurgitation or heartburn.

Most adults with eventration of the diaphragm are asymptomatic. In the newborn infant, however, it can produce profound distress with attacks of severe dyspnea, cyanosis and vomiting which may even lead to death. A similar series of events may occur if the infant is born with a large diaphragmatic hernia. The severity of the symptoms in this condition depends on the rapidity and the degree of herniation of the abdominal contents and the amount of compression of the thoracic viscera. A large diaphragmatic hernia can displace the mediastinum towards the normal side. Dullness to percussion and diminished breath sounds are usually present on the affected side, although a tympanitic note may be elicited if the hernia should contain the stomach or a portion of the bowel.

RADIOLOGICAL MANIFESTATIONS

In the normal anteroposterior chest film the two hemidiaphragms are visible as well-defined, smooth curved lines, with their convexity directed upwards. The summit of the right leaf normally occupies a position about 2 cm. higher than the left. In the lateral view, the summit of the diaphragm occupies an anterior position, and its major portion slopes downwards and backwards. An elevated hemidiaphragm is easily recognized. If a diaphragmatic hernia is present, the contour of the affected diaphragm appears abnormal. The space-occupying abdominal viscus in the lower thorax may be solid or air-containing, and the mediastinum is displaced away from the side of the hernia (Fig. 69). If the diaphragm is depressed, it appears low and flattened and the costophrenic angles are widened. One leaf may be affected in this manner by a pleural effusion, pneumothorax or a localized overdistention of the lung due to a check-valve obstruction of a bronchus. Both hemidiaphragms are usually depressed in cases of chronic obstructive emphysema or during an exacerbation of bronchial asthma.

Diaphragmatic movement is assessed by fluoroscopic examination of the degree of movement during inspiration and expiration. In the lateral view, the posterior part of the diaphragm moves freely, but its summit appears to have very little movement. The smooth contour of a hemidiaphragm may be lost because of adhesions, which appear as irregular peaks between it and the base of the lung. If the hemidiaphragm becomes adherent to the chest wall, the costophrenic angle is obliterated and its outer part does not move during respiration.

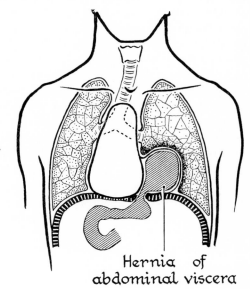

FIGURE 69.   Diaphragmatic hernia.

Hernia of abdominal viscera

When a hemidiaphragm is paralyzed, it is practically motionless during quiet breathing but may move upwards for a short distance when a deep inspiration is made. This is even more effectively demonstrated when the patient sniffs. The sniffing procedure causes the normal diaphragm to descend, whereas a paralyzed diaphragm rises upwards in the chest. This "paradoxical movement" of the paralyzed diaphragm is produced by several factors. Inspiratory elevation of the ribs lowers the intrapleural pressure and this has a sucking effect on the paralyzed diaphragm. In addition, the inspiratory descent of the normal diaphragm increases the intra-abdominal pressure, which is transmitted through the abdominal viscera to the undersurface of the paralyzed diaphragm.

The elevated hemidiaphragm associated with a collapsed lobe of the lung, a pulmonary infarction or a subdiaphragmatic abscess shows considerable restriction in its movement, but it moves in a normal direction. Any condition which produces an increase in the intra-abdominal pressure can elevate both leaves of the diaphragm and restrict their movements, but their movements occur in a normal direction.

FUNCTIONAL MANIFESTATIONS

The effect of a paralyzed diaphragm on the respiratory function depends on the degree of paradoxical movement which takes place. Even bilateral paralysis of the phrenic nerves may produce minimal impairment in function if little or no paradoxical movement is present. If there is considerable paradoxical movement, however, both the vital capacity and the maximal breathing capacity are decreased, the residual volume is increased and an abnormal distribution of inspired air occurs. As a result, hypoxia and, in severe cases, hypercapnia may develop. Of greater importance, however, is the fact that paralysis of the diaphragm reduces the effectiveness of the cough reflex.

When a diaphragmatic hernia is present, the ventilatory function may be impaired. The vital capacity is reduced, the amount of reduction depending on the extent of lung compression. The distribution of gas is impaired, so that ventilation-perfusion ratios are altered and hypoxia is produced. Hypercapnia is unlikely to occur unless the herniation is massive or is associated with bronchopulmonary disease affecting the other lung.

CHAPTER XIII

Diseases of the Chest Wall and Thoracic Cage

ANY DISEASE which interferes with the function of the respiratory muscles or increases the resistance to distention of the chest cage may lead to chronic respiratory failure and cor pulmonale, even though there is no underlying bronchopulmonary disease. In addition, a traumatic injury to the thoracic cage may alter the pulmonary function sufficiently to precipitate acute respiratory failure.

In the early stages of these conditions, respiratory function may be only moderately impaired, so that although hypoxia is present, it is not associated with carbon dioxide retention. Nevertheless, the development of even a minor respiratory infection may precipitate acute respiratory failure with severe hypoxia and hypercapnia. Under such circumstances, the patient may be unable to increase his alveolar ventilation sufficiently to cope with the increased metabolism of the infection and the fever because the work of breathing may become so great that even a slight increase in ventilation elevates the carbon dioxide production to such an extent that the arterial carbon dioxide tension may actually rise. In the later stages of these diseases, alveolar hypoventilation frequently becomes the common denominator, although the mechanisms which produce it may be different in individual cases. If the alveolar hypoventilation should persist for any length of time, retention of bicarbonate and secondary polycythemia occur. In addition, pulmonary hypertension and right-sided heart failure may eventually develop in all of these conditions.

DISEASES AFFECTING THE SKIN AND SUBCUTANEOUS TISSUES

The skin of the chest occasionally becomes so thickened, fibrosed, stiff and difficult to move that the respiratory excursion of the chest wall

279

is limited. As a result, the tidal volume is reduced, and alveolar hypoventilation consequently develops. Such a situation may occur in scleroderma or after the healing of an extensive burn over a considerable area of the chest wall. Although scleroderma may occasionally produce pulmonary fibrosis associated with an "alveolocapillary block," the pulmonary insufficiency which develops in this disease may result entirely from involvement of the extrapulmonary structures. The involved skin not only has a waxy sheen, but it is taut and cannot be lifted from the underlying structures, and the induration of the skin increases its resistance to stretching, thus limiting its motion. As a result, the respiratory excursion of the thorax is impaired, so that alveolar hypoventilation, hypoxia and hypercapnia may develop.

OBESITY

An excess deposition of fat over the chest wall and abdomen may limit the respiratory excursion of the thorax, so that even in the absence of any obvious intrinsic pulmonary or cardiac diseases, the pulmonary function may be altered to such an extent that respiratory and cardiac failure occurs. In severe obesity a syndrome may be observed which consists of cyanosis, twitching, a tendency towards excessive lethargy and drowsiness, and periodic breathing. These features usually develop insidiously and may be present for a long time before the patient or his relatives realize their significance. A similar situation often occurs in myxedema. Functional assessment of such patients has shown that the total lung capacity is frequently reduced, presumably because of an elevation of the diaphragm, and that the vital capacity is low. In addition, there may be alveolar hypoventilation with hypoxia and hypercapnia. In a recent study of a large series of obese subjects with no clinical evidence of pulmonary or cardiac disease, 66 per cent had hypoxia, and 30 per cent had an associated hypercapnia. If hypoxia has been present for a considerable time, secondary polycythemia may become a complication. The pulmonary vascular resistance often increases, presumably because of the vasoconstrictive effect of the hypoxia and hypercapnia and because of the increase in the volume and viscosity of the blood produced by the polycythemia. As a result, the pulmonary artery pressure rises and the work of the right ventricle of the heart increases, in some cases so severely that right-sided heart failure or cor pulmonale may develop in the later stages. In the more advanced stages, right ventricular hypertrophy and congestive heart failure may occur.

Although excessive obesity is considered to be the prime factor in the development of this condition, the exact mechanism by which excessive weight can lead to respiratory failure has not been adequately elucidated. The compliance of the lung-thorax system is considerably lower in the obese subject than in the normal entirely because of a reduction in the compliance of the extra-pulmonary structures, indicating that there is an increase in their elastic resistance to distention. This elastic resistance increases even further when the patient assumes the supine position, a finding which may possibly explain why obese patients are nursed more easily in the sitting position and why their condition tends to deteriorate if they are kept supine.

It is generally accepted that the basic physiologic defect in the obese subject is a reduction in the alveolar ventilation. In addition, it has been shown that the oxygen cost of breathing is approximately three times as great in obese persons as in normals. The oxygen consumption associated with an increase in ventilation in an obese and a nonobese subject is shown in Figure 70. It can be seen that a slight increase in ventilation raises the oxygen consumption considerably in obesity, and that this rise becomes precipitous when the ventilation is increased still further. The high oxygen cost of breathing in obese people may be the

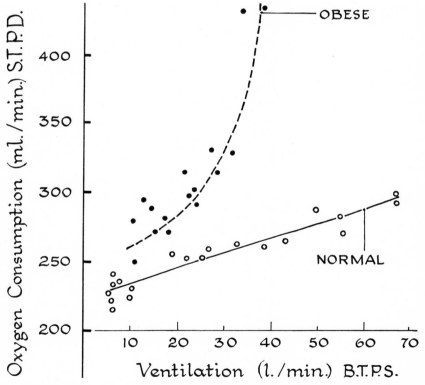

FIGURE 70.   The change in oxygen consumption with increasing ventilation in a normal subject and in an obese subject. (From Cherniack, R. M.: Respiratory effects of obesity. Canad. M.A.J., *80*:613, 1959. By permission.)

result of an increase in the work of breathing, although a reduction in the efficiency of the respiratory muscles has also been demonstrated. This reduced efficiency is similar to that seen in normal subjects who are made to breathe at a lower resting level by applying pressure around the chest.

The high oxygen cost of breathing is of prime clinical importance in obesity, because the level of the arterial carbon dioxide tension is dependent on the ratio between the metabolism and the alveolar ventilation. If the production of carbon dioxide is high in relation to the level of alveolar ventilation, hypercapnia develops. This alveolar hypoventilation is not associated with an increased physiologic dead space, but instead appears to be related to the breathing pattern. An obese person tends to breathe rapidly and shallowly, so that alveolar hypoventilation develops as a result of reduced tidal volume. This respiratory pattern is the type chosen when the work required to overcome elastic resistance is increased, presumably because it is the rate at which the work of breathing is least for that particular alveolar ventilation.

Alveolar hypoventilation is exaggerated if the obese person develops bronchitis or some other pulmonary condition which leads to a further increase in the work of breathing. Likewise, if a patient who is suffering from a chronic bronchopulmonary disease becomes obese, he experiences a further increase in his work of breathing. In both situations there is an increased tendency for alveolar hypoventilation and the consequent development of hypoxia and hypercapnia.

DISEASES AFFECTING THE RESPIRATORY MUSCLES

Any disease process which interferes with the normal function of the respiratory muscles may lead to a serious alteration in pulmonary function and the development of respiratory insufficiency. These disturbances in function may vary from distribution defects due to the unequal expansion of areas of lung tissue, to severe alveolar hypoventilation.

In patients suffering from dermatomyositis, myasthenia gravis or muscular dystrophy, the thoracic muscles may contract asymmetrically because of the varying strength of the intercostal muscles. Different areas of the lung are therefore unequally or asymmetrically inflated, so that the inspired gas is distributed abnormally. Ventilation-perfusion ratios are altered throughout the lung, and hypoxia develops. Occasionally, polycythemia and cor pulmonale may be the presenting clinical features. Carbon dioxide retention does not occur as long as there is hyperventilation of a sufficient number of alveoli. On the other hand, if an excessive muscular weakness should develop, or if an acute respiratory infection should supervene in the above-mentioned conditions, adequate alveolar ventilation may become impossible, with the consequent development of severe hypoxia and carbon dioxide retention.

Adequate inflation of the lungs may become impossible because of the paralysis of the respiratory muscles in patients suffering from poliomyelitis, tetanus, polyneuritis or spinal injuries. As a consequence, severe alveolar hypoventilation with hypoxia and hypercapnia develops, unless artificial respiration is instituted to provide an adequate alveolar ventilation. If hypoxia, either alone or together with hypercapnia, is present for a prolonged period of time in these diseases, it may lead to the development of secondary polycythemia and bicarbonate retention, and pulmonary hypertension and cor pulmonale may follow.

DISEASES AFFECTING THE BONY THORAX

Any condition which increases the resistance of the ribs to movement is liable to produce respiratory insufficiency. Examples are chronic diseases of the thoracic spine such as kyphoscoliosis and rheumatoid spondylitis, and acute conditions such as traumatic chest injuries. If there is a considerable reduction of the chest movements, alveolar hypoventilation becomes a prominent feature, so that severe hypoxia, hypercapnia and cardiac failure may develop.

DEFORMITIES OF THE THORACIC SPINE

Distortion of the chest cage is a frequent consequence of deformities of the thoracic spine. When this occurs it is generally accompanied by a distinctive set of physiological abnormalities which may be present in varying degrees. Severe cardiorespiratory disability develops only in patients who have advanced spinal deformities, such as a kyphosis in which the angle of curvature is greater than 20 degrees, or a scoliosis in which the curvature is greater than 100 degrees. Minor forms of kyphosis and scoliosis do not appear to have any associated cardiorespiratory insufficiency. On the other hand, in kyphoscoliosis the effects of a combination of these two deformities on the circulation and the respiration appear to be additive. In a kyphoscoliosis in which each of these components is only moderate in degree, the alteration of pulmonary function may be equivalent to that produced by a severe form of either kyphosis or scoliosis alone.

When kyphoscoliosis is present, the thoracic cage is distorted and its contents are compressed. An increased elastic resistance to distention of both the lungs and the chest wall results, so that the vital capacity and the total lung capacity are reduced. On the other hand, there is only a very moderate increase in the nonelastic resistance. For this reason, the timed vital capacity and the maximal mid-expiratory flow rate are usually within normal limits. Both the mechanical work of breathing and the oxygen cost of breathing are high because of the raised elastic resistance. The maximal breathing capacity is frequently severely restricted, while the distribution of inspired air is usually only moderately impaired.

The breathing pattern is typically rapid and shallow, presumably because of the increase in the elastic resistance to distention. This particular pattern is probably selected because it requires the least amount of work for breathing. The minute ventilation is often increased. The size of the physiologic dead space is usually unaltered, but alveolar hypoventilation still occurs because of the small tidal volumes, so that hypoxia and hypercapnia develop. Two other factors may aggravate the hypoxia. Although the distribution of inspired air is only moderately impaired, the perfusion is uneven because of the compressed lung, so that the ventilation-perfusion ratios are altered, producing a picture resembling that of venous admixture. In addition, the diffusing capacity is usually reduced, presumably because of a reduction in the size of the pulmonary vascular bed available for diffusion.

In the early stages of kyphoscoliosis the pulmonary arterial pressure is usually normal at rest, but an increased blood flow during exercise may be associated with a considerable rise in the mean pulmonary artery pressure. In the later stages of this condition, pulmonary hypertension may be present even at rest. The increased pulmonary vascular resistance is probably due to mechanical compression of the pulmonary vessels with the consequent reduction in their caliber. A decreased distensibility of some of the vessels, especially those enclosed in airless pulmonary tissue, may also be incriminated. Medial hypertrophy of smaller precapillary vessels similar to that observed in patients who have pulmonary hypertension resulting from an abnormally large pulmonary blood flow probably also aggravates the elevated resistance to blood flow. Hypoxia and hypercapnia, which in themselves produce pulmonary vasoconstriction, are other aggravating factors which increase the pulmonary vascular resistance and lead to pulmonary hypertension.

The work of the right ventricle is increased because of the elevated pulmonary vascular resistance, so that hypertrophy of the right ventricle and eventually right-sided heart failure frequently develop. In severe cases, the chronic hypoxia and hypercapnia may also affect the function of the left ventricle, so that left ventricular failure and pulmonary congestion further complicate the picture.

TRAUMATIC INJURIES TO THE CHEST

Approximately 25 per cent of deaths caused by traffic accidents result from chest injuries. Most such injuries are nonpenetrating, crushing or compression injuries, although occasionally a closed penetrating wound, or very rarely, an open penetrating wound may occur.

Nonpenetrating Injuries. Crush injuries of the chest are usually nonpenetrating. These may consist of a single rib fracture, multiple rib fractures, multiple fractures involving either a single or several ribs, or a fracture of the sternum. The crushing or compression type of chest injury may occur in a variety of ways. There may be a direct crushing or compression beneath a heavy object, such as an automobile, a direct blow to the chest or a deceleration type of compression injury caused by a head-on collision, so that the driver is forcefully thrown against the steering wheel, or his passenger against a seat or panel.

Even though there is no fracture of either the ribs or the cartilages, the chest cage may be compressed in an anteroposterior direction to such an extent that the sternum is practically in contact with the vertebrae. When the compressive force is released, the ribs and the sternum may spring back to their original positions without showing any external evidence of the compression. Multiple hemorrhages throughout the lungs, or rupture of a pulmonary vessel producing a solitary hematoma may occur in such an injury. If any ribs are fractured, they are most likely in the mid-axillary region. If the compressive force is applied in an oblique direction, the rib fractures may be situated posteriorly on one side and anteriorly on the other. Compression of the chest cage, particularly in an elderly person, may result in bilateral fractures of the anterior ends of the ribs, which may or may not be associated with separation of the costochondral or chondrosternal junctions, or even with a fracture of the cartilages.

A "flail" chest results from fractures of multiple ribs or the disruption of several costosternal cartilages. Figure 71 demonstrates that this kind of injury usually causes paradoxical movement of the chest wall at the site of the fractures, so that the affected area is drawn in during inspiration and is pushed out during expiration. When a rib is fractured at two sites, the free fragment of bone is abnormally mobile. As the diaphragm descends and the intrapleural pressure becomes more negative during inspiration, the flail area is pushed inwards by the atmospheric pressure surrounding the chest. During expiration, the intrathoracic pressure becomes greater than that of the atmosphere, causing the flail area to bulge outwards. Because of the paradoxical movement of the affected lung, air may be shunted backwards and forwards from one lung to the other during the phases of respiration so that the patient actually inspires a portion of his expired air. This shunting, called "pendaluft," is equivalent to rebreathing from a dead space. Consequently, the air reaching functioning alveoli has a lower oxygen tension and an elevated carbon dioxide tension. In order to compensate for this, an attempt is made to increase the rate and depth of respiration. Very

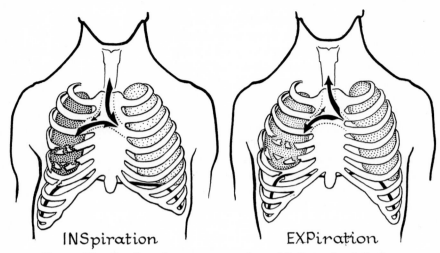

INSpiration   EXPiration

FIGURE 71.   Paradoxical movement and pendaluft in the flail chest.

little benefit is derived from increasing the respiratory rate, however, as most of the movement of air takes place within the dead space. Because of the inadequate alveolar ventilation severe hypoxia and hypercapnia may develop. In severe cases, this paradoxical movement of the chest cage also causes the mediastinum to swing to and fro during respiration, and it interferes with the venous return to the heart. Because the flow of blood into the great veins of the thorax depends to a certain extent on the inspiratory sucking action of the negative intrapleural pressure, the cardiac output may fall, bringing on peripheral vascular collapse.

Penetrating Injuries.   An "open" pneumothorax exists when there is a free communication between the outside air and the pleural cavity through a wound in the thoracic wall. If the wound is wide-open and gaping, air is able to enter the pleural cavity during inspiration and to leave during expiration, causing the mediastinum to shift towards the unaffected side during inspiration and return towards the affected side during expiration. This pendulum movement of the mediastinum may interfere with the normal venous return to the heart and may therefore lead to circulatory failure. In addition, "pendaluft" may occur, air being shunted backwards and forwards from one lung to the other, so that the arterial oxygen tension may fall and the arterial carbon dioxide tension may rise. If this communication should become sealed off, the air in the pleural space constitutes a "closed" pneumothorax.

If the wound remains small and acts as a check-valve, air is able to enter the pleural cavity during inspiration but is prevented from escaping during expiration. The intrapleural pressure consequently rises, producing what is called a "tension" pneumothorax. Because of the elevated intrapleural pressure on the affected side, the mediastinum becomes displaced to the opposite side, resulting in compression of the normal lung. In addition, the raised intrapleural pressure and the deviated mediastinum may impede the venous return to the right side of the heart, resulting in a serious reduction in the cardiac output and hypotension.

Complications of Thoracic Injury. In addition to the severe physiologic imbalances created by the drop in alveolar ventilation, other complications may develop. Pulmonary edema may occur within a few hours after a serious accident. The mechanism of the development of pulmonary edema under such circumstances is not clearly understood. As a further complication, it has been suggested that fracture of even a single rib may cause a measurable reduction of gaseous exchange in the lungs. If the injury has caused a hemothorax or a pneumothorax, the alteration in pulmonary function is greatly aggravated, particularly if air in the pleural space is under tension.

The cough reflex may be affected by the "splinting" of the injured side, making it difficult to expel even normal bronchial secretions. This difficulty may be even further exaggerated by blood or edema fluid in the smaller air passages which may completely obstruct the small bronchi so that the trapped air is absorbed into the pulmonary capillaries with resultant atelectasis of lobules, segments or even lobes of the lung. These atelectatic areas are liable to become infected, especially if there already is sepsis in the tracheobronchial tree.

Laceration of lung parenchyma or tearing of the internal mammary or intercostal vessels may result in serious intrapulmonary bleeding or an intrapleural hemorrhage. Rupture of the tracheobronchial tree, usually near the bifurcation of the trachea or in one of the major bronchi, may take place. A hemothorax, pneumothorax, hemopneumothorax, or occasionally a chylothorax may further complicate the picture.

There may be rupture of one of the chambers of the heart, the aorta, the vena cava, the pulmonary artery or vein, or the azygos vein. Damage to the coronary vessels or the myocardium may also occur. In severe crushing injuries, rupture of the diaphragm may result from the blunt trauma to the chest. This more commonly occurs on the left side and results in protrusion of abdominal viscera into the thoracic space, seriously embarrassing respiration. Rupture of the esophagus rarely takes place, but acute gastric dilatation is a fairly frequent occurrence. The reason for this is obscure but it is seen frequently in any hypoxic insult.

The presence of air in the muscle planes and the subcutaneous tissues is a common accompaniment of nearly all penetrating chest injuries as well as many nonpenetrating ones. The air may track through the subcutaneous tissues over long distances and it may involve the scalp or even the lower extremities.

Mediastinal air results from the rupture of air vesicles within the lung, the escaped air dissecting its way along the pulmonary vessels into the mediastinum and the neck. It may also be produced by rupture of either the trachea or an intramediastinal portion of a bronchus. If mediastinal air is present in large quantities, it may compress the great veins, thereby causing serious impairment of the venous return to the heart. This is usually associated with evident respiratory embarrassment, severe substernal pain and occasionally a "crowing" type of respiration due to compression of the trachea. A crunching sound which is synchronous with the heart beat may be detected by auscultation over the sternum.

An extravasation of blood into the pericardial sac as a result of a rupture or a wound affecting either a chamber of the heart or one of the great vessels within the pericardium may compress the heart and reduce the cardiac output. The venous pressure therefore rises, causing the neck veins to become distended. The jugular venous pressure may rise during inspiration and fall during expiration, probably because of transmission of pressure from the right atrium, which may not be able to enlarge sufficiently to accommodate the increased venous return during inspiration. The blood pressure falls, the pulse pressure becomes smaller, and the cardiac sounds may have a distant quality. In severe cases the patient may lose consciousness as a result of the cerebral hypoxia which develops secondary to the reduced cardiac output.

Clinical Manifestations. In a patient who has suffered a chest injury, there may be local crepitations over the chest wall due to subcutaneous air, or points of tenderness over the fracture sites of the ribs or sternum. If there is an over-riding rib fragment, a localized deformity over the chest wall may be noted. The excursion of the chest wall may lag on one side, or there may be a paradoxical movement which denotes a "flail" chest. If subcutaneous air is present over the base of the neck or in the suprasternal notch, mediastinal air is likely to be present as well. If a pneumothorax or hemothorax is present, the trachea and the apex beat are shifted to the opposite side, and tactile fremitus and breath sounds are absent on the affected side. The percussion note differentiates between pneumothorax and hemothorax since the note is hyperresonant if air is present and dull in the presence of fluid.

Radiological Manifestations. If it is at all possible, x-ray films of the chest with detailed studies of the ribs should be obtained. The number, position and extent of the rib fractures may not be easily determined because of the presence of a hemothorax, subcutaneous air or the lack of displacement of the ribs at the fracture sites. The presence of air or fluid in the pleural space and the shift of the mediastinum are readily apparent.

CHAPTER XIV

Cardiorespiratory Insufficiency

RESPIRATORY insufficiency develops whenever the respiratory apparatus is unable to provide adequate arterial oxygenation or elimination of carbon dioxide. The earliest manifestation of chronic respiratory failure is usually an insufficiency for oxygen exchange; associated insufficiency for carbon dioxide elimination develops later. Severe respiratory insufficiency frequently induces cardiac insufficiency and, conversely, cardiac failure, per se, may also lead to respiratory failure.

RESPIRATORY INSUFFICIENCY

Respiratory insufficiency may develop in patients who are suffering from bronchopulmonary disease, chest wall or thoracic disease, or central respiratory depression. Table 7 illustrates that although the respiratory insufficiency is produced by different mechanisms in these three conditions, the end result is always hypoxia, either alone or in association with hypercapnia.

INSUFFICIENCY OF OXYGEN EXCHANGE

Insufficiency for oxygenation, which produces a fall in the arterial oxygen tension and oxygen content, occurs in patients suffering from pulmonary disease whenever there is a diffusion defect, a venous-to-arterial shunt, unequal ventilation-perfusion ratios or alveolar hypoventilation—or any combination of these conditions.

A diffusion defect occurs when the quality of the membrane is altered, as in pulmonary fibrosis or congestion, or when there is a reduced capillary bed available for diffusion, as in pulmonary emboli, or following pneumonectomy. Carbon dioxide retention does not develop because this gas is able to diffuse across the alveolocapillary membrane 20 times more readily than oxygen. In fact, the arterial carbon dioxide tension is usually low, presumably because of the hyperventilation induced by the

289

TABLE 7

THE MECHANISM OF DEVELOPMENT OF HYPOXIA AND HYPERCAPNIA

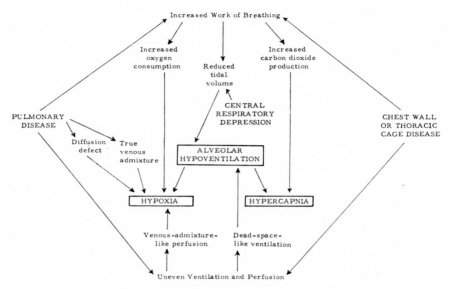

hypoxic stimulus. Consequently, the total carbon dioxide content is low and the pH tends to rise toward alkalotic levels. The inhalation of 100 per cent oxygen completely relieves hypoxia due to this type of disturbance.

In a congenital venous-to-arterial shunt within either the heart or the lungs, there is an admixture of hypoxic, hypercapnic blood with arterialized blood. The altered arterial blood gas tensions induce hyperventilation, and since the lungs are usually healthy, the arterial carbon dioxide tension remains either normal or low, while the pH may tend towards the alkalotic side. Hypoxia is still present, however, for it is not corrected by the hyperventilation. Hypoxia due to this type of disturbance is not corrected by the inhalation of 100 per cent oxygen.

Ventilation-perfusion ratios may vary throughout the lung, because of either uneven ventilation or uneven perfusion, or both. When areas of lung are adequately ventilated but poorly perfused, the air takes little part in gaseous exchange, a condition called dead-space-like ventilation. This in itself does not produce hypoxia, unless the ventilation of the remainder of the lung is inadequate to cope with the increased perfusion. Most patients are usually able to hyperventilate the alveoli that are normally perfused so that the arterial carbon dioxide tension and carbon dioxide content are frequently normal or low, and the pH may tend toward the alkalotic side. If there is perfusion of poorly ventilated alveoli or, in other words, venous admixture-like perfusion, there is a tendency for hypercapnia to develop in association with the hypoxia. Carbon dioxide retention may still not occur if a sufficient number of adequately perfused alveoli are hyperventilated. The hypoxia, however, is not alleviated by the hyperventilation.

INSUFFICIENCY OF BOTH OXYGEN EXCHANGE AND CARBON DIOXIDE ELIMINATION

The amount of carbon dioxide eliminated from the lungs in a minute can be calculated from the formula:

$$\dot{V}_{CO_2} = V_A \times F_{A_{CO_2}}$$

where $\dot{V}_{CO_2}$ is the volume of carbon dioxide eliminated per minute, V_A is the alveolar ventilation per minute and $F_{A_{CO_2}}$ is the concentration of carbon dioxide in the alveoli.

When this formula is rearranged and the concentration of carbon dioxide is converted to its partial pressure, it becomes apparent that the alveolar carbon dioxide tension is intimately related to, and dependent upon, two factors. These are the alveolar ventilation and the metabolic consumption of oxygen or production of carbon dioxide. Thus:

$$pCO_2 = \frac{\dot{V}_{CO_2}}{V_A} \times 0.863$$

or

$$pCO_2 = \frac{\dot{V}_{O_2} \times R}{V_A} \times 0.863$$

where the pCO_2 is either alveolar or arterial, for these are equal; $\dot{V}_{O_2}$ and V_{CO_2} are the oxygen consumption and carbon dioxide production in ml./min.; R is the respiratory quotient; V_A is the alveolar ventilation in l./min., and 0.863 is a correction factor for converting gas volumes to body temperature and the concentration of carbon dioxide to its partial pressure in mm. Hg.

From these formulae it can be seen that retention of carbon dioxide or hypercapnia develops whenever the alveolar ventilation is inadequate relative to the level of the metabolism. Respiratory failure with hypoxia and hypercapnia develops, therefore, whenever the alveolar ventilation diminishes without a proportionate fall in metabolism or there is a rise in oxygen consumption and carbon dioxide production without a proportionate increase in the alveolar ventilation.

Since the tidal volume is composed of both a dead-space component and an alveolar component, alveolar hypoventilation develops if the physiologic dead space is increased or the tidal volume is diminished.

The physiologic dead space is frequently abnormally increased in patients suffering from a variety of bronchopulmonary diseases. A reduced tidal volume is a common finding in patients suffering from bronchopulmonary disease, chest wall and thoracic cage disease, or central respiratory depression, particularly if the work of breathing is increased. Under all of these circumstances, hypoxia is always associated with the hypercapnia unless the patient is inspiring an oxygen-enriched gas mixture.

The responsiveness of the medullary respiratory center to carbon dioxide may be altered under various circumstances. This change may occur in patients suffering from skull injuries, cerebrovascular accidents (particularly if the cerebrospinal fluid pressure is elevated), or overdosage of morphine, barbiturates, tranquilizers or anesthetics. In addition, prolonged hypercapnia due to pulmonary or extrapulmonary disease may in itself lead to central respiratory depression, reduced tidal volume with consequent alveolar hypoventilation, and hypoxia and hypercapnia.

When the partial pressure of carbon dioxide rises because of either a diminished alveolar ventilation or an increased production of carbon dioxide, the arterial pH shifts to the acid side in a manner which is indicated by the Henderson-Hasselbalch equation:

$$\mathrm{pH} = \frac{6.10 + \log \mathrm{HCO_3^-}}{0.0301 \, \mathrm{pCO_2}}$$

This shift results in an accelerated excretion of hydrogen ions and fixed anions and an enhanced renal tubular re-absorption of cations. Consequently, the concentration of buffer anions in the plasma is raised to higher than normal levels. At this time, therefore, the plasma chloride is low, the bicarbonate is elevated, and the pH is nearly normal. The serum sodium is usually normal, while the potassium is frequently elevated.

CARDIAC INSUFFICIENCY SECONDARY TO RESPIRATORY INSUFFICIENCY

Heart failure is a frequent manifestation of severe respiratory disease. Initially, right ventricular failure is usually encountered; left ventricular failure may also develop in the later stages of respiratory insufficiency. The mechanisms by which these conditions are brought about are illustrated in Table 8.

RIGHT VENTRICULAR FAILURE

Right-sided heart failure, a frequent consequence of respiratory insufficiency, develops because of a high pulmonary vascular resistance.

TABLE 8

THE MECHANISM OF DEVELOPMENT OF HEART FAILURE IN RESPIRATORY
DISEASE

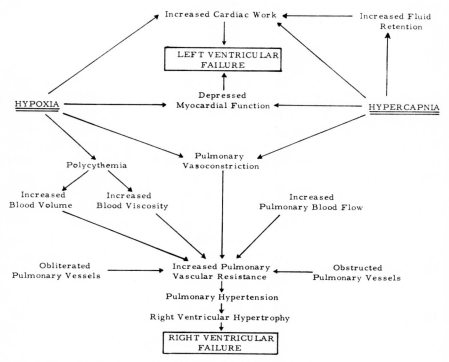

Although the mechanism of production of the increased pulmonary vascular resistance may vary, hypoxia, and in most cases, hypercapnia are the common denominators in all cases of respiratory insufficiency. The altered gas tensions presumably lead to vasoconstriction of the pulmonary vasculature. In addition, the pulmonary vascular resistance may be elevated by the increased blood volume and viscosity due to the secondary polycythemia; by obliteration of pulmonary capillaries, as in kyphoscoliosis, pulmonary fibrosis and chronic obstructive emphysema; or by obstruction of the pulmonary vessels, as in pulmonary embolism. The pulmonary vascular resistance may be further aggravated by the anastomoses which develop between the bronchial and pulmonary circulation in certain pulmonary conditions such as bronchiectasis. Under these circumstances, the high pressure in the bronchial circulation is transmitted to the pulmonary circulation, thereby aggravating the already increased work load of the right side of the heart.

The high pulmonary vascular resistance leads to pulmonary hypertension with subsequent right ventricular hypertrophy and eventual right-sided heart failure. As a result, there are jugular venous distention, hepatic enlargement and peripheral edema. On the other hand, it has been pointed out that edema rarely develops unless the arterial carbon dioxide tension is elevated, and it has been postulated that the consequent compensatory reabsorption of bicarbonate bound to base leads to expansion of the extracllular space and tissue edema.

LEFT VENTRICULAR FAILURE

Although there is no concrete evidence for the development of left ventricular failure in cases of respiratory disease, it probably does occur. With prolonged hypoxia and hypercapnia, the function of the myocardium may be depressed. Autopsies on patients with cardiorespiratory insufficiency have frequently demonstrated multiple fine areas of fibrosis in the myocardium of the left ventricle, probably the result of chronic hypoxia. This, plus the added load of an increased blood volume, may compromise the left ventricle so that it is unable to function efficiently. In those diseases in which excessive bronchopulmonary vascular anastomoses develop, the burden of the collateral circulation falls on the left side of the heart, which may fail. The resultant pulmonary congestion in turn further increases the work of breathing and aggravates the hypoxia so that gross right and left heart failure may be present.

RESPIRATORY INSUFFICIENCY SECONDARY TO CARDIAC INSUFFICIENCY

Just as respiratory failure may lead to left ventricular failure, so primary left ventricular failure may lead to respiratory failure. When the left ventricle fails, as in hypertension or arteriosclerotic myocardial disease, pulmonary congestion develops. As a result, there is an increased barrier to the diffusion of oxygen. If the diffusion defect is predominant, hypoxia and hyperventilation with a normal or low arterial carbon dioxide tension may be encountered. The pulmonary hypertension secondary to the elevated left atrial pressure is aggravated by the hypoxia, so that right ventricular hypertrophy and eventually failure may develop. In fact, left ventricular failure is the commonest cause of right ventricular failure.

THE ASSESSMENT OF

RESPIRATORY

DISEASE

THE CLINICAL ASSESSMENT

THE RADIOLOGICAL ASSESSMENT

THE CLINICAL-PATHOLOGICAL ASSESS-
MENT

THE FUNCTIONAL ASSESSMENT

CHAPTER XV

The Clinical Assessment

FROM THE foregoing sections, it is apparent that the many diseases which affect the respiratory system may alter respiratory function and produce various symptoms. The assessment of the symptoms in their proper chronological sequence, in conjunction with any abnormal physical findings detected during a systematic physical examination, usually establishes the anatomical location and a tentative diagnosis of the particular pattern of disease which is present.

THE HISTORY

In order to obtain a true picture of the various complaints which have led the patient to seek medical advice, it is important that the physician have the patient's complete confidence. The patient should be treated with kindness, consideration and tact, and although specific questions may be necessary at times, it is usually a wise policy to allow the patient to relate his story in his own way, with just enough prompting and guidance on the part of the physician to prevent irrelevancies. The entire historical aspect of the patient's illness is usually recorded under specific headings.

ENTRANCE COMPLAINTS

Before recording the patient's story, it is most important to elicit the primary complaints or the chief symptoms which have caused concern to the patient. These should be enumerated in chronological order and their approximate dates recorded.

THE PERSONAL HISTORY

In addition to a searching and detailed enquiry into the respiratory aspect of the present illness, it is desirable to elicit all of the per-

297

tinent facts about the patient's background, living habits and environment, for these may possibly have some bearing on the development of
the illness. From knowledge of the patient's background and from a
functional review of the nonrespiratory systems, the physician is able to
place the respiratory illness in its proper perspective.

The personal history and habits are of primary importance and
should be investigated in great detail. Some occupations and places of
residence, as well as abnormal dietary habits and improper care, play
important roles in the development of respiratory disease.

Environment. The country of origin and the economic status of
the parents should be recorded. An early life of extreme poverty, with the
associated malnourishment and poor hygienic standards, may predispose
to the development of various diseases such as tuberculosis. The level of
education and the age at which the patient left school often yield considerable information about his insight into his complaints.

Occupation. A detailed and complete occupational history, starting with the patient's very first job, should be elicited and the duration
of each employment should be included. For instance, underground work
in a mine, even twenty or thirty years previously, may be responsible
for the development of pneumoconiosis. Employment in a fluorescent
light factory or residence nearby may result in berylliosis. Other industrial dusts, such as that of asbestos, may also produce pulmonary fibrosis.
Farming may expose a person to several different types of respiratory
diseases. Chicken farming may be the source of histoplasmosis, and
sheep farming may lead to the development of hydatid cysts in the lungs.
A farmer may develop pneumonitis from working in a silo, bronchitis
from the inhalation of fungal spores in a barn, or bronchial asthma as a
result of an allergy to grain dust.

Residence. A detailed chronological account of the specific areas
of each of the countries in which the patient may have resided or visited
in the past should be obtained. Certain countries are notorious for the
prevalence of endemic diseases, especially those which affect the lungs.
In North America, histoplasmosis is endemic in the valleys of the great
rivers, such as the Mississippi, the Ohio and the St. Lawrence, and
coccidioidomycosis is prevalent in the deserts of California and Arizona.
Schistosomiasis is found in Puerto Rico, Central America and Egypt.
Residence in heavy industrial areas may predispose to disease; atmospheric pollution with smoke and fog has been incriminated in the
development and perpetuation of chronic bronchitis and chronic obstructive emphysema.

Personal Habits. The resistance of the patient to disease may be
ascertained from knowledge of his personal habits. Exhausting labor in
poorly ventilated surroundings and insufficient rest are factors which
may play a role in the reduction of resistance to disease. Mental and

financial difficulties as well as continued pressure at work all contribute
to mental fatigue. In addition, malnourishment due to an inadequate
diet increases the susceptibility to disease. This may occur in women
who diet injudiciously in order to lose weight, or in chronic alcoholics
who sacrifice food for alcohol. Gross over-eating and obesity can also
lower the resistance of a person or precipitate cardiorespiratory insufficiency. Excessive cigarette smoking over a prolonged period of time has
been linked to the development of bronchogenic carcinoma and is particularly important in perpetuating chronic bronchitis. Contact with
infected birds and domestic fowl may point to ornithosis, and contact
with dogs, cats or horses may be responsible for attacks of bronchial
asthma.

   Past Illnesses.   An enquiry should be made into the various illnesses which the patient has suffered in the past. In a case of allergic
bronchial asthma, there may be a previous history of infantile eczema,
atopic dermatitis or allergic rhinitis. Measles or pertussis in childhood,
especially if prolonged and associated with pneumonia, may lead to the
development of bronchiectasis. Bronchiectasis should also be suspected
if the patient has had several attacks of pneumonia, especially if they all
affected the same lung or the same lobe of the lung. In the middle-aged
or elderly, repeated attacks of pneumonia involving the same area may
be caused by a bronchogenic carcinoma. A pulmonary abscess should be
suspected if a dental extraction or an operation on the upper respiratory
tract was performed shortly before the onset of the present illness.
Chronic sinus infection with acute episodes may indicate the etiology of
attacks of recurrent bronchitis. Sarcoidosis should be suspected if there
is a history of enlarged painless lymph nodes, dimness of vision in one
or both eyes, a chronic skin eruption or erythema nodosum, all of which
disappeared spontaneously. Pulmonary tuberculosis should be suspected
if the patient has suffered from a draining abscess in a lymph node or
has had an acute attack of serous pleurisy.

FAMILY HISTORY

   An enquiry should be made into all serious illnesses as well as the
cause of any death which may have occurred in the immediate family.
The wife or husband, the children, the siblings and all known relatives
should be included. This is important because it directs attention to
hereditary predispositions to certain diseases, such as mucoviscidosis or
malignancy, or it may indicate contact with an infection such as tuberculosis at some stage in the patient's life. If certain members of the
family have suffered from bronchial asthma or hay fever, the patient
may have inherited an allergic tendency.

REVIEW OF NONRESPIRATORY SYSTEMS

A functional enquiry should be made into the nonrespiratory systems because certain respiratory illnesses may be the consequences of disease processes primarily affecting other organs. For example, a carcinoma of the kidney may have metastasized to the lung, or a pneumonitis may have resulted from aspiration of esophageal contents because of an esophageal stricture.

Nervous System. Cerebral metastasis from a pulmonary neoplasm, a cerebral abscess secondary to bronchiectasis or an attack of tuberculous meningitis may produce symptoms such as a severe intractable throbbing headache, vertigo, diplopia, drowsiness, confusion, disorientation, syncopal attacks and convulsions. However, many of these symptoms may also be caused by carbon dioxide retention. It is not unusual for a patient with severe chronic respiratory insufficiency to be admitted to a neurological ward and investigated for a suspected expanding intracerebral lesion. Paraesthesias associated with muscular wasting and weakness of the limbs may be due to a peripheral neuropathy which occasionally complicates a bronchogenic carcinoma. The development of weakness in a group of muscles in association with respiratory insufficiency may be due to a mild attack of poliomyelitis or infectious polyneuritis.

Emotional disturbances may well be responsible for many of the patient's complaints. Conversely, the thought that the respiratory symptoms are due to some incurable organic disease may engender symptoms of anxiety and apprehension in the patient with respiratory disease, and as a result he may become irritable, depressed and highly emotional and may have difficulty in sleeping.

Cardiovascular System. Symptoms such as exertional dyspnea, palpitation and ankle swelling may point to the development of cor pulmonale secondary to a respiratory disease. The development of orthopnea and an increase in the number of pillows used during sleep suggest the onset of left ventricular failure. A recent attack of severe substernal pain followed by dyspnea suggests a myocardial infarction and possible pulmonary congestion. An attack of pleuritic or anginal chest pain in a patient with heart failure or a swollen, painful and tender limb suggests the possibility of a pulmonary embolus.

Gastrointestinal System. Aspiration of esophageal contents into the tracheobronchial tree may occur when there is difficulty in swallowing, due to either a stricture or a malignant process in the esophagus. A similar situation may arise from a hiatus hernia or a dilated esophagus due to achalasia of the esophageal sphincter.

Anorexia and vague dyspeptic complaints may be associated with toxemia from active pulmonary tuberculosis or any chronic bronchopulmonary disease, such as bronchiectasis. A postprandial epigastric pain which is relieved by the ingestion of food and alkalies suggests peptic ulceration which is occasionally seen in association with chronic obstructive emphysema. Diarrhea may indicate the development of amyloidosis if the patient is suffering from a suppurative pulmonary disease, carcinoid tumor of the bowel, tuberculous ulceration of the bowel or adrenal insufficiency caused by tuberculosis or metastases.

Genitourinary System. Frequency, dysuria and hematuria may be due to tuberculous involvement of a kidney, and hematuria may also be produced by a renal carcinoma. A painful or swollen testicle may indicate tuberculous or malignant involvement. Amenorrhea is not an uncommon accompaniment of pulmonary tuberculosis as well as many other wasting diseases.

Metabolic System. Weakness, fatigability and weight loss are frequently present in most chronic respiratory diseases. A rapid loss of weight may occur in active pulmonary tuberculosis or malignancy. A rapid gain in weight may lead to alveolar hypoventilation and the symptoms related to hypoxia and carbon dioxide retention.

Locomotor System. The presence of clubbing of the fingers since birth or early childhood is significant, as is the onset of acquired clubbing which may have been noticed by the patient. The thickened bones of hypertrophic pulmonary osteoarthropathy may be noted. Painful, tender, discolored areas of erythema nodosum, which commonly occur over the extensor surfaces of the legs, may provide a clue to the possibility of tuberculosis or sarcoidosis. The onset of weakness in specific groups of muscles may suggest poliomyelitis or infectious polyneuritis.

The finding of a tremor may indicate hyperthyroidism as the cause of a complaint of dyspnea. On the other hand, a flapping tremor of the hands, similar to that which occurs in hepatic coma, is also seen in severe carbon dioxide retention.

THE HISTORY OF PRESENT ILLNESS

With the information obtained by judicious questioning as suggested in the foregoing sections, one is equipped to tackle the important part of the history, that which deals with the respiratory illness itself.

A chronological history of the respiratory illness should be obtained, the patient being prodded to begin his story from the time that he last felt "completely well." After the onset of the symptoms has been established, it is essential to obtain a detailed chronological description of the progress of each complaint. The mode of onset of each symptom, whether acute or gradual; its progress, whether continuous or recurrent; its development, whether progressive or stationary, should all be carefully elucidated. If it is an acute illness, a description of the day-by-day or even hour-by-hour events should be elicited. If it is a chronic illness, the progression of events from month to month or year to year is important.

Having obtained this general picture of the illness, the physician next asks for a detailed description of each symptom. The patient usually complains of one or more of the following symptoms: cough, sputum, hemoptysis, dyspnea, chest pain, fever, excess fatigability and loss of weight. The mechanisms of development and the significance of such symptoms have already been discussed in Chapter V. The following discussion deals with the type of questions that should be asked by the historian in order to clarify each of the major symptoms of respiratory disease.

Cough. The date of the onset of the cough and its progression, or even the absence of a cough, should be recorded. Is the cough present relatively constantly, or is it recurrent? What are its characteristics? Is it dry or productive? Does it sound brassy, or is it wheezy? Has it been increasing in severity? What is its chief time of occurrence? Is it related to posture and does it awaken the patient from his sleep? If it is paroxysmal, are there any known precipitating factors? Are the attacks of coughing ever associated with dizziness or fainting spells? How is the cough relieved?

Expectoration. If the cough has become productive, it is important to record the date expectoration began and whether it has increased in amount. The daily volume and the color of the sputum should be ascertained, both when it first developed and during its progression to the time of the examination. Do the volume and the color of the sputum vary during the day, and if so, when is the largest amount expectorated? Is it "hawked up" from the back of the throat, or does it come up from the chest? Does the sputum come up easier in any particular posture? What is the consistency of the sputum; is it thin and watery or thick and viscid? Does it have an odor or a taste? The history of a sudden expectoration of a large amount of foul sputum suggests the possibility of a lung abscess.

Hemoptysis. The date of each hemoptysis should be carefully recorded, with minute detail regarding the amount of blood expectorated during each bout, as well as the nature and consistency of the blood. Occasionally, the patient can actually localize the site of the origin of the blood. Was there any associated bleeding from the nose or gums, or is there a bleeding tendency elsewhere? It is important to enquire whether a hemoptysis was associated with pain in the chest, shortness of breath or fever.

Dyspnea. If dyspnea is present, the date of its onset and its progression, if any, should be noted. Does the dyspnea occur during rest, on exertion, or while the patient is lying down? Does the breathing difficulty occur during inspiration or expiration, and is it constant or recurrent? If the dyspnea is not constant, is it related to exertion or to some other precipitating factor? If it occurs with exertion, what is the exercise tolerance? How far can the patient walk without dyspnea, and how many flights of stairs can he climb? How often do attacks of dyspnea occur, and how long do they last? If there is associated wheezing, when does this begin, and what relieves it? Is it associated with chest pain or coughing spells, and is it relieved by the expectoration of sputum? Is he awakened at night by dyspnea, and if so, what relieves the attack? Does it disappear gradually, or does it improve only after some sputum has been expectorated?

Chest Pain. If there is chest pain, when did it begin, and was its onset sudden or gradual? What is its anatomical location? Does it radiate, and where to? Is it dull and aching or sharp and knife-like? Is it constant or intermittent, and has it increased in severity? What is the effect of coughing, deep breathing, changes in posture, belching or exercise? Is there any associated area of tenderness on the chest wall? How is the pain relieved?

Upper Respiratory Symptoms. Is the upper respiratory tract a possible source of infection in the lungs? Does the patient have frequent head colds, sore throats, hoarseness or plugging of the nose? Are these associated with sinus headaches, a postnasal discharge or nose bleeds? What is the condition of the teeth and gums? Has there been a history of possible aspiration of infected material from the upper respiratory tract?

Constitutional Symptoms. The onset and duration of fever, chills, excessive sweating, anorexia, weakness, excessive fatigue or weight loss and their relationship to the other symptoms should be recorded and assessed. These usually have already been elicited in the functional enquiry.

THE PHYSICAL EXAMINATION

After the complete history has been elucidated, the historian is able to piece the pertinent pieces of information together so that several probable diagnoses are suspected. These suspicions may now be strengthened and consolidated by the physical examination. The following account presents the methods used to examine the patient in order to demonstrate the various abnormal signs produced by respiratory disease. A mastery of these methods is essential in order to arrive at a correct diagnosis. Of equal importance is the attitude of the examiner towards the patient. He should be courteous and considerate and should avoid any unnecessary discomfort for the patient. In addition, the room temperature must be comfortable, the lighting adequate and, above all, the patient co-operative.

Just as a functional enquiry into the nonrespiratory systems is important in the history of the respiratory illness, a thorough and complete physical examination of the entire body is equally important. Although it is not within the scope of this dissertation to cover the complete physical examination, it is obvious from the previous sections that respiratory disturbances may produce signs and symptoms which are referable to other systems. In addition, abnormal physical findings in organs other than the lungs frequently yield valuable clues as to the nature of the respiratory illness. In the following discussion, a detailed description of the examination of the respiratory system is presented. The mode of examination of the remaining systems is not included, and only those findings which may be helpful in assessing findings in the respiratory system are referred to.

The examination should be carried out in an orderly, systematic manner and in exactly the same fashion in every patient, so that no abnormal physical sign is missed. It is through errors of omission that failures in diagnosis occur.

GENERAL OBSERVATION

Inspection of the patient, as the initial phase of the physical examination, should be conducted conscientiously and meticulously before any other attempt is made at eliciting signs of disease. Much that is learned from inspection is acquired automatically and unconsciously. For instance, anyone, no matter what his training has been, can make a fairly accurate guess at the age of a casual acquaintance, but he is quite unable to describe the physical evidence on which that judgment is based. Even lay people habitually scrutinize an associate and decide from what they see that he "looks well" or "does not look well." In a similar way, experienced clinicians unconsciously gather valuable impressions by pure abstraction. This occult faculty largely accounts for what is termed "clinical intuition."

In the following notes some of the common physical abnormalities that may be seen are enumerated and briefly discussed. Any single observation is of little value, but in combination with other signs it may be of extreme value in arriving at a final assessment of the underlying respiratory disease.

THE HEAD

It is impossible to enumerate all the factors that may be detected from even a casual glance at a patient's face. One can usually immediately determine, however, whether or not the patient is in distress and whether the distress is psychical or physical in origin. From the facial expression, one often involuntarily estimates the mental capacity, the general character, the temperament and the mood of the patient. More specific physical facts should also be gathered, particularly whether there is respiratory distress, pallor, plethora, cyanosis, pigmentation, rash, jaundice, edema, venous dilatation, emaciation and obesity.

It is extremely important to note the presence or absence of respiratory distress when evaluating respiratory disorders. Does the patient look as though he is having difficulty breathing, and are the accessory muscles of respiration being used? Widening of the alae nasae during inspiration points to a difficulty in breathing. Is the respiratory difficulty chiefly during either inspiration or expiration, or both, and is there audible wheezing? The breathing pattern should also be noted. Normal persons breathe at a rate of twelve to eighteen respirations per minute. An increased rate of breathing is called *tachypnea,* and a slower than normal rate is called *bradypnea.* A slow, deep, regular type of breathing, called *Kussmaul breathing,* is seen in patients suffering from metabolic acidosis. In addition, the respiratory rhythm may be abnormal. Several types of irregular breathing are frequently encountered in disease states. The commonest irregularities are *Cheyne-Stokes respiration*— a cyclical waxing and waning in the intensity of the respiratory movements—and its variant, *Biot's respiration*—a short, rapid breathing interrupted by complete pauses. Although these respiratory arrhythmias are occasionally seen in normal persons during sleep and in the very obese even while awake, their development in the presence of respiratory, cardiovascular or renal disease is usually of grave significance.

Localized neurological signs may be suggestive of a cerebral abscess secondary to a pulmonary abscess or bronchiectasis, or a metastasis from a bronchogenic carcinoma. A toxic delirium may occur in the severe acute respiratory infections. Confusion, irrational behavior and hallucinations may be caused by severe respiratory insufficiency and carbon dioxide retention. Tuberculous meningitis may develop in association with miliary tuberculosis. Although pneumococcal meningitis occurs very rarely, meningismus may occur in pneumococcal pneumonia.

The Eyes. The finding of exophthalmos in a dyspneic patient may be due to either hyperthyroidism or compression of the trachea by a substernal toxic thyroid gland. Argyll Robertson pupils, which are indicative of syphilis, may be associated with an aneurysm of the aorta compressing a bronchus. A unilateral Horner's syndrome can be produced by a bronchogenic carcinoma involving the cervical sympathetic ganglia on the same side.

The Upper Respiratory Tract. As has been described earlier, diseases affecting the upper respiratory tract either may be the sole cause of or may play a contributory role in the production of respiratory symptoms. Whether this part of the respiratory tract is healthy or not may be determined largely by inspection. A searching examination of the mucous membranes of the nose, the mouth, the tongue, the gums, the pharynx and the larynx should, therefore, precede the examination of the lungs. Inspection of these mucous membranes may reveal cyanosis or the reddish purple color associated with polycythemia.

The patency of each nasal passage should be tested by having the patient sniff through one while the other is obstructed. In addition, a nasal speculum should be used to examine the interior of the nose. The appearance of the nasal mucosa and the character of any nasal discharge should be noted. In the presence of inflammation, the mucosa is redder than normal, and the discharge may be purulent. In allergic rhinitis, the mucosa is boggy and pale, the discharge is thin, watery and clear, and the passageway is frequently obstructed. Nasal polyps are often associated with this condition. The appearance and position of the nasal septum should also be noted, for a deviated septum may lead to nasal obstruction and subsequent infection. The presence of a purulent exudate in one or both passages or a purulent postnasal discharge may indicate chronic purulent sinusitis. This may be the factor involved in recurrent bronchitis or exacerbations of infection in bronchiectasis. Fresh blood in one of the passages may indicate the origin of a recent hemoptysis.

The buccal mucosa should be carefully examined for eruptions, petechiae and pigmentation. An odorous breath, particularly if it is offensive, may result from improper oral hygiene and pyorrhea or from a chronic infection of the tonsils, the adenoids or the nasal mucosa. In addition, any septic diseases of the lungs, such as bronchiectasis and lung abscess, or pyloric obstruction secondary to a duodenal ulcer or gastric carcinoma may make the breath malodorous. The condition of the gums and teeth should be checked, for poor dental care and pyorrhea may be the factors in the development of bronchopulmonary diseases. The presence (or absence) of a postnasal discharge and whether it is mucoid or purulent should be noted. In a child, hypertrophied adenoids, especially if associated with chronic tonsillar infection, may cause a recurrent bronchitis, and an abnormally lengthened or inflamed uvula may be the cause of a persistent cough.

Inspection of the larynx is not usually a part of the routine physical examination. However, it is essential that it be performed if the patient complains of hoarseness, a croupy cough or aphonia. Although this examination should be made by direct laryngoscopy, it is more frequently done indirectly with a laryngeal mirror.

THE NECK

Inspection of the neck may yield important clinical information. Engorgement of the veins of the neck or visible pulsations in these veins in a patient who is propped up at an angle of 45 degrees, so that the veins are at a higher level than the right auricle, are abnormal and indicate that the venous pressure is increased. Bilateral jugular venous distention is usually due to congestive heart failure, although it may also be produced by obstruction of the superior vena cava when it is associated with visible collateral veins over the neck and anterior chest wall. Distention of both jugular veins, particularly during expiration, is not an unusual finding in patients suffering from severe obstructive bronchiolar disease.

A painful stiff neck due to cervical disc degeneration may be associated with irritation of the cervical nerve roots and upper chest pain. A swelling due to enlarged cervical nodes or thyroid gland may be quite evident. An enlarged, hard, fixed thyroid gland may be carcinomatous and may be the source of pulmonary metastases. Lymphadenopathy may be due to tuberculosis, malignancy, sarcoidosis, infectious mononucleosis or one of the lymphomas. Scars on the neck may be the result of draining sinuses or operative removal of a tuberculous adenitis.

Palpation is used to determine the position, the resiliency, the consistency, the size and the anatomic relations of the various masses or lumps that may have been discovered by inspection. It serves to differentiate whether various masses in the neck are lymph nodes, the thyroid gland or soft tissue. Lymph nodes should always be searched for in the jugular region, the supraclavicular areas, the axillae and the epitrochlear and inguinal regions. The finding of an enlarged supraclavicular node may frequently aid in the diagnosis of bronchogenic carcinoma and may serve as a guide to its operability.

CLUBBING OF DIGITS

Inspection of the hands and feet for the presence of clubbing is an absolutely essential part of the physical examination for disorders of the respiratory system. Clubbing of the fingers and toes is an important manifestation of respiratory disease, and its presence is therefore of great diagnostic significance.

When the lateral aspect, or profile, of the terminal phalanx of a finger of a healthy person is examined, the proximal end of the nail forms an obtuse angle of approximately 160 degrees with the soft tissues covering the root of the nail. The earliest sign of digital clubbing is hypertrophy of these soft tissues, so that this "base angle" is gradually obliterated and becomes 180 degrees or greater. Obliteration of the "base angle" is a constant feature throughout the progress of the condition. The normal "base angle" and that seen in digital clubbing are shown in Figure 72.

The further progression of this condition is shown in Figure 73.

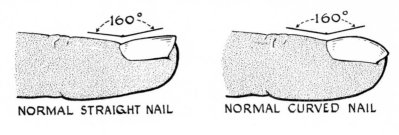

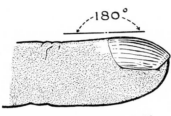

NORMAL STRAIGHT NAIL   NORMAL CURVED NAIL

CLUBBED NAIL, EARLY

FIGURE 72. The "base angle" in a normal digit, in a digit with a curved nail and in a clubbed digit.

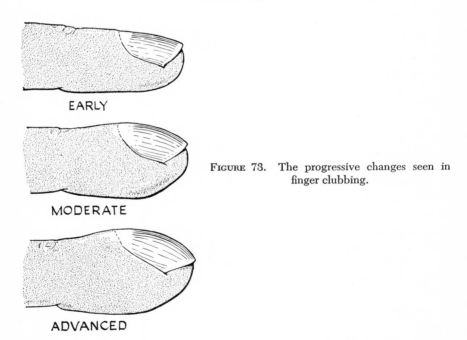

EARLY

MODERATE

FIGURE 73. The progressive changes seen in finger clubbing.

ADVANCED

As the clubbing becomes more severe, the skin overlying the nail bed becomes stretched and glistening and loses its normal wrinkles, so that it looks as if it had been polished by a nail buffer. The nail itself then

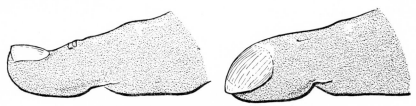

FIGURE 74.   A normal and a clubbed big toe.

gradually thickens, becoming curved and developing longitudinal ridges. At the same time, the pulp of the terminal phalanx enlarges and eventually becomes blunted and bulbous. In the advanced stage, the nail is thickened, ridged and curved both in its longitudinal and transverse planes, and the distal end of the nail overrides the end of the finger so that it resembles a parrot's beak. The nail itself is easily moved by pressure and gives the impression of lying on a bed of fluid.

It is important that clubbing of the digits should not be confused with the curving of normal nails occasionally found in perfectly healthy people. As is seen in Figure 72, it superficially resembles moderately advanced clubbing and is frequently mistaken for it, because the nails are curved in both longitudinal and transverse directions and may even be thickened. Their distinguishing feature, however, is the "base angle" which, in contrast to digital clubbing, is normal, always remaining at 160 degrees.

The thumb and index finger are usually first affected, and the other fingers become involved later as the condition progresses. The condition is usually bilateral, although unilateral clubbing in which the digits of only one hand are affected may also occur. Unidigital clubbing, in which only one finger of a single hand is involved, has also been described. As the terminal phalanges of the toes are normally misshapen, clubbing of these digits is not as obvious as that which takes place in the fingers. The appearance of the terminal phalanx of the big toe more closely approximates that of the fingers, however, and it is this digit which should be examined for clubbing. The appearance of the normal and the clubbed big toe is shown in Figure 74.

With further progression of the condition, hypertrophic pulmonary osteoarthropathy may develop. This is suggested by the presence of thickening and tenderness of the ankles and wrists in the presence of gross digital clubbing.

THE CHEST

In order to proceed with the examination of the chest, a knowledge of the boundaries of the thoracic contents is essential. With this knowledge, the examiner is able to have a mental picture of what lies directly beneath his examining fingers or the stethoscope.

Surface Anatomy. Certain conventional topographical lines are used to demarcate various areas on the chest wall. The *mid-clavicular line* runs vertically downwards over the anterior chest wall from the middle of the clavicle to the lower costal margin. The *mid-axillary line* runs vertically downwards over the lateral area of the chest wall from the middle of the apex of the axilla to the lower costal margin. When the arms hang by the side, the *mid-scapular line* runs vertically downwards from the middle of the inferior angle of the scapula to the kidney angle.

There are also certain important landmarks on the surface of the chest wall which help to orientate the examiner regarding the position of the underlying thoracic contents. These are principally the spinous processes of the thoracic vertebrae, which are easily palpable along the whole course of the thoracic spine. When the patient is erect with his head bent slightly forward, the first thoracic spine is easily recognized since it is the lower one of two prominent projections at the junction of the neck and the thorax, the upper projection being the spinous process of the seventh cervical vertebra. When the patient is in an erect position with the arms hanging loosely by the side, the third thoracic spine is situated at the level of the root of the spine of the scapula, and the seventh thoracic spine lies at the level of the inferior angle of the scapula. The *kidney angle,* which is at the junction of the posterior end of the costal margin and the sacrospinalis muscle, is situated at the same level as the twelfth thoracic spine.

The *sternal angle,* or *angle of Louis,* which marks the sternal attachment of the second and, rarely, the third costal cartilage, is situated in the front of the chest at the same level as the fifth thoracic spine and the lower border of the fourth thoracic vertebra. The sternal angle, which also lies at the same level as the bifurcation of the trachea, indicates the approximate upper level at which the lungs meet anteriorly and the upper limit of the auricles of the heart. In order to demonstrate the presence of an increased venous pressure, therefore, the arms must be elevated above the level of the sternal angle. The veins collapse when the arms are elevated to this level if the pressure is normal.

When the arms are held at the sides, the hilum of the lung, which lies posteriorly in the chest, corresponds to a rectangular area on the surface of the chest between the spine and the vertebral border of both scapulae at the level of the fourth, fifth and sixth vertebrae. The apices of both lungs lie in the root of the neck and are closely covered by pleura. The apex of each lung occupies an area which starts at the lower end of the sternoclavicular junction, curving upwards to about one inch above the clavicle and then descending to the lower end of the clavicle, at the junction of its lateral and middle thirds.

The anterior border of the right pleural space can be indicated by a line drawn from the sternoclavicular joint to the center of the angle of Louis and then straight down the sternum as far as the xiphisternal joint. The surface markings of the anterior border of the right lung correspond almost exactly to that of the right pleura, for the lung lies just a little inside it.

On the left side, the anterior border of the pleura corresponds to a line drawn from the left sternoclavicular joint to the center of the angle of Louis and then down to the level of the fourth costal cartilage, where it turns laterally to the left border of the sternum, and then runs downwards to the seventh costal cartilage. The anterior border of the left lung occupies a position slightly inside the pleura until the fourth left costal cartilage is reached, when it turns laterally along the fourth costal cartilage to a point about 3 cm. from the left sternal border. From here it again turns downwards and ends at the sixth costal cartilage, about 2.5 cm. from the border of the sternum.

The inferior borders of both pleural spaces correspond to a line starting at the lower ends of both anterior margins and then running backwards, crossing the sixth ribs at the mid-clavicular line, the eighth ribs in the mid-axillary line and the twelfth ribs in the mid-scapular line, finally ending about 2.5 cm. lateral to the twelfth thoracic spine. The posterior part of these lines is fairly horizontal and passes through

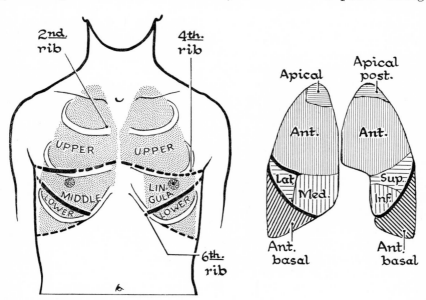

SURFACE MARKINGS

FIGURE 75. Surface markings of the lungs (anterior aspect).

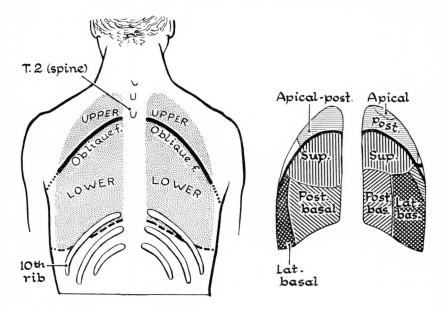

SURFACE MARKINGS

FIGURE 76.   Surface markings of the lungs (posterior aspect).

the kidney angle, ending at the medial ends of the twelfth ribs. The inferior borders of both lungs correspond to those of the pleura in its anterior part, crossing the mid-clavicular and mid-axillary lines at the sixth and eighth ribs, respectively. Thereafter, they cross the mid-scapular line at the tenth rib posteriorly and end at the level of the tenth thoracic spine. The posterior borders of the pleurae and lungs run parallel to one another, that of the lung being just lateral to the pleural border, which lies about one inch from the thoracic spinous processes. These borders start at the posterior ends of their inferior margins and run upwards as high as the seventh cervical spine.

The situation of the various lobes of both lungs is illustrated in Figures 75 to 77. The major, or oblique, fissures in both lungs form the lower and upper borders, respectively, of the upper and lower lobes. Similarly, the transverse fissure of the right lung separates its upper lobe from the middle lobe.

THE OBLIQUE FISSURE.   The oblique fissures run identical courses in both lungs. Their projection on the surface of the chest wall can be mapped out by marking a line starting at the second thoracic spine posteriorly and running obliquely downwards, curving around the chest wall over its posterior, lateral and anterior aspects. It crosses the mid-axillary line at the fifth rib and ends anteriorly at the inferior border of the sixth costal cartilage, midway between the mid-sternal and mid-clavicular lines. If the patient stands erect and places his hands behind his neck, the position of the scapulae is such that their vertebral borders correspond to the posterior parts of the oblique fissures.

THE TRANSVERSE FISSURE. The minor or transverse fissure, which is present only in the right lung, forms the upper border of the middle lobe and separates it from the upper lobe. The lingular segment of the left upper lobe corresponds morphologically to the right middle lobe and it possesses its own bronchus, although a true fissure is generally absent. The transverse fissure is outlined on the chest wall by a line starting at the anterior border of the lung at the level of the third or fourth intercostal space. It then passes laterally, in a slightly upward direction, ending at the point where the oblique fissure crosses the mid-axillary line.

THE BRONCHOPULMONARY SEGMENTS. The bronchopulmonary segments correspond to certain areas over the chest wall within the confines of the boundaries of the lobes.

The anterior segment of the upper lobe of the right and left lungs covers an area over each upper anterior chest between the levels of the clavicle and the transverse fissure. The apical segment of the right lung occupies the area of the lung above the clavicle anteriorly, as well as a small area posteriorly in the apex of the lung. The remainder of the

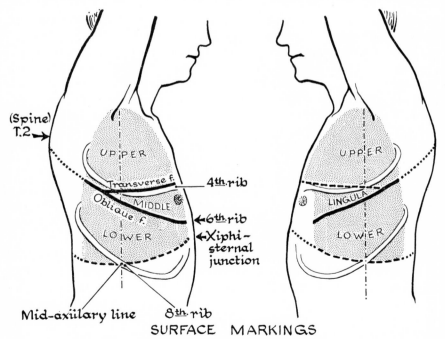

SURFACE MARKINGS

FIGURE 77. Surface markings of the lungs (lateral aspect).

whole of the posterior aspect of the right upper lobe is occupied by its posterior segment. The apical-posterior segment of the left upper lobe occupies an area similar to that occupied by the apical and posterior segments of the right upper lobe.

The right middle lobe is divided into medial and lateral segments which are of approximately equal size. The medial segment is situated over that part of the middle lobe which occupies the anterior surface of the chest, and the lateral segment occupies the remaining area of the middle lobe, lying over the anterior portion of the axilla. The lingular segment of the left upper lobe lies under an area over the left anterior chest wall which is identical to that of the middle lobe of the right lung. It has two bronchopulmonary segments, a superior and an inferior. The superior segment, as the name implies, is situated above the inferior segment, occupying approximately the upper half of the lingular area.

The surface anatomy of the bronchopulmonary segments of the two lower lobes is very similar. The superior or apical segment occupies the upper part of the posterior aspect of the lower lobe, its upper boundary being the oblique fissure and its lower boundary corresponding approximately to the spinous process of the seventh thoracic vertebra. The remainder of the posterior aspect of the lower lobe is occupied by the posterior basal segment. The axillary aspect of the lower lobe is occupied by the lateral basal segment, and that part of the lower lobe on the anterior surface of the chest wall is occupied by the anterior basal segment. The medial basal segment of the right lower lobe, which lies next to the mediastinum, has no comparable area over the surface of the chest wall.

THE HEART.   The apex beat of the heart, which corresponds to the apex of the left ventricle, can be felt and frequently can also be seen. It is normally situated in the fifth left intercostal space, 3.5 inches from the mid-line of the sternum. The left border of the heart, which is formed by the appendage of the left atrium superiorly and by the left ventricle, starts one inch from the left border of the sternum at the level of the second costal cartilage and runs convexly to the left as far as the apex of the heart. The right border of the heart, which is formed entirely by the right atrium, corresponds to a line which is slightly convex to the right running between the third and sixth costal cartilages, about one-half inch from the right border of the sternum. The superior border of the heart, which is formed by the right and left atria, corresponds to a line drawn between the upper ends of the left and right borders. The inferior border of the heart, which is formed chiefly by the right ventricle and partly by the left ventricle, is located by a line joining the lower ends of the left and right borders and passing over the xiphisternal joint. Normally, the borders of the pericardial sac correspond to those of the heart.

Inspection of the Chest. Much valuable information suggestive of underlying respiratory disease can be gained by careful inspection of the chest. There are wide variations in the general contours of normal thoracic cages, but the bony structure of the chest cage is normally symmetrical. Its symmetry is largely related to a straight thoracic spine, so that deformities of the thoracic spine can produce corresponding alterations in the chest cage. These may be easily overlooked unless the thoracic spine is routinely examined, both by inspection and palpation of the spinous processes.

Scoliosis, kyphosis and kyphoscoliosis should be carefully looked for. In scoliosis with convexity to the right, the lateral margins of the thoracic vertebrae become more widely spaced on the right, or convex, side. As a result, the ribs are diverged on the convex side and are converged on the concave, or left, side. Thus, the right side of the chest is more prominent, the left side of the chest is retracted, and the sternum is deviated from its mid-line position towards the left. The extent of disfiguration which the chest undergoes varies with the degree of deformity of the thoracic spine.

Other deformities of the thorax which should be looked for are funnel-chest and pigeon-breast. The funnel-chest deformity consists of an abnormal depression of the lower end of the sternum and the costal cartilages in that region. The pigeon-breast deformity consists of a protrusion of the lower part of the sternum with its attached cartilages. These deformities of the thorax are usually of no serious significance, although severe grades of funnel-chest may so distort and compress the mediastinum that cardiac and respiratory embarrassment may develop in later years.

THORACIC MOVEMENT. There is no absolute standard of normal chest movement, so that only a definite departure from the average can be regarded as significant. In generalized obstructive disease of the bronchi, the chest is frequently barrel-shaped, tending to move up and down "as a whole" during breathing. An inequality of movement of the two sides of the chest is most important, for it suggests that there is some underlying disease in the side which moves less. Although the costal margin normally moves outwards during inspiration, it may occasionally move paradoxically inwards during inspiration and outwards during expiration. This may occur in conditions in which the diaphragm has been pushed down, so that it loses its dome-shape.

An additional very important observation is the presence of "indrawing," which is frequently seen over the lower lateral part of the chest cage. In this condition the intercostal spaces are sucked in during inspiration, usually because of fibrosis and retraction of the lung or chronic obstructive emphysema. If the indrawing is sudden in onset it is usually due to acute bronchial obstruction with subsequent atelectasis.

THE APEX BEAT. If the cardiac impulse is visible, its character, exact position and extent should be noted. The position of the apex beat is extremely important in the differential diagnosis of the underlying respiratory disease, and the character of the impulse may suggest right or left ventricular enlargement.

COLLATERAL VEINS. The presence of engorged superficial veins over the chest wall usually indicates the presence of partial or complete obstruction of the superior vena cava. If the vena azygos is still patent, the veins are dilated only over the upper half of the anterior chest wall. Dilated veins are found over the lower chest as well if the vena azygos is also obstructed.

Palpation. POSITION OF MEDIASTINUM. An alteration in the size of the lungs is reflected by a shift of the mediastinum from its normal mid-line position. When such a shift takes place, it is indicated by a similar change in the position of the trachea and the apex of the heart.

In order to locate the apex beat, the third, fourth, fifth and sixth left interspaces should be explored from the mid-axillary line to the sternal edge, using the tip of one finger. It is the point furthest to the left and downward at which a definite systolic impact can be felt. The normal position of the apex is in the fifth left interspace 3.5 inches from the mid-sternum. If the apex beat is lateral to this, the heart is either hypertrophied or displaced. The apex beat frequently cannot be found, especially in sthenic or obese subjects. With hyperinflation of the lungs, the apex beat may not be palpable, although the action of the heart may be seen and felt in the epigastrium.

The intensity of the cardiac impulse is noted by placing the palm of the hand firmly over the left inframammary region. A localized systolic thrust is felt in a normal heart, but a heave is imparted to the ribs if there is left ventricular hypertrophy. If there is right ventricular hypertrophy, a thrust may be felt just to the left of the sternum, and a simultaneous retraction occurs over the left ventricle, so that a rocking motion is produced.

The trachea is a more sensitive guide to the position of the mediastinum than is the apex beat because the heart, which is filled with blood and therefore is a comparatively heavy organ, does not move as easily as does the trachea, which lies in the least anchored portion of the mediastinum. The position of the trachea is determined by insertion of the fully extended index finger into the patient's suprasternal notch, just medial to one sternoclavicular joint, as shown in Figure 78. The tip of the finger is then pressed gently back towards the cervical spine. The procedure is then repeated on the other side, using the same finger. It is important that the trachea be palpated at a level no higher than the suprasternal notch, since this is the upper limit of its mediastinal portion. Small deviations of the position of the mediastinum may be reflected at this level and yet may not be obvious at a higher level. If the trachea is in its normal mid-line position, the finger slides along the lateral borders of the trachea and strikes only soft tissue on both sides. If the trachea is deviated from its normal mid-line position, the examining finger encounters the cartilaginous rings of the trachea on the side to which the mediastinum has shifted and only soft tissue on the other side.

The trachea and apex beat may be displaced by an abnormality of the bony thoracic cage, a lesion of the lung parenchyma, a disease of the pleural space or an abnormality of the diaphragm. In chest cage deformity they are displaced to the side of the compressed lung. In a pulmonary condition such as atelectasis or a local fibrosis they are displaced to the side of the lesion, but in pleural effusion or pneumothorax they are shifted to the opposite side. When there is herniation of abdominal contents into the thorax, the mediastinum is also shifted to the opposite side. It is important to realize that the trachea may normally be shifted to the right in elderly people as a result of the pressure of an elongated arteriosclerotic arch of the aorta. The finding of a centrally placed trachea and a shift of the apex beat to the left is in all probability due to left ventricular hypertrophy.

MOVEMENT OF THE CHEST CAGE. A reduced distensibility of a portion of a lung is reflected by a diminished movement of the overlying

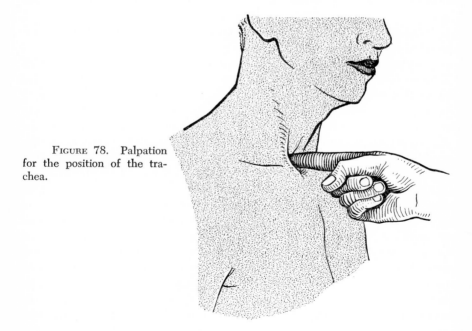

FIGURE 78. Palpation for the position of the trachea.

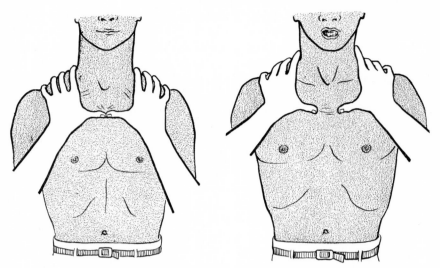

FIGURE 79.   Examination of the movement of the upper lobes.

portion of the chest cage. By eliciting diminished movement of a portion of the chest cage, the examiner acquires the first hint that some patho-logical process is present in either the underlying pleura or the lung. This finding is of prime importance because diminished movement of the chest wall is the earliest evidence of pulmonary disease, often de-veloping before any alteration in density occurs in the affected area of the lung.

The upper anterior chest wall overlying the upper lobes moves forward during inspiration because the anterior ends of the first four ribs are elevated. The method of examining movement in the upper lobes is illustrated in Figure 79. The examiner places the palms of both his hands symmetrically over the patient's upper anterior chest wall, with his extended fingers overlying both trapezius muscles. The skin is then stretched downwards by dragging the hands until both palms lie in the infraclavicular areas, and the fingers are situated over the supraclavicular regions. With the thumbs fully extended, both hands are then pulled towards the sternum until the tips of the thumbs meet in the mid-sternal line. The patient is asked to inspire deeply, and while the chest grad-ually expands the examiner allows his hands to follow the movement of the patient's skin, which is stretched under his palms. The movement of the hands may be magnified if the examiner allows his shoulders to act as a fulcrum. As the patient's chest expands the examiner's hands move laterally and upwards, away from each other. Provided that both upper lobes are healthy, each thumb moves an equal distance from the mid-sternal line, but if one of these lobes is diseased the distances moved are unequal. The actual extent of the movement of the hands varies from subject to subject and is of no importance as long as the hands move equally.

The middle lobe of the right lung and the lingular segment of the left upper lobe underlie the corresponding fifth and sixth ribs and are expanded by their inspiratory elevation. Expansion of this portion of the chest wall takes place in both an anteroposterior and a lateral direction. As shown in Figure 80, it is primarily the lateral expansion of these ribs which is tested by the examiner. Both hands, with all the fingers widely outstretched, are placed along the rib interspaces high in the axillae, and the palms are kept flat against the chest wall. The underlying skin on the patient's chest is then pulled medially until both outstretched thumbs meet in the mid-line over the sternum. When the patient inspires deeply the thumbs move away from each other for an equal distance from the mid-sternal line if the underlying lung parenchyma is normal.

Both lower lobes underlie the corresponding seventh to the tenth ribs. Expansion of this part of the chest cage during inspiration takes place entirely in a lateral direction. As shown in Figure 81, movement of the lower lobes is assessed on the posterior aspect of the chest cage by placing the outstretched fingers of both hands in the axillae, while firm pressure is exerted on the chest with the palms. Both hands are then drawn medially, pulling the underlying skin with them until the outstretched thumbs meet in the mid-line over the vertebral spinous processes. When the patient inspires deeply the thumbs separate, the extent of the movement of both sides being equal if the underlying lower lobes are normal.

The lower lobes differ from the other lobes of the lungs in that

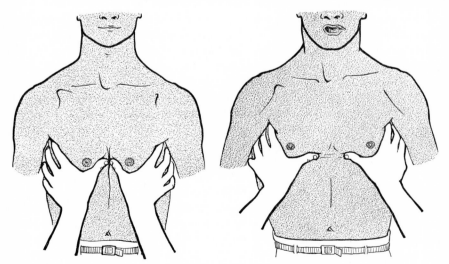

FIGURE 80.   Examination of the movement of the middle lobe and lingula.

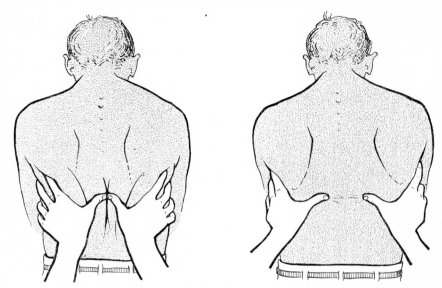

FIGURE 81. Examination of the movement of the lower lobes.

in addition to inspiratory expansion in a lateral direction, there is also vertical expansion by the downward excursion of the diaphragm. The vertical movement of the diaphragm may be assessed by percussion, a procedure which is discussed later. The diaphragm also assists in the elevation of the lower ribs during inspiration. In examining for this action of the diaphragm, the examiner stands beside the supine patient and places both his hands lightly over the lower ribs. Both thumbs are then placed along the costal margins, their tips almost meeting in the mid-line over the xiphoid process. As shown in Figure 82, the examiner's thumbs follow the movement of the costal margins when the patient inspires deeply. If the diaphragmatic pull is normal, the angle at the xiphoid increases equally on both sides.

If the diaphragm were simply a flat sheet of muscle, its fibers would contract in a straight line between its attachments to the costal margin and the central tendon, and the lower ribs would move inward in a medial direction. This is what happens when the diaphragm becomes flattened by some disease process in its neighborhood, such as hyper-inflation of the lungs, or fluid or air in the pleural space. If the diaphragm is elevated because of either an enlarged liver or a collection of pus beneath it, its dome shape becomes exaggerated, and the outward movement of the affected costal margin may increase.

VOCAL FREMITUS. Vocal fremitus is produced by vibrations over the thoracic wall during the production of vocal sounds. *Tactile fremitus* is the vibration felt by the examiner's hand while the patient slowly repeats a combination of words, such as "one-two-three" or "ninety-nine."

Auditory fremitus is the vibration heard by means of a stethoscope applied to the patient's chest wall when a combination of words is spoken.

When vocal fremitus is assessed, it is essential that both lungs be compared with one another in order to detect any local abnormality. The intensity of vocal fremitus is normally uniform over both healthy lungs, except over the apex of the right lung, where its intensity is frequently increased because the larger bronchi are closer to the chest wall in this area. It increases whenever the density of the underlying lung is altered and decreases when fluid, air, excessive muscle or fat is interposed between the lung and the palpating hand. Vocal fremitus is less intense in women and children than in men, probably because their voices are less resonant.

If the subject whispers words instead of speaking them, the vibrations created have a very high frequency. As long as the underlying lung parenchyma is healthy no sounds are heard on the chest wall because they are damped by the selective transmitter property of the alveoli. If the underlying lung tissue is diseased, however, and its "selective transmitter" quality is lost, the whispered sound is transmitted to the chest wall with great clarity. This *whispering pectoriloquy* is a very helpful sign in the detection of consolidation, particularly when there are small patchy areas, such as those which develop in lobular pneumonia.

Percussion. An alteration of the density of the lung may be discovered by percussion of the chest wall. The position of the fingers during the act of percussion is shown in Figure 83. If the examiner is right-handed, the left middle finger is used as the pleximeter. The terminal phalanx and interphalangeal joint should be applied to the patient's chest wall with very little pressure, the rest of this finger and the remaining four fingers being slightly raised; if this is not done, the percussion note is dampened. The striking, or plexor, finger is the middle

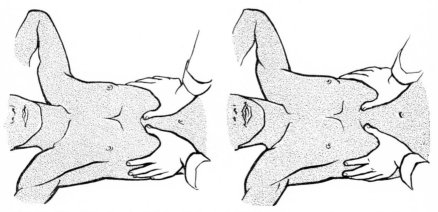

FIGURE 82. Examination of the action of the diaphragm on the costal margins.

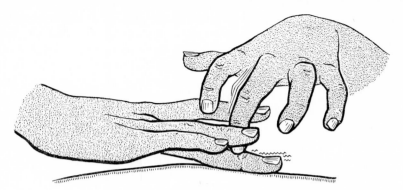

FIGURE 83.   Percussion of the chest.

finger of the other hand. The wrist is used as a fulcrum, and the plexor finger is brought down sharply at a right angle to tap the terminal interphalangeal joint of the pleximeter finger. The blow should be short, sharp and light, and the recoil of the finger should be instantaneous. If the recoil is slow, the sound may be dampened. If the percussion is too forceful, large areas of the chest may be made to vibrate, so that underlying pulmonary lesions may be missed. If the lesion is situated more than 2 inches from the chest wall, its presence may not be detected by percussion because of the overlying healthy parenchyma.

The pleximeter finger should be placed along the line of either the ribs or the interspaces, and whichever is chosen should be used systematically throughout the examination. Comparable areas on both sides of the chest should be examined consecutively, interspaces being compared with interspaces, or ribs with ribs. In this way one is able to localize a lesion and to define its borders.

By noting the pitch of the sound produced during percussion, the examiner is able to determine the ratio of air-containing tissue to solid tissue in the area directly beneath the percussing finger. Well-aerated lung parenchyma produces a low-pitched sound, similar to that of a muffled drum. A sound that is higher in pitch and dull or flat indicates that there is an increased amount of solid tissue under the percussing finger. Provided that it is not due to an exceedingly muscular or obese chest wall, this kind of sound indicates either that the lung is more dense because of atelectasis, fibrosis or consolidation, or that fluid has accumulated in the pleural space.

The downward excursion of the diaphragm may be assessed by means of percussion. Because the vertical movement of the diaphragm is greater in the posterior aspect of the chest, this examination is made over the lower posterior surface of the chest wall while the patient is sitting. The pleximeter finger must be placed in a horizontal position, so that it is parallel with the plane of diaphragmatic dullness. It is easier to detect the abrupt change in note while passing from resonance to dullness. The examiner should therefore percuss lightly over the lower lobe of the lung, moving the pleximeter finger downwards for short distances until the abrupt, flat note produced by the solid intra-abdominal contents is reached. This level indicates the position of the diaphragm. The procedure is also carried out while the patient is holding his breath after both a full expiration and a full inspiration. All these levels can be marked on the chest wall and the diaphragmatic excursion on the two sides compared. The extent of diaphragmatic movement varies in different persons, but it is normally equal on both sides.

Auscultation. The technique of interpreting the type of breath sounds and adventitious sounds which are detected by means of a stethoscope is called auscultation. This should be carried out over the entire chest so that all areas of the lungs are investigated.

BREATH SOUNDS. It is imperative that abnormal breath sounds be recognized and their significance appreciated. As has already been pointed out, in the normal "vesicular" breath sound the inspiratory phase is easily heard; the expiratory phase is fainter and approximately one-third as long as the inspiratory phase. Vesicular breath sounds are heard everywhere over healthy lungs, except over the apex of the right lung, where the sound has a bronchovesicular quality because the bronchi are closer to the chest wall. In this site the expiratory phase is longer, louder and higher in pitch than that of the vesicular sound. When this bronchovesicular sound is heard anywhere except over the right apex, it implies that the underlying lung parenchyma has become affected by a disease process which has altered its "selective transmitter" properties. As a result, more of the higher frequency vibrations pass through the chest wall to the stethoscope.

If the inspiratory and expiratory notes are equal in pitch, intensity and duration, and if there is a silent interval, or gap, between the end of inspiration and the beginning of expiration, the breath sound is called "bronchial." It means that the disease process has become so extensive that solidification of lung parenchyma has developed around a patent bronchus. The intensity of the breath sound itself depends on the diameter of the bronchus underlying the solid portion of lung. Conversely, if the bronchus which underlies the solidified parenchyma is not patent, so that there is no air movement in it, the breath sound may be faint or even absent.

ADVENTITIOUS SOUNDS. Adventitious sounds are not normally heard. When present, they act as clues to the type of pathological process in the diseased portion of the lung.

Rhonchi are prolonged musical or whistling notes which are produced only within the lumen of the tracheobronchial tree. They are indicative of increased turbulence, presumably because the lumina of the

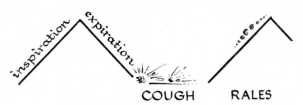

FIGURE 84.   Post-tussic rales.

tubes are narrowed. Rhonchi therefore become more pronounced during the expiratory phase of respiration, and especially during the expulsive phase of coughing. If the bronchial obstruction is very slight, however, rhonchi may be elicited only by a special maneuver. One can either have the patient cough, or still better, have him expire forcibly for as long as possible while the examiner manually compresses the lower part of the chest. A persistent rhonchus which is localized to one portion of the chest wall is a very important finding, for it may signify a new growth, a bronchostenosis or an aspirated foreign body.

The pitch of the rhonchus depends on the diameter of the bronchus in which the sound is produced. A rhonchus which has a low-pitched quality is produced in one of the larger bronchi, in contrast to one produced within a terminal bronchiole, which has a very high-pitched note. Similarly, medium-pitched rhonchi are likely produced within the medium-sized bronchi.

In contrast to rhonchi, *rales* are moist, short, disconnected, bubbling sounds which are heard most readily during inspiration. The pitch of a rale depends on the size of the chamber involved, as well as on the type of lesion. Rales may be classified according to their pitch and position during inspiration, which, in turn, yield information about their site of production. Low-pitched, coarse rales heard in the initial third of inspiration suggest that there is exudate in the large and medium-sized bronchi. Medium-pitched rales heard during the middle third of inspiration suggest that the smaller bronchi are involved, and high-pitched or fine rales in the terminal third of inspiration suggest that the lung parenchyma is involved.

If the disease in the alveoli is very slight, rales may not be elicited by an ordinary deep inspiration. They can often be brought out, however, by having the patient inspire and expire deeply and then produce a short cough. As seen in Figure 84, a shower of very fine rales may be then heard during the next inspiration. These *post-tussic rales* are probably produced by the separation of sticky alveolar walls which have become adherent during the compressive phase of the cough. Conversely, rales which have been heard on ordinary breathing may disappear following a cough, indicating that the secretion producing the rales is situated in the bronchi or bronchioles and that it has been moved up higher in the bronchial tree by the act of coughing.

A creaky, interrupted, dry sound which characteristically extends uniformly throughout the whole of inspiration and of expiration suggests that there is fibrosis of lung parenchyma or the peribronchial tissues.

A *pleural rub* is a creaking, leathery sound which seems to be close to the examining ear. It is a very coarse, loud, grating sound heard at the end of inspiration and at the beginning of expiration (Fig. 85). The rub is diagnostic of pleural irritation, for the sound is produced by the inflamed surfaces of the two pleural layers rubbing against one another during respiration. Since the excursion of the pleural surfaces is greatest over the lower lobes, friction rubs are most frequently detected in the lower parts of the chest; they are only very occasionally heard over the upper areas.

The *coin click test* is performed by having an assistant place a coin over the anterior part of the chest and clicking it with another coin while the examiner auscultates over the posterior part of the same side of the chest. The sound that is heard over a normal chest is muffled and faint, but it has a metallic quality which comes through clearly if a large pneumothorax is present.

When air and free fluid are both present in the pleural cavity, a splashing sound may be produced which is easily detected by the stethoscope. This *succussion splash* is demonstrated by shaking the patient while the examiner listens to the chest. If a bronchopleural fistula is present, one often hears a gurgling sound, which is caused by air escaping from the fistula into the fluid.

Signs of Pulmonary Heart Disease. Respiratory disease may lead to an increase in the pulmonary vascular resistance, with consequent pulmonary hypertension and right ventricular hypertrophy. Evidence of increased pulmonary vascular resistance can be elicited only by examining the heart. In the following discussion only the methods of examination of the heart which are pertinent to the signs of increased pulmonary vascular resistance are presented.

CARDIAC IMPULSE. The position and character of the cardiac im-

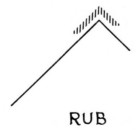

RUB

FIGURE 85. The pleural rub.

pulse, if it is visible, should be noted during inspection of the chest. In this way right or left ventricular hypertrophy may be suspected. The character of the cardiac impulse is as important as its location, for a steady heave over the right ventricle at the left parasternal line is frequently felt in cases of right ventricular hypertrophy and pulmonary hypertension. There is often an associated conspicuous retraction over the left ventricle, which gives the precordium a characteristic rocking motion. In addition, dilatation of the pulmonary artery may produce a visible pulsation over the pulmonic area.

THE HEART SOUNDS. The heart sounds usually yield valuable information about the presence of pulmonary hypertension. The second heart sound is due to aortic and pulmonic valve closure. The aortic element is best heard in the aortic area and at the apex of the heart, and the pulmonic element is best heard in the pulmonic area. On palpation, particularly over the pulmonic area, vibrations associated with an accentuated second pulmonic sound and a systolic ejection click indicate that pulmonary hypertension is present. On auscultation, the intensity of the second pulmonic heart sound should be noted, because it increases when pulmonary hypertension is present. The pulmonic second sound is normally split. The split is accentuated during inspiration, because of a prolongation of the systole of the right ventricle resulting from increased filling during inspiration. If the split does not widen during inspiration it further suggests the presence of pulmonary hypertension. Prolonged splitting of the second pulmonic sound during inspiration is probably due to a delay in closure of the pulmonary valve, which is usually caused by either a bundle branch block or a mild pulmonary stenosis.

A systolic ejection click in the pulmonic area is also indicative of pulmonary hypertension. This occurs during systole just after the opening of the pulmonary valve, at the end of the period of isometric contraction. It is probably due to accentuated ejection vibrations, and is almost invariably found in patients with large left-to-right shunts, mild pulmonary stenosis or dilatation of the pulmonary artery.

The presence of heart murmurs may yield evidence for the source of respiratory symptoms. The typical apical diastolic murmur of mitral stenosis may indicate the possible origin of a recent hemoptysis, or auricular fibrillation may explain the cause of a pulmonary infarction.

THE ABDOMEN

The abdomen should be palpated for abnormal masses and enlargement of the liver or spleen. An enlarged liver may be caused by congestive heart failure, metastatic infiltration from a bronchogenic carcinoma, one of the lymphomas, or an amebic abscess. A palpable spleen is found in association with one of the lymphomas or sarcoidosis, as well as with septicemia or sub-acute bacterial endocarditis. A malignant condition involving the stomach, bowel, kidney or one of the ovaries may produce a palpable mass. A benign tumor of the ovary may be the cause of Meig's syndrome, a condition in which ascites and a unilateral hydrothorax develop. A hard, fixed, nodular prostate indicates a malignant process which may be the source of pulmonary metastases. A carcinoma of the rectum is easily accessible to the examining finger. A fistula-in-ano should make one suspect a tuberculous etiology if a pulmonary lesion is present.

EXTERNAL GENITALIA

The scar of an old primary chancre due to syphilis suggests the possibility of an aortic aneurysm, as does the finding of an enlarged nontender syphilitic orchitis. A tuberculous epididymitis makes one suspect the possibility of active pulmonary tuberculosis.

THE SKIN

Anemia is almost always suggested by the presence of pallor in the palms and finger pulps. For many reasons, this is a much safer guide to the hemoglobin content of the blood than the color of the face, for the latter may be weather-beaten or disguised by cosmetics. The presence of cyanosis should be particularly noted. In addition, pigmentation in the skin creases suggestive of Addison's disease should be looked for.

In an allergic state, atopic dermatitis or urticaria may be present. Erythema nodosum may occur in association with a streptococcal sore throat, tuberculosis, sarcoidosis or coccidioidomycosis. Metastases from a bronchogenic carcinoma may develop in the subcutaneous tissues, where they may be felt as firm, nontender nodules. Chronic infiltrations in the skin may occur with sarcoidosis, fungus infections and histiocytosis "X." Icterus may be associated with a pulmonary infarct.

THE EXTREMITIES

A painful, tender, thrombosed vein due to thrombophlebitis may account for the source of a pulmonary infarction. Congestive heart failure causes bilateral pretibial edema. A peripheral neuropathy develops on rare occasions as a complication of a bronchogenic carcinoma. Enlarged tender shafts of the long bones due to hypertrophic pulmonary osteoarthropathy, in association with digital clubbing, indicate the presence of a bronchogenic carcinoma, one of the suppurative lung diseases or congenital heart disease. A diffuse pulmonary fibrosis is occasionally associated with the typical deformed joints of rheumatoid arthritis. The presence of degenerative arthritis of the large joints, together with Heberden node formation on the distal phalanges of the fingers, suggests the possibility of similar degenerative changes in the thoracic spine, which may be the cause of chest pain.

SUMMARY

It must be emphasized that the abnormal findings which are elicited during the clinical examination of the chest indicate only that certain pathological processes have taken place, as well as their approximate location. These findings do not yield any information about the exact type of disease process which has produced the changes. This can be inferred only when the abnormal physical findings are taken in conjunction with the history of the illness. It is only by making a thorough enquiry into the chronological development of the symptoms, the duration of the illness and the nature of its progress, together with a careful, complete general physical examination, that it is possible to arrive at a presumptive clinical diagnosis of the disease.

When the history and physical examination are completed and recorded, a paragraph should follow summarizing the salient signs and symptoms, and another listing the various possible diagnoses, in the order of their preference, under the heading of "Differential Diagnosis."

CHAPTER XVI

The Radiological Assessment

AFTER the examiner has obtained a complete history from the patient and has performed a thorough physical examination, he is usually able to arrive at a tentative diagnosis of the pulmonary lesion. Further valuable information leading to a more definitive diagnosis can now be obtained by a radiological assessment of the patient's chest. Although there are many bronchopulmonary diseases in which the x-ray examination is entirely noncontributory, most pulmonary lesions can be demonstrated radiologically long before their presence is detected by the usual clinical methods of examination. It therefore follows that a radiological examination is an integral part of the assessment of a patient suffering from a respiratory disease. Apart from the place of radiography in the initial detection of disease, x-ray films and fluoroscopic examination also serve as a standard for following the course of disease and its response to therapy.

The radiological examination may be considered as a twofold assessment. The static assessment consists of x-ray films of the thorax taken in the posteroanterior and lateral positions and, in addition, more detailed and specialized techniques when they are indicated. By this means the anatomical position of a lesion and frequently the pathological diagnosis may be established. This information may be supplemented by fluoroscopy of the heart and lungs during normal respiration and various breathing maneuvers, which yields valuable information regarding the dynamic function of the lungs.

THE RADIOLOGICAL APPEARANCE OF THE NORMAL CHEST

The thorax is an ideal region for a radiological examination. The aerated lung parenchyma offers very little resistance to the passage of roentgen rays and it therefore produces very radiant shadows. On the other hand, the soft tissues of the thoracic wall, the mediastinum, the heart and great vessels, and the diaphragm do not permit the rays to pass through to as great an extent and therefore appear as denser opacities on the x-ray film. The bony structures of the thorax, the ribs, vertebrae and sternum, are even less readily penetrated and their shadows are consequently even more dense.

The appearance of the normal x-ray film of the chest must be clearly understood before any attempt can be made to determine the existence of abnormalities or disease processes, particularly since normal x-ray findings vary considerably with age, sex and habitus, and under different conditions of respiration in the same individual. The examiner must learn all the various appearances which may be considered normal by studying large numbers of x-ray films, just as he can learn to recognize normal breath sounds only by repeated stethoscopic examination.

THE LUNGS

The radiological appearance of the normal lungs is shown in Figure 86. The trachea is a horizontal translucent shadow situated in the mid-line, overlying the cervical vertebrae. The hila or lung roots are poorly defined areas of increased density in the medial part of the central portion of the lung fields. These are made up of the pulmonary blood vessels, the bronchi and a group of lymph nodes. The left hilum is partially obscured by the overlying shadow of the heart and great vessels, and it lies at a slightly higher level than the right hilum. In the middle third of the lung fields there is a series of linear reticular shadows which are wider and denser in the region of the hila, progressively decreasing as they move out toward the periphery. These linear markings are principally formed by arteries, but veins and lymphatics also contribute to them. A bronchus, seen end-on, forms a ringlike area of increased density with a central translucency, but a blood vessel seen end-on appears as a round solid shadow. In the peripheral portions of the lung these linear markings are much less obvious. They are usually similar in both lungs, but those on the left side are obscured by the heart.

The lobes of the lungs cannot normally be distinguished. It is of utmost importance, however, to have clearly in one's mind the anatomical location of each of the lobes, and the delineation of the various bronchopulmonary segments. The major or oblique fissures of both lungs are usually seen only in the lateral view as a very thin dense line. The minor or transverse fissure on the right side is normally seen on the postero-anterior film as a fine hairlike line running transversely in either the third or the fourth intercostal space, and on the lateral view it runs horizontally from the hilum to the anterior margin of the chest cage. The position of these fissures is frequently of diagnostic value. For instance, if the right upper lobe is contracted or atelectatic, the fissure is drawn up; if the middle lobe is atelectatic, it is drawn downwards. Similarly, when

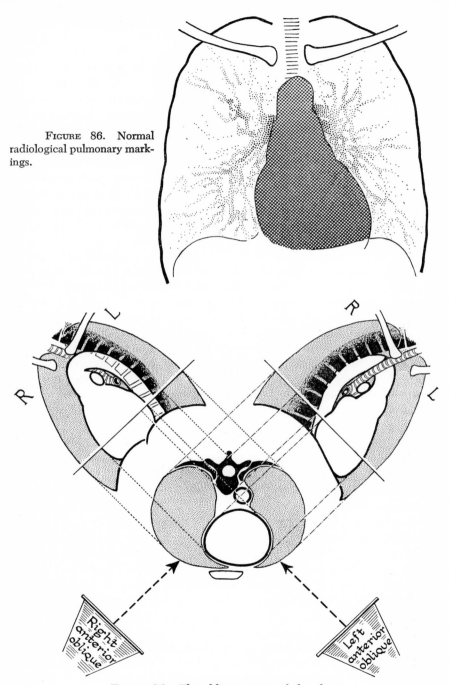

FIGURE 86. Normal radiological pulmonary markings.

FIGURE 87. The oblique views of the chest.

the lower lobe is collapsed, the major fissure is drawn downwards and posteriorly.

The upper lobes mainly lie anteriorly. The lower lobes occupy the posteroinferior aspects of the chest. The right middle lobe lies in the inferior portion of the anteromedial aspect of the chest. The lobes overlap each other considerably, however, so that a clear localization of each lobe is not possible in the posteroanterior view of the chest. For this reason, a lateral view and occasionally oblique views are essential in order to delineate accurately the lobes of the lungs and their various bronchopulmonary segments. The appearance of the chest film in the two oblique positions is shown in Figure 87. In addition, a transection of the chest is shown in order to visualize the portions of the lung and heart which are seen in both the right and left oblique views. The oblique views are taken with the corresponding shoulder against the x-ray cassette. In a right anterior oblique view, therefore, the right lower lobe is situated posteriorly, and the lingula of the left lung is delineated anteriorly. In the left anterior oblique view, the left lower lobe is situated posteriorly, and the right middle lobe is located anteriorly.

THE HEART

On the posteroanterior x-ray film, the heart shadow comprises a series of arcs or curves which represent the margins of the various chambers and the great vessels (Fig. 88). On the left side, the edge of the left ventricle begins at the diaphragm and extends upwards to the upper one-third of the cardiac outline. Above this there is a short arc which is formed by the left auricular appendage. The pulmonary artery is visualized as a small curved area which is situated immediately superior to this shadow. The uppermost aspect of the silhouette on the left is composed of the aortic knob and the margin of the descending aorta, and occasionally the subclavian artery. On the right side, there are two curves along the border of the heart shadow, the lower one representing the right auricle, and the upper one the superior vena cava and perhaps a portion of the ascending aorta. If the x-ray film is taken during a deep inspiration, the inferior vena cava may be visualized as a triangular shadow lying between the diaphragm and the right auricle.

On a lateral x-ray film of the chest, the posterior mediastinum is visualized as an area of radiolucency between the posterior border of the heart and the anterior aspect of the spine. The descending aorta is outlined in this space.

In the right anterior oblique position, the posterior border of the heart shadow is made up of the left and right auricles, with the superior vena cava above. The anterior border of the heart shadow is formed by the right ventricle.

The left anterior oblique position is particularly valuable for the

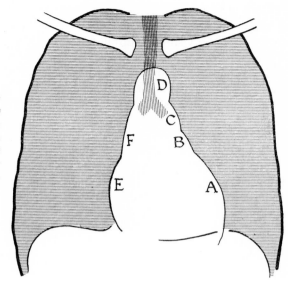

FIGURE 88. The radiological appearance of the heart: A, left ventricle; B, left auricular appendage; C, pulmonary artery; D, aortic knob and margin of descending aorta; E, right auricle; F, superior vena cava.

visualization of the right ventricle, which lies along the diaphragmatic and the inferoanterior portion of the cardiac outline. The left auricle and the left ventricle form the posterior portion of the silhouette.

THE DIAPHRAGM

The two hemidiaphragms are rounded, smooth, sharply defined shadows, the right one being normally situated one interspace higher than the left. The right leaf of the diaphragm merges with the shadow of the liver. The costophrenic angles are moderately deep and they are approximately equal in size on the two sides.

BONY STRUCTURES

The ribs, the clavicles, the scapulae and portions of the humeri are reasonably clearly outlined on most x-ray films of the chest. Abnormalities in these structures should be carefully sought, for they are important aids in diagnosis. For instance, notching of the ribs is an important manifestation of coarctation of the aorta.

EXAMINATION OF THE X-RAY FILM OF THE CHEST

It is important that the x-ray film should not be either overexposed or underexposed. The patient should be well centered before the exposure is made, so that the sternal notch overlies the vertebrae. The outline of the vertebral column should be just visible through the heart shadow. The ribs should show good bony detail and the vascular markings should be visible from hilum to periphery. The cardiac outline, and if possible the transverse fissure, the left subclavian artery and the inferior vena cava, should be sharply defined.

It is essential that the examiner study an x-ray film of the chest in a systematic fashion. The actual sequence followed is probably not important, as long as it is systematic and thorough. The examiner should determine the size of the cardiac shadow and of the mediastinum, as well as their contours. The position of the trachea and its branches and, if possible, their contours should be assessed. Note should be made of the position and the shape of the two hemidiaphragms, the depth, clarity and position of the two costophrenic angles and the appearance of the lateral borders of the lungs. The size, shape and position of both hilar shadows should be noted. It is difficult to differentiate definitely between a normal and a pathologically enlarged hilum, unless there are gross abnormalities. Enlargement of both hila suggests either that there is diffuse pulmonary disease which has led to an increase in the pulmonary artery pressure or that the lymph nodes in both hilar regions have become enlarged. A malignant disease should be considered if only one hilum is enlarged, particularly in association with a pulmonary lesion in an elderly patient. When the hila are enlarged and butterfly-shaped and there are associated increased pulmonary markings, the likely cause is pulmonary congestion. The size and extent of the pulmonary markings and the appearance of the lung fields bilaterally should then be examined, with special reference to any abnormal shadows. If a lesion is seen, it is important to localize it to the particular bronchopulmonary segment which is involved. A lesion of the right middle lobe and the medial basal segment of the right lower lobe usually obliterates the cardiac border, whereas lesions of the posterior basal segment of the right lower lobe do not. The bony structure should then be studied for the appearance of the ribs bilaterally, the vertebrae, both clavicles, scapulae and humeri.

An assessment of the x-ray film in this manner usually confirms the diagnosis which has been established previously by the history and physical examination. It may, in addition, reveal the presence of pulmonary disease which has not been suspected. On the other hand, further special radiographic techniques may be required in order to establish the diagnosis.

SPECIAL RADIOGRAPHIC TECHNIQUES

INSPIRATION-EXPIRATION FILMS

X-ray films taken during both inspiration and expiration can supply information which would otherwise be gained only by fluoroscopy. The extent of diaphragmatic motion, the aeration of the lungs during inspiration and their emptying during expiration, as well as the presence of a mediastinal shift can be assessed. Similarly, films taken during the Valsalva and Mueller maneuvers may reveal the vascular nature of a pulmonary lesion. Unlike fluoroscopy, these films provide a record which can be filed for future reference.

LATERAL DECUBITUS FILMS

If the presence of fluid in the pleural space is suspected but it is not grossly evident in the ordinary film, it may become apparent on a film taken in the lateral decubitus position, with the patient lying on the suspected side. If a pleural effusion is present, the fluid shifts to the most dependent position.

LORDOTIC FILMS

A pulmonary lesion may be obscured on the conventional postero-anterior chest film because of the overlapping of the ribs. An abnormal shadow may be made more distinct if the film is taken in the lordotic position.

TOMOGRAPHY

Tomography is a technique by which the x-ray beam is focused at various depths within the lung. A series of films of the lung can be obtained which are taken at various planes as little as 1 cm. in depth. By this means one can study pulmonary lesions which are ordinarily obscured by bone, soft tissues and other shadows. In addition, one is able to delineate the characteristics of a radiological shadow, particularly when it is deep-seated. Full chest tomography, in which the x-ray beam is focused on the mid-sagittal plane of the whole chest, has been used to study the status of the pulmonary vasculature. In normal subjects, the pulmonary vessels can be followed out to the periphery, but in patients with chronic obstructive emphysema in which there has been vascular obliteration, the peripheral vessels are attenuated or absent.

STEREOSCOPIC FILMS

Stereoscopic films may also be used to localize pulmonary lesions. In this technique, two x-ray films of the chest are taken at the same time and, by making them overlap, a three dimensional impression of the chest is obtained when they are viewed stereoscopically.

BRONCHOGRAMS

An x-ray film of the chest made after either iodized oils or water-soluble iodized solutions are instilled into the tracheobronchial tree is called a bronchogram. The radio-opaque iodized substances reveal in great detail the size and the appearance of the tracheobronchial tree. From knowledge of the segmental anatomy of the lung, the exact location of the bronchial disease can be established. In addition, bronchograms demonstrate the form of the bronchi and test their patency, as evidenced by their ability to conduct the oil to the periphery of the lungs.

In a normal bronchogram, the bronchi beyond the early segmental branches divide at intervals of about 1 cm. The final branches lie about 1 to 2 mm. apart and are 1 to 3 mm. long. The filling terminates at about 3 mm. from the edges of the ribs in the posteroanterior view and at the same distance from the interlobar septa in the lateral view. The walls of the peripheral branches are parallel and the lumen decreases in caliber after branching.

In bronchiectasis, on the other hand, the bronchi are dilated, have an irregular outline and may be unable to conduct the oil to the periphery of the lungs because of obstruction by secretions, organic narrowing or obliteration. Only the larger bronchi or more proximal branches become filled, and a local dilatation of the proximal bronchus of the first to the fifth generation following the lobar division is usually found. The dilatation may be fusiform, tubular or cystic and may be slight in extent or quite gross.

In chronic bronchitis, the bronchial filling usually reaches further towards the periphery, and the changes are generally found in smaller bronchi and bronchioles. Dilatation of a peripheral bronchiole shows up as a circular shadow 1 to 3 mm. in diameter at the end of a small branch. There may be few or many such shadows.

ESOPHAGOGRAM

The esophagogram is an x-ray film of the chest taken while the patient drinks a mixture of barium. This is a very useful procedure, particularly when involvement of the mediastinum by a pulmonary malignant process is suspected. In such a situation, displacement of the esophagus may indicate the presence of enlarged mediastinal lymph nodes or metastatic involvement of the esophagus.

ANGIOGRAPHY

This is a technique whereby a radio-opaque substance is injected into the blood stream and x-ray films are taken during its passage through the right side of the heart, the pulmonary circulation, the left side of the heart and then the aorta. It is a very valuable procedure in the diagnosis of cardiopulmonary disorders, particularly when there is a right-to-left shunt of blood.

FLUOROSCOPIC EXAMINATION OF THE CHEST

When a pulmonary abnormality is found and when some disability has resulted, no matter how minor, fluoroscopy should be performed. Before the fluoroscopic assessment is begun the examiner's pupils must be well dilated and dark-adapted. This requires a period of at least twenty minutes if the examiner wears special red goggles or ten minutes in a totally dark room.

Since fluoroscopy has serious potentialities as far as radiation is concerned, the physician who is performing this procedure should exercise the utmost precautions and use adequate protective devices. Even though much can be learned by fluoroscopy, it should not be relied upon as the only means of detecting or excluding pulmonary disease. It should be considered only as an adjunct to the diagnostic radiograph, providing particular information about the function of the respiratory system.

This examination yields the most information if a systematic and detailed plan is followed. Although it is obvious that much can be learned about the heart, this will not be discussed except as it is related to respiratory disease.

GENERAL SURVEY OF THE CHEST

The fluoroscopic examination should be carried out with the patient standing facing the examiner. The entire chest should first be examined for any abnormalities and obvious gross parenchymal lesions. The position of the trachea and the butterfly-shaped hilar markings should be noted. The lowest portion of the trachea may be normally displaced to the right by an elongated aorta in an elderly person. As mentioned earlier, the left hilum is usually a little higher than the right. The pulmonary markings are more prominent near the hila and fade out towards the periphery. The right hemidiaphragm is normally higher than the left, possibly because it is pushed up by the liver.

Normally, both lung fields are equally illuminated, the amount depending on the phase of respiration, being more translucent during inspiration and darker during the expiratory phase. Aeration and deflation of the lungs should be assessed during quiet breathing, during deep breathing and during a cough. If the lungs do not become less translucent during expiration, there may be either a loss of elasticity or a generalized partial bronchiolar obstruction of the check-valve type. If this finding is localized in one area of the lung, there may be obstruction of a bronchus by a malignant process or a foreign body.

DETAILED EXAMINATION OF THE LUNG FIELDS

Following the general survey, the shutters of the fluoroscopic screen should be narrowed down and small areas of both lungs then separately examined from the apex to the base. When there is a possibility that a lesion may be vascular, such as an arteriovenous fistula, both the Valsalva and the Mueller maneuvers should be performed. In the former, the patient makes a deep inspiration and then attempts to expire forcibly against a closed glottis. This elevates the intrathoracic pressure so that any thin-walled vascular structure, such as a vein, is emptied and diminished in size. In the Mueller maneuver, the patient is instructed to exhale and then attempt to inhale forcibly against a closed glottis. This causes a fall in the intrathoracic pressure resulting in distention of any thin-walled vascular structures. Strong pulsation of the hilar vessels may indicate that there is an insufficiency of the pulmonary valve, a patent ductus arteriosus, or some other disease which causes an increased pulmonary artery blood flow.

THE DIAPHRAGM AND MEDIASTINUM

The resting level of the diaphragm at the end of a quiet expiration should be noted. In addition, the movement of the diaphragm on both sides should be assessed during quiet breathing as well as during a deep inspiration. The normal diaphragm moves about 1 inch during quiet breathing and 2 to 3 inches during a deep inspiration. Diminished movement of the diaphragm may be associated with either localized or diffuse pulmonary disease. The diaphragms are depressed and show restricted movement in chronic obstructive emphysema.

If a hemidiaphragm does not move at all, it is important to determine whether it is paralyzed. Paralysis of the diaphragm is usually determined by the "sniff test." The diaphragm is apparently essential for the production of a sniff, and when it is bilaterally paralyzed, as it may be in poliomyelitis, the patient is unable to sniff. If the phrenic nerves are intact, a sniff results in a sharp downward movement of the diaphragm. If one of the leaves of the diaphragm is paralyzed, a sniff or even a normal inspiration may result in a paradoxical movement of the diaphragm. In such a situation, the normal hemidiaphragm descends while the paralyzed one rises during inspiration, being pushed upwards by the increased intra-abdominal pressure.

The costophrenic angles should be examined for movement. They normally enlarge during inspiration and narrow during expiration. The costophrenic angles can be obliterated by small quantities of pleural fluid or by diaphragmatic adhesions.

A shift of the mediastinum towards one side during respiration means that the intrathoracic pressure on the affected side is less than it is on the other. Because this is most commonly seen when a bronchial obstruction is present on one side, it is often associated with failure of the lung fields on the affected side to darken during expiration.

THE CONTOUR OF THE HEART

It is important to assess the status of the pulmonary circulation during the fluoroscopy of a patient who is suspected of suffering from some form of pulmonary disease. The region of the pulmonary artery and the right side of the heart should be carefully examined. If the curve of the pulmonary artery is enlarged, some degree of pulmonary hypertension is suggested. In both the left anterior oblique and the right anterior oblique positions the right ventricle forms the anterior border of the heart. If this should be enlarged, it may fill the entire lower anterior portion of the chest in these oblique views.

By studying the variation of the chest from normal as it appears on the x-ray film and on the fluoroscopic screen, the examiner is able to recognize any abnormality, and from a knowledge of the anatomy of the lungs, he is able to establish its exact location. The x-ray film provides a static picture of the anatomy and pathologic condition of the lungs during life, and the fluoroscopic examination yields information about the functional aspects of a respiratory disease process, especially with reference to the heart, mediastinum and diaphragm. Apart from the place of radiography in the initial detection of disease, x-ray films and fluoroscopic examination also serve for following the course of a disease and its response to therapy.

CHAPTER XVII

The Clinical-Pathological

Assessment

FROM the clinical and radiological assessment, a presumptive diagnosis of the pathological pattern caused by a particular respiratory disease can usually be established. Confirmation of the clinical diagnosis and identification of the responsible agent require the expert assistance of the bacteriologist and the pathologist.

Although a considerable number of laboratory examinations can be carried out to investigate a respiratory disease, only a small proportion of these are essential in the determination of the etiological diagnosis. The most important studies are the bacteriological and cytological examination of abnormal secretions and the histological examination of diseased tissues. No respiratory illness can be considered to be adequately assessed if these tests are omitted.

Only the more important laboratory studies are discussed in the following section and these are considered particularly with regard to their diagnostic value. Textbooks of bacteriology and clinical pathology should be consulted for a description of the procedures of the various tests.

ABNORMAL SECRETIONS

The abnormal secretions most commonly examined are sputum, pleural fluid and the discharge from draining sinuses.

SPUTUM

Abnormal bronchial secretions result from inflammation in either the lung parenchyma or the tracheobronchial tree, or both. These secretions are usually expectorated as sputum, swallowed and found in the gastric contents, or aspirated from the bronchial tree by suctioning through a catheter or bronchoscope.

Collection. The ideal time for the collection of sputum is shortly after awakening, for abnormal bronchial secretions tend to accumulate during a night's sleep. Care must be taken to reduce contamination with organisms which normally inhabit the oropharynx. Postnasal secretions can generally be "hawked up" and discarded before a specimen is collected. In addition, the patient should brush his teeth, wash his mouth and gargle with a good antiseptic. Then he should cough vigorously and expectorate the sputum into a sterile container.

The sputum should be sent to the laboratory with a minimum of delay. If the container is not sterile, and the specimen is allowed to remain at room temperature, there may be an overgrowth of saprophytic organisms. Thus the culture may be contaminated and the antibiotic sensitivity tests invalidated.

Occasionally a patient may be unable to expectorate sputum because he is too ill, too elderly or too young to be cooperative. In such cases, a satisfactory specimen may be obtained by deliberately inducing the cough reflex through application of a sterile cotton applicator or laryngeal mirror to the base of the tongue, or by inserting a sterile suction catheter into the trachea.

BRONCHOSCOPIC ASPIRATION.   Secretions may be aspirated directly from the affected bronchus through a bronchoscope. This procedure obviously has a therapeutic as well as a diagnostic value. Bronchoscopic aspiration is particularly valuable for demonstrating malignant cells, tubercle bacilli and fungi.

GASTRIC ASPIRATION.   Considerable quantities of sputum are unknowingly swallowed by patients. For this reason, the aspiration of gastric contents in the fasting state shortly after awakening is a valuable procedure, particularly for the detection of tubercle bacilli. As acid-fast saprophytic bacilli may be found normally in the gastric contents, however, significant information can be obtained only by culturing the material or inoculating it into a guinea pig.

Macroscopic Examination. VOLUME.   The amount of sputum expectorated during a twenty-four hour period often provides useful information about the nature of the disease as well as its course and prognosis. A daily volume of over 100 ml. may be expectorated in such diseases as bronchiectasis, lung abscess and occasionally chronic bronchitis. A change in the amounts of sputum expectorated from day to day can be informative. The daily volume should gradually decrease if recovery is taking place. If it remains unchanged or increases in amount, it may indicate that the disease is progressing unfavorably. A sudden decrease in volume may be due to obstruction of the draining bronchus, an event usually associated with a deterioration in the patient's condition. A sudden increase in volume may indicate rupture of a pulmonary abscess or an empyema into the bronchial tree.

COLOR AND CONSISTENCY. Mucoid sputum is translucent and glairy, has a viscid, tenacious consistency, and is often gray among city dwellers and cigarette smokers. In acute pulmonary edema the sputum is pinkish, watery and frothy. Purulent sputum is generally yellow or green, and the color and consistency of mucopurulent sputum, which consists of a mixture of mucus and pus, depends on the proportions of these ingredients. If a large collection of purulent sputum is allowed to stand in a conical glass, it often tends to separate into three layers. The top layer is usually frothy and discolored, the middle layer tends to be cloudy and watery, and the lower layer generally consists of a thick sediment of pus.

Blood in the sputum is easily recognized, and may be in the form of streaks or small clots mixed in the sputum. In hemoptysis, the expectoration consists entirely of blood. The color of the blood depends on the interval between the actual bleeding and the expectoration of the sputum. Fresh blood is bright red, but it becomes dark if it is not immediately expectorated.

ODOR. The odor of the sputum should always be noted. Most specimens are odorless. Purulent sputum may occasionally have a sweetish odor. A rotten, decomposed stench is indicative of an anaerobic putrefactive process, and infections caused by certain coliform organisms occasionally also produce a foul odor.

ABNORMAL SUBSTANCES. Occasionally foreign material which is related directly to the underlying disease may be expectorated, either alone or mixed with the sputum. Such substances can occasionally be recognized by their macroscopic appearance, but it is usually necessary to identify them microscopically or chemically.

The sputum of city dwellers is polluted with carbon particles, and the sputum of coal miners is commonly stained by particles of coal dust or may be practically black if the miner is suffering from severe anthracosis.

Particles of calcium known as broncholiths may be found in the sputum. These usually originate from calcified tuberculous hilar lymph nodes which have eroded through the wall of a bronchus into its lumen or from calcium deposits in the lung parenchyma, as in silicosis and histoplasmosis. These calcium particles, usually minute and sandlike in size, are generally irregular, stony-hard and grayish white.

Dittrich's plugs may occasionally be found in the purulent sputum of chronic suppurative diseases, such as bronchiectasis and lung abscess. These yellow-white masses are inspissated, disintegrated, purulent material, consisting of fatty acids and fat globules. They possess an extremely putrid odor and vary in size from that of a pin head to a pea.

Microscopic Examination. The various cells, organisms and minute abnormal substances that may be present in sputum can be identified only microscopically.

CYTOLOGICAL EXAMINATION. This examination helps to determine whether the specimen is derived from the oropharynx or from the lower respiratory tract. Secretions from the upper respiratory passages contain flat polygonal epithelial cells. Large round or oval histiocytes, often filled with carbon particles, are frequently seen in secretions from the bronchial tree. Ciliated, columnar cells which have been shed from the bronchial mucosa are often seen as well.

The sputum of a tuberculous infection contains numerous lymphocytes, whereas that of a nontuberculous bacterial infection contains predominantly polymorphonuclear neutrophils. Many eosinophils are frequently present in the sputum of bronchial asthma. Large numbers of erythrocytes in the sputum are indicative of either a recent hemorrhage, as in the hemorrhagic sputum of pulmonary tuberculosis, or an exudation of blood, as in the rusty sputum of pneumococcal pneumonia.

In bronchogenic carcinoma, the sputum often contains malignant cells which have been exfoliated into the bronchial tree by the neoplastic process. The identification of these cells in the sputum is difficult and can be made only by a technician who has been specially trained in cytological examinations. Failure to demonstrate malignant cells does *not* exclude the presence of a bronchogenic carcinoma.

ABNORMAL SUBSTANCES. Purulent material should be routinely examined for elastic fibers, which indicate active destruction of pulmonary tissue such as may occur in pulmonary tuberculosis, bronchiectasis, lung abscess and pulmonary malignancy. To demonstrate these fibers, a fleck of purulent sputum is mixed with sodium hydroxide, which dissolves all the cellular material, thus allowing any elastic fibers to become visible under the low power objective. They are slender, wavy, highly refractile threads of uniform diameter and of varying lengths, with split or curled ends. They are usually seen either singly or grouped together in small bundles.

The detection of oil droplets in bronchial secretions suggests lipid pneumonia or fat embolism. The oil droplets may be in the cytoplasm of macrophages or may be extracellular. They are easily recognized microscopically because they readily absorb a scarlet-red dye such as Sudan III. Osmic acid stains vegetable and animal oils black and liquid petrolatum yellow.

Asbestos bodies are frequently found in the sputum of asbestosis. These slender, elongated structures with bulbous ends range from 10 to 180 microns in size and stain a brilliant blue with potassium ferrocyanide. They are formed by the deposit of an iron-containing protein on an asbestos fiber.

Rupture of a pulmonary hydatid cyst into a bronchus frequently causes a sudden expectoration of a large quantity of a clear, salty, alkaline fluid. This usually contains components of the larval stage of the *Echinococcus granulosus,* such as scolices and hooklets, as well as bits of membrane from the wall of the cyst. An amebic abscess in the liver may rupture through the diaphragm and perforate through the lung parenchyma into the bronchial tree, producing a thick chocolate-brown sputum, which occasionally contains the motile form of the *Endamoeba histolytica* and its cysts. On rare occasions, *Ascaris lumbricoides* larvae may be found in the sputum. During their life cycle the larvae burrow out through the pulmonary capillaries into the alveoli, after which they slowly move up the length of the trachea and may be swallowed with the sputum.

BACTERIOLOGICAL EXAMINATION. This is one of the most important studies that can be carried out on bronchial secretions. The direct microscopic examination of a stained smear indicates whether the organisms are predominantly gram-positive or gram-negative, or it may reveal tubercle bacilli. An unstained smear may occasionally demonstrate fungi, such as *Actinomyces bovis.* The proper identification of pathogenic organisms can be carried out only by cultural methods, and in the case of the tubercle bacillus, by animal inoculation as well. This technique will be discussed in detail in a later section.

PLEURAL FLUID

The character of fluid in the pleural cavity can be ascertained only by aspiration and laboratory examination. A thoracentesis must be performed in every case of pleural effusion, and when feasible, as much fluid as possible should be aspirated. A representative sample of fluid may be aspirated for purely diagnostic purposes. In that case, at least 100 ml. should be obtained, so that the various laboratory procedures may be carried out with accuracy. Just as with sputum, pleural fluid should undergo a macroscopic and microscopic examination.

Macroscopic Examination. VOLUME. If the amount of aspirated fluid represents the total quantity in the pleural space, it yields valuable information concerning the extent of the underlying pathological process.

NAKED-EYE APPEARANCE. A transudate is usually watery, pale yellow and either clear or slightly hazy. An exudate is generally deep yellow and turbid, and feels thicker and stickier because of its higher protein content. The turbidity of pleural fluid depends upon the number of formed particles it contains, and it may vary from cloudiness to a thick, creamy pus. When red blood cells are present, the color of the fluid varies from a reddish tinge to dark red. Fresh blood in the pleural fluid is generally the result of trauma, pulmonary infarction or a neoplastic process. An empyema fluid may vary from brown to yellow or green. Chylous fluid has a milky turbidity.

COAGULABILITY. The degree of spontaneous coagulation of the pleural fluid after its aspiration depends on the amount of fibrin present. A transudate rarely coagulates, but exudates and neoplastic effusions can coagulate fairly rapidly.

ODOR. Transudates and exudates are usually odorless, but the fluid may have a putrid stench if the pleural effusion is secondary to putrefactive changes in the lung.

Chemical Examination. SPECIFIC GRAVITY. The specific gravity of the aspirated fluid helps distinguish between a transudate and an exudate. The specific gravity of a transudate is usually between 1.006 and 1.018; that of an exudate, because of its larger protein content, is generally considerably higher than 1.018.

PROTEIN CONTENT. The protein content of pleural fluid may vary from 0.1 to 8.0 gram/100 ml. The protein content of a transudate is usually well under 2.5 per cent, but that of an exudate is always higher than 2.5 per cent.

Microscopic Examination. CYTOLOGICAL EXAMINATION. The cellular content of pleural fluid is of considerable importance. Although not diagnostic by itself, the predominant cell type may suggest the probable causative disease. The finding of numerous polymorphonuclear neutrophils is indicative of a pyogenic infection. Numerous lymphocytes are suggestive of tuberculosis, although these can also be found in any chronic pleural effusion. Numerous eosinophils may be found in fluid caused by a parasitic infection, such as hydatid disease. Numerous erythrocytes may be found in pleural fluids caused by trauma, tuberculosis and malignant conditions. Transudates usually contain very few cells, and these are chiefly endothelial cells shed from the pleural membrane. Malignant cells may be present if a neoplastic process is involving the pleural surfaces, but these are generally difficult to recognize unless mitosis is present or unless the cells are arranged in a tissue pattern. Chylous fluid can be recognized by oily droplets which stain readily with Sudan III.

BACTERIOLOGICAL EXAMINATION. The centrifuged sediment of all pleural fluids should be smeared, stained and examined microscopically for bacteria. The identity of the various bacteria that may be present can be established only by cultural methods. If tuberculosis is suspected, animal inoculation is of still greater value. This is discussed in the following section.

BACTERIOLOGICAL DIAGNOSIS

The bacteriological examination of sputum, pleural fluid and material from draining sinuses is of tremendous importance in the definitive diagnosis of bronchopulmonary infections. The responsible organism can be determined, and the correct antimicrobial therapy can be instituted when indicated.

The bacteriological diagnosis is made by direct microscopy, certain cultural procedures and animal inoculation. The direct examination of the stained smear is particularly important for the detection of tubercle bacilli. In nontuberculous bacterial infections, this procedure only determines whether the organisms in the sputum are predominantly gram-positive or gram-negative. Nevertheless, with this knowledge, the appropriate antibiotic therapy can be instituted provisionally before the results of the sputum culture and the sensitivity tests are available.

The implantation of abnormal secretions on an appropriate artificial medium results in the growth of a variety of organisms. The sensitivity of the pathogenic bacteria that are isolated to various antibiotics is then assessed. The bacteriologist's report should always be assessed critically and in the light of the clinical picture. It should be remembered that the bacteria that are grown may be only secondary invaders and not actually responsible for the disease and that organisms which grow profusely when cultured may be present only in small numbers in the bronchial secretions.

Animal inoculation is used primarily in the diagnosis of an active tuberculosis. The guinea pig is the animal of choice, as it is extremely sensitive to both the human and bovine types of tubercle bacillus. This procedure determines the pathogenicity of an acid-fast bacillus if this is in doubt, thus precluding the possibility of a wrong diagnosis.

TUBERCULOUS INFECTION

The tuberculous origin of a pulmonary lesion can be proved only by the demonstration of tubercle bacilli in the bronchial secretions. As the radiological opacities produced by pulmonary tuberculosis can mimic those caused by many nontuberculous diseases, it is imperative that the sputum of all forms of bronchopulmonary diseases be examined repeatedly for tubercle bacilli, no matter how obvious the diagnosis may be.

Tuberculous sputum possesses no special characteristics which distinguish it from that produced in nontuberculous pulmonary diseases. It is usually mucopurulent, but it may be mucoid, hemorrhagic or purulent if it is associated with cavitation. The sputum of all the varieties of active pulmonary tuberculosis, even the frank hemoptysis, always contains a variable number of tubercle bacilli. For this reason, if the clinical picture suggests pulmonary tuberculosis, it may be necessary to examine many specimens of sputum over a period of even months before the diagnosis can be finally excluded. Tubercle bacilli are usually readily demonstrated in active disease, but if the disease is chronic and indolent, the organisms may be found only after repeated and persistent searching.

Direct Examination of the Stained Smear. The detection of acid-fast bacilli, morphologically resembling tubercle bacilli, by the direct microscopic examination of a smear stained by the Ziehl-Neelsen method is generally accepted as positive proof of the diagnosis of pulmonary tuberculosis. However, it has been estimated that at least 100,000 bacilli must be present in 1 ml. of sputum before a single organism can be detected by the direct examination.

If direct examination has repeatedly failed to demonstrate tubercle bacilli in the sputum, despite clinical and radiological evidence strongly favoring the diagnosis of active pulmonary tuberculosis, success may be possible when a large collection of sputum is concentrated. Sodium hydroxide is added to the sputum because it is bacteriocidal to micro-organisms other than tubercle bacilli, dissolves cellular material and reduces the viscosity. The specimen is then centrifuged, and the sediment is stained by the Ziehl-Neelsen method and examined for acid-fast bacilli. It can be cultured and inoculated into a guinea pig as well.

Guinea Pig Inoculation. Since the sensitivity of the various procedures used to detect tubercle bacilli depends on the number of organisms in the bronchial secretions, guinea pig inoculation is the most certain method. An injection of as little as 10 tubercle bacilli can cause a generalized tuberculous infection in the guinea pig. Prior to inoculation, the sputum is treated so as to kill contaminating organisms and to prevent a pyogenic infection. The material is then injected either subcutaneously into the flank or intramuscularly into the thigh. The animal is killed after a period of six to eight weeks, or earlier if it appears ill, and an autopsy is performed. If there is generalized tuberculosis, caseous lesions are found at the site of inoculation as well as in the inguinal, mesenteric and mediastinal lymph nodes, and numerous miliary, yellowish, caseous lesions are present in the spleen and the liver, very few being found in the lungs. These lesions are always smeared and stained for acid-fast bacilli.

Culture. Culture of the sputum on a suitable artificial medium is probably as efficient a procedure as animal inoculation for the demonstration of tubercle bacilli. The only possible advantage it has over animal inoculation is that a shorter time is required for the organisms to grow on an artificial medium. Although tubercle bacilli grow on a variety of culture media, a solid medium containing a mixture of egg and potato flour or starches is commonly used. The specimen is inoculated directly on the culture medium and is incubated at 37° C. A dry, wrinkled, yellowish and warty growth appears in four to six weeks.

Another group of acid-fast bacteria on extremely rare occasions is capable of producing a chronic pulmonary disease which closely mimics tuberculous disease. It has been suggested that they are saprophytic organisms which become pathogenic to man under unusual circumstances. These organisms are distinguished from the tubercle bacillus by cultural methods. They are not pathogenic to the guinea pig, and are able to grow at room temperature. In addition, the culture colonies are pigmented pale yellow to deep orange and have smooth and glistening surfaces.

Tuberculin Skin Test. In general, diagnostic skin tests are used to determine whether there is hypersensitivity to a specific antigen due to previous contact with either a bacterial protein or toxin. Hypersensitivity that is not associated with the formation of antibodies produces a delayed type of skin reaction which is usually manifest in 48 hours. This is the type of reaction which occurs in tuberculous infection and a few mycotic diseases.

The culture medium in which tubercle bacilli are grown contains an active substance which consists of tuberculoprotein and degradation products of the organism. This material, known as Old Tuberculin, is capable of producing a hypersensitivity reaction in persons who have been infected with the tubercle bacillus. The active principle of Old Tuberculin is known as purified protein derivative, or P.P.D. This is the antigen of choice, for it is 200 times as potent by weight as Old Tuberculin and has a more constant composition.

The tuberculin test can be carried out by two different techniques. The one most commonly used is the intracutaneous Mantoux test. The second method, the patch test, consists of the application of Old Tuberculin on the unbroken skin. This method, although painless and therefore favored for testing infants and young children, is inefficient because false-negative reactions occur frequently. The skin reaction is interpreted 48 hours after the injection, although occasionally a positive reaction may develop after 72 hours. A positive skin reaction consists of an area of edema surrounded by a zone of erythema. The edematous area is the only significant part of the skin reaction. The test is reported as negative if there is no reaction or if erythema develops without edema. If the area of edema is less than 5 mm. in diameter, the reaction is doubtfully positive, but if the diameter is over 5 mm. the reaction is read as positive.

A positive tuberculin reaction implies that the tissues of the patient have been infected by the tubercle bacillus at some time in either the distant or recent past, but it does not indicate that tuberculous disease is necessarily present. The strength of the reaction bears no relationship to the activity of the tuberculous focus. An active tuberculous lesion may produce a weakly positive reaction; conversely, a strongly positive reaction does not necessarily indicate that an active tuberculous focus is present. Persons who have never been infected are absolutely insensitive to even enormous doses of tuberculin.

It has been estimated that a period of three weeks to three months is required following the development of a primary tuberculous infection before the tissues become sufficiently sensitized to show a measurable reaction to the injection of tuberculin, depending on the size of the infecting dose and the response of the subject to the infection. In most circumstances the tuberculin reaction remains positive throughout the patient's life.

A negative tuberculin reaction can be of great diagnostic significance. Under such circumstances one can confidently assume that the pulmonary lesion is not tuberculous in origin, provided the tests have been performed with dilutions up to 1:100 of Old Tuberculin and the patient is not critically ill, so that the anergy associated with tuberculous meningitis, tuberculous pneumonia and miliary tuberculosis is excluded. In addition, a positive reaction may be temporarily abolished if the patient is markedly debilitated or is running a high fever, even though he is suffering from active tuberculosis. Certain nontuberculous conditions such as undulant fever, measles and Hodgkin's disease may also temporarily abolish the tuberculin reaction.

NONTUBERCULOUS BACTERIAL INFECTION

The pathogenic bacteria responsible for a bronchopulmonary infection can be isolated only by culturing the sputum and other abnormal secretions. The direct examination of a smear stained by the Gram method does not delineate the organisms present but only indicates whether they are predominantly gram-positive or gram-negative. When the secretions are cultured, however, the organisms can be identified by subculturing the colonies and carrying out special tests. Organisms may also be grown by culturing the blood, for bacteremia is frequently present, particularly in pneumonia.

The culture medium generally used is meat-infusion agar containing fresh blood. The secretions are smeared unevenly on a culture plate so that various concentrations of the inoculum are made on different parts of the medium. When a growth appears, the different types of bacteria are subcultured on separate plates. At the same time, antibiotic sensitivity tests are carried out on the individual plates by placing paper discs impregnated with one of the available antibiotics on the smears. The relative sensitivity of a colony is indicated by the size of the zone of inhibited growth around each disc. If no zone is present, the organisms are considered to be resistant. These findings assist the clinician in deciding on the appropriate antibiotic, if such a therapeutic measure is indicated.

The saprophytic bacteria which normally inhabit the oropharynx are frequent contaminants of sputum. Most of these commensal organisms have never been incriminated in respiratory infections. A few are potentially pathogenic and may invade the tracheobronchial tree when its defense mechanisms break down, as in a viral infection or some debilitating disease. These organisms include the pneumococcus, hemolytic streptococcus, *Staphylococcus aureus,* Friedländer's bacillus and *Hemophilus influenzae.*

The pneumococcus is by far the commonest cause of bacterial infections of the respiratory tract. Of the seventy-five types that form this group of organisms, the most serious infections are produced by types II, III, V and XIV. Differentiation of the various types is no longer necessary, however, since the advent of antibiotic therapy. Blood cultures should be carried out in all cases of pneumococcal pneumonia. Bacteremia, a complication which considerably worsens the prognosis, may be present in about 40 per cent of cases.

The hemolytic streptococcus is the second commonest cause of bacterial infections. Although it may produce a primary type of pneumonia, it generally acts as a secondary invader following in the course of some other infection such as influenza or measles.

Staphylococcus aureus also acts most commonly as a secondary invader, although it does so much less frequently than the hemolytic streptococcus. Staphylococcal pneumonia most frequently develops during the course of influenza or some debilitating disease. It may also develop as a result of the invasion of the blood from a primary focus in some other part of the body, such as a perinephric abscess, the pneumonia then being a part of a widespread infection.

Friedländer's bacillus is a very rare cause of pneumonia. It is occasionally found in the healthy oropharynx where it behaves as a saprophyte, but it can become pathogenic if the body's resistance is lowered. *Hemophilus influenzae* generally produces a primary pneumonia in infants and children, and it is frequently demonstrated in the sputum of patients with chronic bronchitis.

VIRAL INFECTION

A number of the known filterable viruses have been definitely implicated as the etiologic agents of certain acute respiratory infections. In addition, there is a group of acute epidemic respiratory infections which are presumed to be caused by viruses, even though no bacterial or viral agent has been isolated. Of the known filterable viruses that are capable of causing pneumonia in man, the most important ones are the influenza and the psittacosis-ornithosis groups.

Influenza virus can be grown by inoculating the patient's throat washings, which are obtained during the early phase of the illness, into an embryonated egg, as well as into ferrets or mice. The disease can be diagnosed by the virus neutralization test, which demonstrates the presence of antibodies capable of neutralizing the influenza virus in the serum. Specimens are obtained as early as possible after the beginning of the illness, about fourteen days later, and about four weeks after the onset of the disease. The etiology can also be established by the hemagglutination inhibition test, which is based on the ability of the influenza virus to agglutinate erythrocytes, a reaction which can be inhibited by a specific antiserum. Although the influenza virus has been shown to cause pneumonia in experimental animals, its role in the etiology of pneumonia in man is not clear, as it has been isolated from human lungs only on very rare occasions. On the other hand, bacteria such as the hemolytic streptococcus, pneumococcus, *Staphylococcus aureus* and *Hemophilus influenzae* are very common secondary invaders in most cases of influenza, and these organisms are probably the cause of the pneumonia.

The group of primary atypical pneumonias is considered to be caused by a filterable virus, for the disease can be reproduced by inoculating filtered nasal washings into voluntary subjects. A few of the adenoviruses and a large virus known as the Eaton agent have been implicated in some cases of this disease. An interesting serologic feature of primary atypical pneumonia is that in over half the cases a substance capable of agglutinating human Group O erythrocytes appears in the serum at low temperatures, but not at room or body temperature. These cold-agglutinins are found in the pneumonia caused by the Eaton agent but not in that caused by the adenoviruses. The demonstration of a rising titer of those agglutinins during the course of the disease is helpful in arriving at a diagnosis. In many cases of primary atypical pneumonia the serum also contains antibodies against a single type of nonhemolytic streptococcus, the Streptococcus MG, although this organism does not appear to play any part in the causation of the disease.

The causative organism of psittacosis-ornithosis is a large virus which can infect wild and domestic birds as well as man. The virus is shed in the excreta and nasal discharge of infected birds, and humans are infected by the inhalation of the dried excretions. The virus can be isolated by injecting sputum, blood or throat washings into a mouse or the amniotic sac of a chick embryo. A rise in the complement-fixing antibodies in the serum tested in the early acute phase of the disease and again during the convalescent period is helpful in making a diagnosis as well.

MYCOTIC INFECTION

Although mycotic infections of the respiratory tract are very rare in relation to other pulmonary infections, they do occur with sufficient frequency to warrant consideration in the differential diagnosis of an obscure pulmonary lesion. This is particularly true if the patient is known to have resided in a geographical area in which a particular fungus infection is endemic.

An accurate diagnosis of the mycotic infection can be established only by the isolation and identification of a fungus. This may be done on bronchial secretions in the form of sputum, fasting gastric contents or bronchoscopic aspirate, or from the histological examination of diseased tissues.

The presence of fungi in the sputum does not necessarily imply that these organisms are the primary or sole cause of the disease. They may be saprophytic, having accidentally contaminated the specimen, or they may have invaded some other pre-existing disease secondarily. This particularly applies to yeasts, which are frequently found in the sputum of patients with such chronic diseases as pulmonary tuberculosis, bronchiectasis and bronchogenic carcinoma. On the other hand, certain other fungi, when isolated from the bronchial secretions, can definitely be considered primarily responsible for disease, particularly *Actinomyces bovis, Coccidioides immitis,* and *Blastomyces dermatitidis.*

Candida albicans and other members of the Candida family are normally inhabitants of the mouth. For this reason, the diagnosis of candidiasis is often difficult, especially since the advent of the widespread use of antibiotics and corticosteroids, which has increased their incidence in sputum cultures.

Actinomyces bovis is present in the form of "sulphur granules," which consist of a dense tangle of gram-positive mycelia in the bronchial secretions and the discharge from sinuses. These whitish yellow amorphous masses are often visible to the naked eye if the pus is shaken in normal saline and examined against a dark background. Although *Actinomyces bovis* is normally saprophytic and may be found in the mouths and throats of healthy persons, it can become pathogenic if it gains a foothold in devitalized tissues. The organism can be grown only under anaerobic conditions, a feature which distinguishes it from *Nocardia asteroides,* which can be grown only under aerobic conditions. *Nocardia asteroides* is normally a saprophyte as well, inhabiting the soil as well as dead organic matter, but it may infect man by being inhaled into the lungs or inoculated into the skin.

Aside from *Actinomyces bovis* and *Nocardia asteroides,* most pathogenic fungi can be identified only by cultural methods. They are isolated by culturing the sputum on either Sabouraud's agar at room temperature or blood agar at 37° C.

Blastomyces dermatitidis, the fungus responsible for North American blastomycosis, is a large, yeast-like cell which produces pulmonary lesions closely resembling pulmonary tuberculosis, bronchogenic carcinoma and other fungus infections. Most cases are found in North America, particularly in the southern United States and in the Mississippi Valley.

Coccidioides immitis, the cause of coccidioidomycosis, exists in nature in a mycelial form, but it becomes a large spherule once it invades the tissues. It is endemic in the semi-arid areas of the southwestern United States. Although most infections are mild or unapparent, a fatal disseminated form of the disease can occur.

Histoplasma capsulatum, which is responsible for histoplasmosis, differs from all the other pathogenic fungi in that it is an intracellular organism. It is confined to the cells of the reticuloendothelial system and so is rarely found in the sputum. The disease may vary in severity from a mild or unapparent respiratory infection to a rapidly fatal disseminated disease. Humans are probably infected by inhaling soil dust which contains the spores of Histoplasma and chicken droppings have been implicated as a source of infection. The disease is endemic in the valleys of large rivers, such as the Mississippi, the Ohio and the St. Lawrence.

Fungus Skin Tests. Infection by pathogenic fungi causes a hypersensitivity of the tissues of the host to subsequent invasion by either the same fungus or the proteins characteristic of that particular organism. This reaction resembles the hypersensitivity reaction of the tissues to tuberculin, in that an intradermal injection of the appropriate antigen results in a delayed reaction. The antigen usually employed is a sterile filtrate of a synthetic broth medium in which one of the fungi has been grown. The only antigens which are of diagnostic value are those produced by *Coccidioides immitis, Histoplasma capsulatum* and *Blastomyces dermatitidis,* which are called coccidioidin, histoplasmin and blastomycin. Unfortunately, there are no standard methods of preparation of these antigens as yet, and no purified standardized fractions of the fungi have been developed. Cross reactions may occasionally occur between these antigens. Histoplasmin may cross-react with both coccidioidin and blastomycin, particularly with the latter. Nevertheless, the specific antigen for the fungus causing the disease generally produces the strongest reaction.

A positive intradermal reaction implies that infection with a particular fungus has occurred, but it does not indicate whether this happened in the remote or very recent past. In addition, a positive reaction is not diagnostic and does not necessarily indicate that the pulmonary disease under study has been caused by the fungus whose antigen produced the reaction. A negative intradermal reaction is of greater diagnostic value, for it indicates that the body has not been infected by that particular fungus. Occasionally anergy may develop in a patient who is seriously ill so that no skin reaction occurs after the intradermal injection of the antigen even though he is suffering from that particular fungal disease.

Serologic Tests. The complement fixation and precipitin tests may be helpful in establishing the diagnosis of mycotic infection. These tests become positive only after the development of a hypersensitivity reaction in the tissues. The complement-fixating antibodies appear later than the precipitins and persist for a longer time, so that the precipitin test is of more value in the early phase of the disease. A negative reaction to either test, however, does not necessarily imply that a mycotic infection is not present.

RICKETTSIAL INFECTION

Rickettsia are rarely responsible for the pneumonia which develops in such rickettsial infections as typhus fever and Rocky Mountain spotted fever, the commonest cause being secondary bacterial invaders. On the other hand, it is rickettsia which are responsible for the pneumonia in Q fever. This is a worldwide disease, caused by *Coxiella burnetii*, which infects wild animals and cattle. It is probable that humans are infected through the ingestion of infected meat and milk and by the inhalation of infected dust. The rickettsia can occasionally be isolated by the injection of the patient's blood or urine into a guinea pig or into the yolk sac of a chick embryo. The diagnosis is usually made serologically by the complement-fixation and agglutination tests using *C. burnetii* yolk sac antigen. Complement-fixating antibodies usually appear during the first week of the illness, and agglutination antibodies usually appear during the second or third week. The Weil-Felix reaction, an agglutination test using Proteus Ox19, Ox2 and OxK, is frequently positive in most rickettsial diseases except Q fever.

HISTOLOGICAL DIAGNOSIS

In some cases, an accurate diagnosis of the respiratory disease can be established only by histological examination of diseased tissues, if such material is available. Especially in malignant disease, a biopsy of the tumor is the most certain diagnostic procedure. Biopsy material from the bronchi is obtained through a bronchoscope. Excision of an enlarged peripheral lymph node may be extremely helpful in the diagnosis of metastatic carcinoma, lymphoma and leukemia. A needle biopsy of the liver may demonstrate the typical tubercles of sarcoidosis. In other cases, it may be necessary to resort to different procedures, such as surgical excision of impalpable scalene lymph nodes, needle aspiration of lung tissue or a biopsy of the lung through an open thoracotomy.

BRONCHOSCOPY

A bronchoscope is a speculum which enables the examiner to inspect the interior of the tracheobronchial tree. This examination is restricted to the trachea, the major bronchi and the orifices of their larger subdivisions. The smaller bronchi and their peripheral radicles cannot be visualized. Nevertheless, it is still possible to obtain information about the smaller branches by aspiration of their secretions for bacteriologic and cytologic studies. Bronchoscopy enables the examiner to inspect the pathological changes which may be present in the larger bronchi. It is possible to obtain specimens of abnormal tissue or to aspirate abnormal secretions for laboratory examination. In addition, bronchial drainage can be improved by the removal of abnormal tissue or a foreign body obstructing a bronchus, or by the dilatation of a bronchial stricture. The bronchoscopic aspiration of viscid bronchial secretions is often a life-saving procedure.

Bronchoscopy is indicated whenever there are any symptoms or signs of a localized bronchial obstruction, whether incomplete or complete. It is imperative if there is the least suspicion of a bronchogenic carcinoma, for over 50 per cent of these tumors can be seen by means of the bronchoscope, and many more are diagnosed from the malignant cells which are exfoliated into the aspirated bronchial secretions. The procedure is of particular value in determining the source of a hemoptysis, especially if surgical extirpation of the pulmonary lesion is being contemplated.

SCALENE NODE BIOPSY

The scalene nodes are deep, impalpable lymph nodes situated in a pad of fat which lies anterior to the scalenus anticus muscle in the neck. Those on the right drain the lymph from the entire right lung and the left lower lobe. Lymph from the left upper lobe goes to the left scalene nodes. The middle part of the left lung may drain to either side.

Since the scalene nodes are connected with the mediastinal nodes, a scalene node biopsy determines not only whether a pulmonary neoplasm is present, but whether it has metastasized. It is assumed that the finding of a pathological process in the scalene nodes indicates that it is also present in the mediastinal nodes, suggesting that the disease has progressed to the extent that it is no longer operable. The procedure can also be of value in the diagnosis of sarcoidosis, tuberculosis and the lymphomas. On the other hand, it should be pointed out that a pathological process found in a scalene lymph node need not necessarily reflect the disease that is present in the lung.

NEEDLE BIOPSY OF THE LUNG

This procedure can be helpful in the diagnosis of a large solitary lesion in the lung or occasionally in diffuse infiltrations. A standard liver biopsy needle is used.

The usefulness of a needle biopsy is marred by the fact that the needling is carried out blindly and that any tissue obtained is often inadequate for a proper histological diagnosis. In addition, there is always the hazard of causing a pneumothorax, a hemothorax or a hemorrhage in the lung, and if there is a malignant lesion, it is theoretically possible that malignant cells may be implanted along the track of the needle into the healthy lung tissue, pleura and chest wall.

OPEN LUNG BIOPSY

The open biopsy of diseased lung tissue is the most direct approach to the correct histological diagnosis of a pulmonary lesion. This procedure is of particular value in determining the cause of obscure, diffuse, bilateral pulmonary infiltrations. The procedure is considerably less radical than the conventional open thoracotomy, and it can be performed even on a seriously ill patient with a low pulmonary reserve. After a small incision is made in the anterior chest wall, usually between the fourth and fifth ribs, the anesthetist inflates the lung, causing a portion of lung to protrude through the opening. This is then excised for histological examination.

PLEURAL BIOPSY

In most cases, the disease process responsible for a pleural effusion can be determined by the clinical assessment of the patient's illness and the laboratory examination of the fluid. In a significant number of patients, however, the cause cannot be elicited, particularly in young adults with acute serous pleurisy. In former years active pulmonary tuberculosis frequently developed within five years in a large percentage of cases. For this reason, if the tuberculin test was positive, such cases were considered to be tuberculous until proved otherwise.

An aspiration biopsy of the pleura by means of a specially designed needle at the time the fluid is being aspirated may yield the diagnosis. Because it is a blind procedure, a pleural biopsy may pick up a relatively normal area and miss a pathological lesion, so that negative findings are not uncommon. In certain selected cases, it may be necessary to carry out an exploratory thoracotomy, enabling the surgeon to visualize the diseased areas in the pleura and to detect a significant pulmonary lesion which may have been overlooked.

SKIN TESTS

THE NICKERSON-KVEIM SKIN TEST

The Nickerson-Kveim skin test is a valuable diagnostic procedure, for it is a specific reaction to the intracutaneous injection of sarcoid antigen, which is present only in patients suffering from active sarcoidosis. This is a systemic, granulomatous disease of unknown etiology which primarily affects the reticuloendothelial system. The diagnosis is generally made by the histological demonstration of the characteristic noncaseating epithelioid cell granuloma in biopsy tissues of the lymph nodes, skin, liver, lung and conjunctiva. The diagnostic value of the skin test is limited because it often requires weeks or even months before a positive reaction appears. This consists of a cutaneous papule at the injection site, which, when examined, is histologically consistent with the typical granulomatous lesions of sarcoidosis. A negative reaction occurs in patients who are free from disease.

The antigen, which is crude and unstandardized, is made by emulsifying sarcoid tissues in physiologic saline. It is important that the tissue be involved by active sarcoid disease; otherwise the antigen may be ineffective. It may lose its potency or even its specificity if kept over a long period of time.

The procedure consists of the intracutaneous injection of 0.2 ml. of the antigen into the flexor surface of the forearm. The injection site chosen should be one that is easily identified at a later time. The patient should be seen at weekly intervals, and when a reddish papule appears, it is excised for histological examination. If no papule should appear after a period of eight weeks, the apparently healthy skin of the injection site should be excised, for granulomas may be found on microscopic examination.

One of the criteria for the diagnosis of sarcoidosis is a persistently negative or slightly positive reaction to the intradermal injection of large doses of tuberculin. This occurs even in patients who are known to have had a positive tuberculin reaction in the past. This loss of hypersensitivity to the injection of tuberculin is a nonspecific one, for it is accompanied by a failure of the skin to react to the intradermal injection of other antigens.

THE CASONI SKIN TEST

A positive Casoni skin test is considered to be diagnostic of hydatid disease. Once the skin test becomes positive, it remains so for the remainder of the patient's life. A negative reaction generally means that the patient has not been infected by the Echinococcus. The antigen consists of fluid from an uncomplicated hydatid cyst which has been passed through a Berkefeld or Seitz filter for sterility. The test is performed by the intradermal injection of 0.25 ml. of this antigen into the flexor surface of the forearm so that a good sized wheal is raised. A similar amount of normal saline is injected into the opposite forearm as a control. There are two varieties of positive reaction. First, there is an immediate response of the allergic type which reaches its maximum level within half an hour after the injection. In this reaction the wheal enlarges in size, develops pseudopodia and is surrounded by a zone of erythema. This is followed by a late response which occurs about 24 hours later and consists of an indurated area surrounded by an erythematous zone.

ALLERGIC SKIN TESTS

The allergens responsible for bronchial asthma, allergic rhinitis and other related diseases produce a hypersensitivity of the tissues which is associated with the production of antibodies. The reaction of the skin to the intradermal injection of these allergens consists of an immediate edematous wheal. Allergens can be classified as ingestants, injectants, inhalants and contactants. Unfortunately, reaction to most of these materials is nonspecific. A careful interrogation is often of greater value in eliciting the nature of the particular antigen responsible for the disease than are the intradermal tests. Nevertheless, reaction to a single specific allergen is likely to be highly significant.

SWEAT CHLORIDES

Most patients suffering from mucoviscidosis show a marked elevation of the sodium and chloride levels in the sweat due to an inability of the sweat glands to conserve salt. This electrolyte abnormality has been found also in untreated adrenal insufficiency, and it is being found with increasing frequency in patients who have bronchiectasis. Many patients with mucoviscidosis also have pancreatic insufficiency, with absence of trypsin, lipase and amylase in the duodenal contents and an excess of fat and nitrogenous matter in the feces.

SPECIAL TESTS IN BLOOD

The demonstration of peculiar cells in special preparations of bone marrow and blood, called L. E. cells, establishes the diagnosis of systemic lupus erythematosus, a collagen disease in which interstitial pneumonitis and pleural involvement are frequent.

Measurements of the serum enzymes can be of diagnostic importance in respiratory disease. Those most extensively studied have been the glutamic oxalacetic and glutamic pyruvic transaminases and lactic dehydrogenase. These tests are of particular value in pulmonary embolism and infarction, which causes an elevation of lactic dehydrogenase but does not affect the transaminases. This is a distinguishing feature from acute myocardial infarction, in which both the lactic dehydrogenase and the transaminases are elevated. The mechanism for the changes in the enzyme levels has not been elucidated.

Although bronchopulmonary syphilis is extremely uncommon, this disease should be excluded by serological tests. A false-positive test for syphilis may occasionally occur in lupus erythematosus. It has been suggested that this is caused by the attachment of gamma globulin to the phospholipids of the antigen used in the Wassermann test.

NONSPECIFIC TESTS

Various tests, even though not diagnostic, provide useful information for the assessment of respiratory illness. It is not necessary to describe the tests in any detail here; instead, brief comments on the findings or their interpretation are presented in the following paragraphs.

HEMATOLOGY

Anemia may result from the accelerated blood destruction which occurs in certain bacterial infections, particularly those caused by the hemolytic streptococcus. A chronic infection, such as tuberculosis, may produce anemia as a result of depression of the bone marrow. A neoplasm which has metastasized to the bone marrow may cause anemia by mechanical interference with blood formation. Secondary polycythemia may occur in diseases with associated chronic hypoxia.

A neutrophilic leukocytosis is generally present in acute infections produced by pyogenic organisms, such as *Staphylococcus aureus,* hemolytic streptococcus and pneumococcus. The degree of leukocytosis is governed by the resistance of the patient as well as the virulence and the number of the invading organisms. A severe leukocytosis called a leukemoid reaction may occasionally be seen in malignant pulmonary conditions, particularly those with associated infection and necrosis.

An eosinophilic leukocytosis most commonly occurs in allergic disease and is particularly severe in the migratory pulmonary infiltrations of Löffler's syndrome. It may accompany parasitic infestations such as ascariasis, amebiasis and hydatid disease. It may also be a feature of periarteritis nodosa and of Hodgkin's disease.

A relative lymphocytosis may occasionally be seen in diseases with associated generalized lymphadenopathy, such as Hodgkin's disease and lymphosarcoma, and a high degree of relative lymphocytosis may be found in pertussis.

Various degrees of neutropenia may be found in such viral diseases as measles and influenza, as well as in some overwhelming bacterial infections, probably because of depression of the bone marrow by the organisms or their toxins.

The erythrocyte sedimentation rate frequently provides an indication of the activity of the disease process. An accelerated rate is an important finding, especially if it is known that the rate had been normal in the past. A normal rate, however, does not necessarily mean that the disease is inactive. In acute infective processes, the sedimentation rate is accelerated in the early part of the disease and gradually falls to normal levels as recovery takes place.

BLOOD CHEMISTRY

The blood urea nitrogen may be elevated because of the functional impairment of the kidneys in chronic nephritis. Hyperglycemia is found if diabetes mellitus is present. Hypercalcemia may be a feature of active sarcoidosis. Significant elevation of the serum acid phosphatase is indicative of prostatic carcinoma which has metastasized. Hyperglobulinemia may be present in chronic diseases such as bronchiectasis, tuberculosis and sarcoidosis, as well as lupus erythematosus and periarteritis nodosa. Amyloidosis, a complication of longstanding suppuration, can be demonstrated by the intravenous injection of Congo red, a dye which has an affinity for amyloid tissue.

URINE

The urine should be routinely examined, and if the disease is a chronic one, the examination should be repeated periodically. A small percentage of patients suffering from pulmonary tuberculosis develop genitourinary tuberculosis, particularly when the disease has apparently become inactive. Chronic suppurative diseases may become complicated by the development of renal amyloidosis. Carcinoma of the kidney may metastasize to the lungs or may produce a secondary polycythemia. Patients suffering from diabetes mellitus are more liable to develop pulmonary tuberculosis. The urinary findings of chronic nephritis or congestive heart failure may account for a pleural effusion.

ELECTROCARDIOGRAPHY

The typical electrocardiographic changes of right ventricular hypertrophy and strain and "P pulmonale" may be found in patients suffering from chronic pulmonary diseases who have developed an increased pulmonary vascular resistance. This examination should be repeated at yearly intervals to detect any progression in these changes.

CHAPTER XVIII

The Functional Assessment

FROM the clinical, radiological and clinical-pathological assessment, the clinician is usually able to establish the etiology and anatomical location of the underlying respiratory disease. It is then most important to determine the degree of functional impairment which the disease is producing. Tests of function enable the physician not only to follow the progress of the disease but also, because of his knowledge of the disturbances in pulmonary function, to prescribe the proper therapy and to assess its effects objectively. Since only one aspect of pulmonary function may be altered by some diseases, these studies may occasionally assist in establishing the correct diagnosis of the respiratory condition. In a case of pulmonary disability in which surgery is planned, particularly operative removal of lung tissue, measurements of pulmonary function help to assess the patient's ability to tolerate an anesthetic and narcotics or the removal of lung tissue. In addition, these studies serve as a guide to the preoperative preparation and the postoperative care of the patient.

The tests used to determine the pulmonary function comprise two general groups, tests relating to the ventilatory function of the lungs and the chest wall, and those relating to the gaseous exchange.

VENTILATORY FUNCTION

LUNG VOLUMES

Pulmonary ventilatory function takes place within certain compartments in the lungs, called lung volumes. The total lung capacity can be calculated from a knowledge of the vital capacity and the residual volume. Aside from the residual volume, which is the air remaining in the lungs after a maximal expiration, all of the compartments of the lung may be measured by means of a simple recording spirometer.

The functional residual capacity is determined by a dilution technique which utilizes either an open or closed circuit method, with either helium or nitrogen as the reference gas. In the open-circuit technique, and using nitrogen as the reference gas, the volume and nitrogen concentration of the expired gas are measured after 100 per cent oxygen has been inhaled for seven minutes. The total amount of nitrogen washed out of the lungs represents the nitrogen originally present in the lungs at the end of a normal expiration. From this the functional residual capacity can be calculated. The residual volume can then be estimated by subtracting the expiratory reserve volume, which is measured with a spirometer. In a healthy person, the residual volume is usually less than 30 per cent of the total lung capacity. The residual volume is decreased in diffuse fibrosis of the lungs, as well as in those pulmonary conditions in which the alveoli are either occluded or fail to communicate with the airways. For many years, a ratio greater than 30 per cent was believed to be indicative of chronic obstructive emphysema. However, an increase in residual volume indicates only that the lungs are hyperinflated. The increase may be due to a loss of lung elasticity, as in chronic obstructive emphysema, but it may also be produced by any diffuse obstruction of the airways, as in bronchial asthma. In addition, the residual volume normally increases with age, so that the ratio of residual volume to total lung capacity may be as much as 50 per cent in an elderly healthy person.

The ventilatory function of the lungs and the chest wall may be altered by changes in either the elastic or the nonelastic properties of the respiratory system.

ELASTIC PROPERTIES

A study of the elastic properties of the respiratory system yields information about its distensibility or compliance. The distensibility of the lungs and the chest wall, either together or separately, is determined by the simultaneous measurement of the distending pressure and the resultant volume displacement at a time when there is no movement of air. In practice, the distensibility of the respiratory system is assessed indirectly by determining the vital capacity with an ordinary spirometer, the subject being asked to make a maximal inspiration followed by a forceful deep expiration. The vital capacity varies according to age, body size and sex. Although it has been said to be of limited value as an isolated measurement, it does offer information about the distensibility of the respiratory system if properly performed. Figure 89 illustrates that the volume of the vital capacity correlates with measurements of the compliance of the lung and thorax, the vital capacity decreasing as the total compliance decreases. Thus, the vital capacity is reduced in any condition in which the compliance of the lung is decreased, such as pulmonary fibrosis or congestion, or in which the compliance of the chest wall is decreased, such as obesity or kyphoscoliosis.

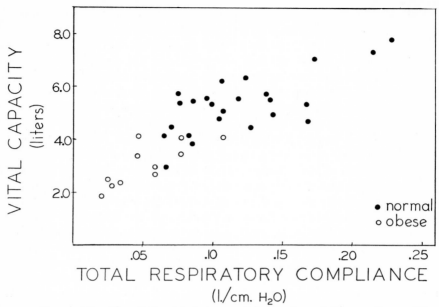

FIGURE 89.   The relationship between vital capacity and the compliance of the lung and thorax. (From Naimark, A. and Cherniack, R. M.: The compliance of the respiratory system and its components in health and obesity. J. Appl. Physiol., *15*:377, 1960. By permission.)

On the other hand, a reduced vital capacity does not necessarily indicate respiratory disease. A great deal depends on the co-operation of the patient. It is essential that the test be repeated several times in order to be certain that the maximal value has been obtained. Conversely, since the volume of the vital capacity is related only to the distensibility of the respiratory system, a patient may be suffering from severe pulmonary disability and yet have a vital capacity well within the normal range. This situation is frequently encountered in patients with an increase in nonelastic resistance due to severe obstructive disease of the airways.

NONELASTIC RESISTANCE

The nonelastic properties of the respiratory system are related to the rate of the change in the tidal volume. The nonelastic resistance during breathing may be assessed by measuring simultaneously the pressure within the lung and the rate of air flow at the mouth. In practice, considerable information about the nonelastic resistance can be obtained by observing the rate at which both an inspiratory and an expiratory vital capacity take place.

The assessment of the expiratory nonelastic resistance is usually carried out in two ways. The vital capacity maneuver is performed and the amounts of air expelled during the first, the second and the third seconds are calculated. This is called the *timed vital capacity.* Normally, 80 per cent of the total vital capacity is expelled in one second, 90 per cent in two seconds and 95 per cent at the end of three seconds. In patients with airway obstruction, these volumes, particularly that of the first second, are sharply reduced. In the second procedure, the rate of air flow during the middle half of the full expiration is determined. This is measured by delineating the volume and duration of the middle half of the expired vital capacity curve. The volume is then divided by the time interval, and the result is called the *maximal mid-expiratory flow rate.* The normal values range from 2 to 5 liters/sec., but in chronic obstructive emphysema and severe bronchial obstruction the flow rate is usually less than 1.0 liter/sec. On the other hand, in patients with a reduced compliance but no associated airway obstruction, as in diffuse pulmonary fibrosis, the timed vital capacity and maximal mid-expiratory flow rate are usually normal.

A simple bedside test may be used to assess expiratory obstruction. The patient, with his mouth opened widely, attempts to blow out a match which is held three to four inches away. If the obstruction to the flow of air is severe, he may be unable to extinguish the flame even though it is held directly in front of his mouth.

Inspiratory obstruction to air flow is also often present and may be extremely severe in patients with chronic bronchial obstruction. An inspiratory vital capacity may be analyzed for the maximal flow rate during the middle half of the full inspiration taken after a maximal expiration, in the same manner as the maximal mid-expiratory flow rate. The maximal mid-inspiratory flow rates are normally greater than those of expiration, and range from 3 to 8 liters/sec.

It should be pointed out that, while the measurements of both the inspiratory and the expiratory rates of air flow are very useful clinically, the rate of air flow which is achieved depends upon the force applied by the subject during inspiration and expiration. Ideally, both the maximal flow rates and the force producing them, or in other words, the intrathoracic pressure, should be assessed.

OVER-ALL VENTILATORY FUNCTION

The alteration in elastic and nonelastic properties of the lungs which takes place in various pulmonary diseases can be determined by means of the pressure-volume loop, which is derived from simultaneous measurements of the intrathoracic pressure and the volume of air displaced during breathing. From this loop can be calculated the work required to overcome the elastic and the nonelastic resistances, as well as the total work carried out on the lungs during either a single breath or in the space of a minute. Unfortunately, no direct method is available for measuring the total work of breathing required to overcome the resistance of both the lung and the chest wall. In practice, the effects of any alterations in the mechanical properties of the lungs and chest wall are assessed by determining the *maximal breathing capacity,* which is also called the *maximum voluntary ventilation.* This is the maximal volume of gas that can be breathed during the period of a minute. The patient is instructed to breathe as hard and as fast as he can for twelve seconds, and the volume of air which is being either inspired or expired is collected in a spirometer. This volume of air is then expressed in liters per minute. The normal values range from 70 to 120 liters/min. in females to 100 to 180 liters/min. in males, but they vary with the age, body surface area and the position of the body. For this reason, the maximal breathing capacity is usually assessed while the subject is standing.

Because maximal ventilation can be attained only by voluntary effort, the subject must be encouraged constantly during the performance of the test. It is essential that the examiner be convinced that the patient has made a maximal effort before a low value is interpreted as being abnormal. Since the rate of air flow is markedly increased during the performance of the maximal breathing capacity, this test is particularly affected by alterations in the nonelastic resistance and to a much lesser extent by changes in the elastic resistance. Thus there is no apparent correlation between the maximal breathing capacity and the vital capacity, but there is a moderately good relationship between the maximal breathing capacity and the maximal mid-expiratory flow rate.

Another over-all effect of altered mechanical properties is an abnormal distribution of air within the lung. The manner in which inspired air is distributed to the alveoli is particularly affected by a local alteration in the physical properties of the lung and thorax, such as an unevenly distributed airway obstruction or a local loss of elasticity. Clinically, uneven ventilation may be recognized by diminished or absent breath sounds over an area of the chest or by unequal translucency of the lungs under fluoroscopy. The manner in which the inspired air is distributed within the lung is measured with a relatively insoluble reference gas. Two types of tests are frequently used. In one, the rate of dilution of nitrogen within the lung during the inhalation of either oxygen or a helium-oxygen mixture is estimated. In the other, the rate at which the lungs and a spirometer reach equilibrium with respect to a foreign gas, such as helium or hydrogen, is determined. The use of helium or hydrogen may result in an inaccurate assessment, however, for the density of these gases is less than that of air so that there is less turbulent resistance while they are being breathed.

The simplest technique is the one which studies the elimination of nitrogen from the lungs while the subject breathes 100 per cent oxygen. The nitrogen concentration in the last portion of a maximal expiration at the end of a period of seven minutes of oxygen breathing, in other words, the alveolar sample, is called the *index of intrapulmonary mixing.* If this value is greater than 2 per cent, it is considered to be indicative of an abnormal distribution of gas. The amount of nitrogen left in the lungs at the end of this test depends, however, upon the rate and depth of breathing as well as on the functional residual capacity. Although a patient may have an impaired distribution of gas, he may dilute the nitrogen in the lung to less than 2 per cent by taking rapid deep inspirations. The rate and depth of breathing should, therefore, be monitored, while the breath to breath wash-out of nitrogen is assessed by means of an instantaneously recording nitrogen meter. If the mean nitrogen concentration of each expired breath is plotted serially on semi-logarithmic paper, either against time or against the number of breaths, the points form an exponential curve. In a normal subject, this curve is made up of two components coming from different spaces, one of which is well or rapidly ventilated and the other poorly or slowly ventilated. When there is an impaired distribution of gas, the volume of the poorly or slowly ventilated space increases, and the number of contributing "slow" spaces may also increase.

In clinical practice, alterations in the ventilatory function of a patient suffering from respiratory disease are usually assessed by measuring the vital capacity, the maximal mid-expiratory flow rate, the maxi-

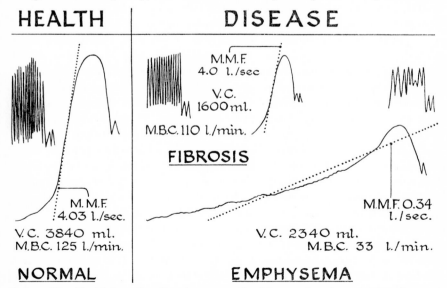

HEALTH	DISEASE

M.M.F.
4.0 l./sec

V.C.
1600 ml.

M.B.C. 110 l./min.

FIBROSIS

M. M.F.
4.03 l./sec.

V.C. 3840 ml.
M.B.C. 125 l./min.

NORMAL

M.M.F. 0.34
l./sec.

V.C. 2340 ml.
M.B.C. 33 l./min.

EMPHYSEMA

FIGURE 90. Ventilatory function in a normal subject and patients with pulmonary fibrosis and chronic obstructive emphysema.

POLIOMYELITIS

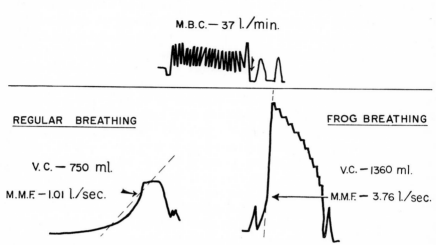

M.B.C.— 37 l./min.

REGULAR BREATHING   FROG BREATHING

V. C. — 750 ml.   V.C. — 1360 ml.

M.M.F. — 1.01 l./sec.   M.M.F. — 3.76 l./sec.

FIGURE 91.   Ventilatory function in a patient with poliomyelitis. The vital capacity has been performed with and without "frog breathing."

mal breathing capacity and the distribution of inspired gas. In this way, the clinician is able to assess qualitatively the mechanical properties of the respiratory system and the over-all effects of these alterations.

Figure 90 shows the types of records of ventilatory function obtained from a normal subject and two patients suffering from pulmonary disease.

In the patient suffering from pulmonary fibrosis, the vital capacity is markedly reduced, while the maximal breathing capacity and maximal mid-expiratory flow rate are very well maintained. From these measurements one may infer that the distensibility or compliance of the lung is reduced and that the airway resistance is essentially normal. Since the increase in elastic resistance is usually diffuse and relatively uniformly distributed, the inspired air is usually distributed uniformly.

In the patient suffering from chronic obstructive emphysema, both the maximal breathing capacity and the maximal mid-expiratory flow rate are markedly reduced, while the vital capacity is only slightly impaired. In addition, because of the increased nonelastic resistance, the maximal breathing capacity is performed at an inspiratory position, in which the resistance is easier to overcome because the bronchi are wider and the elastic recoil is greater. From these tests, one may infer that there is little increase in elastic resistance but that there is a marked increase in the resistance to air flow, which is usually distributed nonuniformly so that the distribution of the inspired air is impaired, the index of intrapulmonary mixing being greater than 2 per cent.

The ventilatory function is also reduced in patients with an increased elastic resistance of the chest cage, as in obesity or kyphoscoliosis, and in patients whose respiratory muscles are unable to perform normally because of neuromuscular disease or paralysis. A record obtained in a patient suffering from poliomyelitis is illustrated in Figure 91. The vital capacity is very low, but it is considerably increased when the maximal expiration follows a large inspiration carried out by means of glossopharyngeal breathing or "frog breathing," by which air is lapped into the tracheobronchial tree with the tongue and cheeks. These findings indicate that the reduced vital capacity may be related to the muscular paralysis rather than to reduced distensibility. The maximal breathing capacity is also reduced because of the paralyzed muscles. The inspired gas is frequently distributed normally, although occasionally nonsymmetrical paralysis leads to poor distribution.

It is essential that diffuse obstruction to air flow be recognized, both by clinical and spirometric means, and it is necessary to determine whether this can be improved by the administration of a nebulized bronchodilating agent. If, following the inhalation of a nebulized bronchodi-

EMPHYSEMA

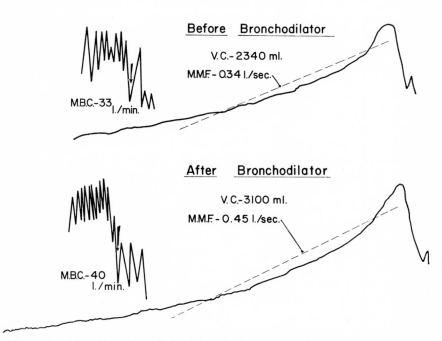

FIGURE 92. The effect of a nebulized bronchodilator on the ventilatory function in a patient with chronic obstructive emphysema.

lator, such as epinephrine, the ventilatory function studies improve by more than 10 per cent, the bronchial obstruction is at least partially reversible. Figure 92 is a record obtained, before and after the administration of nebulized epinephrine, from a patient suffering from diffuse bronchial obstruction. It can be seen that the bronchodilator produced an increase in vital capacity, maximal mid-expiratory flow rate and maximal breathing capacity. The increase in vital capacity suggests that the elastic resistance is decreased, perhaps because of the opening up of completely obstructed airways, and the increase in maximal mid-expiratory flow rate and maximal breathing capacity indicates that the nonelastic resistance has diminished.

GASEOUS EXCHANGE

The presence of cyanosis in a patient may lead the clinician to suspect that the gaseous exchange is inadequate. However, the detection of cyanosis is notoriously difficult and uncertain and, besides, severe pulmonary insufficiency may exist without producing cyanosis. Patients with respiratory disease may suffer from insufficiency of the exchange of either oxygen or both oxygen and carbon dioxide. Carbon dioxide retention is always associated with hypoxia, unless the subject is breathing higher concentrations of oxygen than that present in room air. Whenever there is a reason to doubt the adequacy of gaseous exchange, one should determine the arterial oxygen and carbon dioxide tensions rather than rely on the presence or absence of cyanosis.

Since most patients have disability on exertion, but not while resting, gaseous exchange may be only slightly altered at rest. It is therefore important to assess the gaseous exchange by the simultaneous collection of arterial blood and expired gas while the patient is exercising as well as when he is resting.

The arterial blood is usually collected through an indwelling needle in the brachial artery into a heparinized syringe, without the blood being exposed to air. The oxygen and carbon dioxide content of the blood is usually determined by vacuum extraction. The oxygen and carbon dioxide tensions can be measured directly or, if the arterial pH is measured as well, they can be calculated from the oxyhemoglobin dissociation curve and the Henderson-Hasselbalch equation. The expired air is analyzed for its gas concentrations so that the respiratory quotient may be determined. This is done to insure that the patient is in a "steady state" during the test. In addition, it allows the effective alveolar oxygen tension to be calculated, and thereby the gradient between this and the arterial oxygen tension.

Because of the relative inadequacy of methods of estimating oxygen saturation, the arterial oxygen tension is a more sensitive indicator of hypoxia than is the oxygen saturation. Low arterial oxygen tension in patients with cardiopulmonary disease is likely to be due to one of the following causes. (1) The alveolar ventilation may be inadequate to cope with the level of metabolism. In this situation, the hypoxia is always associated with carbon dioxide retention. (2) There may be uneven ventilation-perfusion ratios in different areas of the lungs. Under such circumstances, the arterial carbon dioxide tension may be decreased, normal or increased, depending on the ability of the remainder of the lungs to compensate by hyperventilation. (3) Venous to arterial shunts, either intrapulmonary or intracardiac, may be present. In this case, the arterial carbon dioxide tension is usually normal or decreased, because the lungs are frequently capable of compensatory hyperventilation. Finally, (4) there may be an impairment of diffusion. In this situation, the arterial carbon dioxide tension is frequently low because of compensatory hyperventilation.

ALVEOLAR HYPOVENTILATION

Although an inadequate alveolar ventilation is the most important functional disturbance encountered in respiratory disease, it is not easily recognized clinically unless it is extremely gross.

It is virtually impossible to assess the adequacy of the alveolar ventilation by means of a physical examination alone. A definitive answer can be obtained only by the direct or indirect measurement of the arterial carbon dioxide tension. The arterial carbon dioxide tension can be determined directly by means of either the bubble technique or the carbon dioxide electrode, or indirectly from the Henderson-Hasselbalch equation after measuring the arterial pH and total carbon dioxide content or from the rebreathing carbon dioxide tension.

If the lungs are healthy, the alveolar or end-tidal carbon dioxide tension may be used as an index of the arterial. The use of an alveolar sample is not applicable in pulmonary diseases, however, because there is a great disparity between the arterial and the end-tidal carbon dioxide tensions when the lungs are diseased. On the other hand, the arterial carbon dioxide tension can be estimated by a rebreathing technique in both normal subjects and those suffering from pulmonary disease. A mixture of carbon dioxide and oxygen is rebreathed from a bag until the carbon dioxide in the bag comes into equilibrium with the mixed venous blood. The equilibrium is recognized by the plateau which develops when the carbon dioxide concentration at the mouth is recorded with a rapid analyzer. The mixed venous carbon dioxide tension can also be measured without a rapid gas analyzer by having the subject provide the necessary oxygen-carbon dioxide mixture himself. This is done by having him rebreathe about a liter of 100 per cent oxygen for two minutes. This rebreathed mixture is later rebreathed again for 15 to 20 seconds and then it is analyzed for carbon dioxide. A maximum of only 20 seconds is allowed because it takes about this time for blood which has been unable to give off carbon dioxide to the alveoli to reach the tissues and return again with its carbon dioxide tension still further elevated. Utilizing this technique, it is relatively easy to assess the adequacy of alveolar ventilation in patients suffering from respiratory disease and to recognize respiratory failure with carbon dioxide retention.

An elevated arterial carbon dioxide tension indicates that the level of the alveolar ventilation is inadequate to cope with the metabolic production of carbon dioxide. This situation is encountered in conditions in which the total ventilation is decreased, as in barbiturate poisoning or muscular paralysis; in which the dead space ventilation is increased, as in chronic obstructive emphysema; or in which the work of breathing or the total body metabolism is disproportionately increased.

ALTERED VENTILATION-PERFUSION RATIOS

Although the ratio of the total alveolar ventilation to the total pulmonary blood flow may be normal, the blood is not maximally arterialized unless the same ratio exists in all parts of the lung. The manner in which the inspired gas is distributed is moderately easy to assess, but distribution of the pulmonary blood flow is not.

A qualitative assessment of an alteration of ventilation-perfusion ratios can be obtained from an analysis of the gas tensions of the arterial blood and the expired air. From these data, the physiological dead space/tidal air ratio, the effective alveolar oxygen tension and the alveolo-arterial oxygen tension gradient can be calculated.

If there is poor distribution of blood to alveoli which are well ventilated, or if there is overventilation of alveoli which are normally perfused, the composition of the gas leaving these alveoli is close to that of the inspired air. The amount of ventilation of poorly perfused alveoli is determined by an analysis of the physiological dead space. This is normally less than 30 per cent of the tidal volume; if it is greater than 30 per cent, it suggests that nonperfused or poorly perfused alveoli are being ventilated.

Perfusion of poorly ventilated alveoli results in the admixture of blood which is venous in type with arterialized blood. The amount of venous admixture is determined by an analysis of the alveolo-arterial oxygen tension gradient at high and low levels of oxygenation. When the patient is at rest and breathing room air, a large gradient is usually due to venous admixture. Normally about 5 per cent of the cardiac output is presumably shunted through the bronchial and thebesian veins and this acts as venous admixture. A venous admixture of greater than 5 per cent of the cardiac output suggests that there is either perfusion of poorly ventilated or nonventilated alveoli, or that there is a "true" right-to-left shunt of blood. If the impaired function is entirely due to altered ventilation-perfusion ratios, the arterial oxygen saturation should rise to 100 per cent when pure oxygen is breathed.

TRUE VENOUS ADMIXTURE

The presence of an anatomical right-to-left shunt or a "true" venous admixture is determined by measuring the arterial oxygen saturation while the patient breathes 100 per cent oxygen. If there is a true shunt, the arterial oxyhemoglobin saturation does not rise to 100 per cent, even though pure oxygen is being inhaled, because blood which has not been in contact with alveolar air is added to arterialized blood. Though usually due to an arteriovenous aneurysm or a defect in the heart, failure to attain full saturation of the hemoglobin may also occur if areas of lung are completely obstructed so that they are perfused but not ventilated. Under these circumstances true venous admixture can still be ruled out by dye curves, which are obtained by the injection of dye into the venous system and noting its appearance time in a peripheral artery. If a true shunt is present, the dye appears early, but if there is perfusion of nonventilated areas, the appearance time is normal.

DIFFUSION DEFECT

An alteration in the diffusing capacity of the lungs is assessed by using either oxygen or carbon monoxide as the reference gas. When oxygen is used, the alveolar-arterial oxygen tension gradient is determined while the subject breathes two oxygen-nitrogen gas mixtures. The mixtures selected are one which results in an approximately normal arterial oxygen saturation and another which results in an oxygen saturation of approximately 70 per cent. The mean partial pressure gradient for oxygen between the alveoli and the capillaries is then estimated by a trial and error method from the alveolo-arterial gradient at the two levels of oxygenation. When a low percentage of oxygen is inhaled, the oxygen content of the pulmonary capillaries is almost the same as that of the mixed venous blood, so that the effect of venous admixture becomes insignificant. Under these circumstances, almost the whole of the alveolo-arterial oxygen tension gradient must be due to a difference between the oxygen in the alveolus and in the capillary. A large gradient means that a diffusion defect must be present.

Because of the technical difficulties of the oxygen method, the diffusing capacity for carbon monoxide is most frequently utilized as a measure of the diffusing capacity. There are several techniques of estimating the diffusing capacity for carbon monoxide. The single-breath method is the easiest to perform, but it may not be physiological and cannot be carried out during exercise. The normal values for the diffusing capacity of carbon monoxide range from 15.4 ml./mm. Hg/min. by the single-breath technique, to 15 to 30 ml./min. by the steady-state technique. Because of the difference in the diffusing characteristics of oxygen and carbon monoxide, the diffusing capacity of oxygen is approximately 1.23 times that of carbon monoxide.

The breath-holding method is a single-breath technique in which the subject follows a full expiration by a rapid inspiration of a gas mixture containing a low concentration of carbon monoxide. The mixture usually used consists of approximately 0.4 per cent carbon monoxide, 10 per cent helium, 20 per cent oxygen and the remainder nitrogen. The subject holds his breath for about ten seconds and then expires maximally. A sample of gas is collected from the last part of the expiration, the alveolar sample. The concentrations of carbon monoxide and helium in the inspired and in the alveolar gas samples are then determined. Since helium is an inert gas and relatively insoluble in blood and tissue, its dilution in the alveolar sample is the same as the dilution of the inspired carbon monoxide. The initial concentration of carbon monoxide in the alveoli is determined and the volume of carbon monoxide which has diffused across the alveolocapillary membrane is then calculated. The mean gradient for carbon monoxide is simply the mean alveolar carbon monoxide tension, because there is virtually no partial pressure of carbon monoxide in the plasma. It should be pointed out, however, that the mean alveolar carbon monoxide tension is not the arithmetical mean of the initial and final carbon monoxide tensions, since the tension of this gas in the alveoli falls exponentially during breath-holding. The diffusing capacity of the lung for carbon monoxide is calculated from the formula:

$$D_{CO} = \frac{\text{alveolar volume}}{(\text{barometer pressure} - 47 \text{ mm. Hg})} \times \text{natural logarithm } \frac{(\text{initial pCO})}{(\text{alveolar pCO})}$$

where D represents diffusing capacity, and p the partial pressure of carbon monoxide. The alveolar volume is equal to the residual volume, since the inspiration started from the residual volume.

In the steady-state carbon monoxide method, the patient breathes air containing a low concentration of carbon monoxide for several minutes, until a steady-state condition of carbon monoxide exchange is reached. The expired gas is then collected and analyzed for carbon monoxide, carbon dioxide and oxygen. The amount of carbon monoxide transferred from the alveolar gas to the capillary blood per minute is then calculated. The mean alveolar carbon monoxide tension is determined by either measuring the end-tidal carbon monoxide tension or calculating it from the physiological dead space and the carbon monoxide tension in the expired gas. Since the physiological dead space for both carbon dioxide and carbon monoxide are considered to be equal, the formula is:

$$V_E \times \frac{P_{A_{CO_2}} - P_{E_{CO_2}}}{P_{A_{CO_2}}} = V_E \times \frac{P_{A_{CO}} - P_{E_{CO}}}{P_{A_{CO}} - P_{I_{CO}}}$$

and

$$P_{A_{CO}} = P_{I_{CO}} - \frac{P_{A_{CO_2}}}{P_{E_{CO_2}}} (P_{I_{CO}} - P_{E_{CO}})$$

where V is the ventilation, P the partial pressure, and the subscripts A, E, and I are the alveolar, expired and inspired gases.

Since the arterial carbon dioxide tension is equal to the alveolar and is more reliable than the alveolar, particularly in patients suffering from pulmonary disease, it is substituted for alveolar carbon dioxide tension in the above equation.

The blood of normal healthy subjects always contains a small amount of carbon monoxide-hemoglobin because of the polluted atmosphere in which we live, so that there is a small partial pressure of carbon monoxide in the blood, even in healthy nonsmokers. Occasionally, the value of the plasma carbon monoxide tension must be subtracted from the alveolar carbon monoxide tension in order to determine the diffusing capacity of the lung for carbon monoxide. This is particularly true in heavy smokers as well as in the steady-state technique, in which carbon monoxide is breathed for a period of time.

The maximal diffusing capacity decreases with age, perhaps because of a diminution in the vascular bed or because of some qualitative change in the alveolocapillary membrane. A low diffusing capacity of the lung is encountered in patients with a qualitative change in the alveolocapillary membrane, as in diffuse fibrosis of the lungs. It is also diminished in those cases in which there has been a reduction in the amount of capillary bed available for diffusion due to an obliteration of the pulmonary vasculature, as in pulmonary emboli, or in which a large amount of lung tissue has been destroyed by disease or removed by surgery. It is unaltered in bronchial asthma but becomes markedly reduced in the later stages of chronic obstructive emphysema, probably because the amount of lung surface available for diffusion is diminished. This has been attributed to a loss of lung elastic tissue, with the destruction of the alveolar walls and their capillaries.

An estimate of a diffusion difficulty can be made indirectly. The finding of a low arterial oxygen tension with a normal or reduced carbon dioxide tension suggests that the hypoxia is due to either a diffusion defect or an arteriovenous shunt. The inhalation of 100 per cent oxygen completely corrects the arterial unsaturation if a diffusion defect is present, but unsaturation is not completely corrected when the hypoxia is due to true venous admixture.

SUMMARY

From the above discussion, it is apparent that a single pulmonary function test is of no value by itself. Each of the tests measures some particular aspect of pulmonary function. In clinical practice, limited studies of pulmonary function, such as ventilatory function studies, usually suffice. In those cases that warrant it, the quantitative functional assessment of a patient with respiratory disease should include tests of gaseous exchange, at rest and during exercise, in addition to the ventilatory function tests. It is only with a thorough understanding of the pathophysiology of the respiratory disease and the existing disability that proper therapy can be instituted.

SUGGESTED ADDITIONAL READING

SECTION 1. Basic Considerations.

Adams, W. and Veith, I.: Pulmonary Circulation. New York, Grune & Stratton, 1959.

Brodovsky, D. M., Macdonell, J. A. and Cherniack, R. M.: The respiratory response to carbon dioxide in health and emphysema. J. Clin. Invest. 39:724, 1960.

Campbell, E. J. M.: The Respiratory Muscles. London, Lloyd-Luke, 1958.

Campbell, E. J. M., Westlake, E. K. and Cherniack, R. M.: Simple methods of estimating the oxygen consumption and efficiency of the breathing muscles. J. Appl. Physiol. 11:303, 1957.

Campbell, E. J. M., Westlake, E. K. and Cherniack, R. M.: The oxygen consumption and efficiency of the respiratory muscles of young male subjects. Clin. Sc. 18:55, 1959.

Cherniack, R. M.: The oxygen consumption and efficiency of the respiratory muscles in health and emphysema. J. Clin. Invest. 38:494, 1959.

Cherniack, R. M.: The physical properties of the lung in chronic obstructive pulmonary emphysema. J. Clin. Invest. 35:394, 1956.

Cherniack, R. M., Farhi, L. E., Armstrong, B. W. and Proctor, D. F.: A comparison of esophageal and intrapleural pressure in man. J. Appl. Physiol. 8:203, 1955.

Cherniack, R. M. and Snidal, D. P.: The effect of obstruction to breathing on the ventilatory response to CO_2. J. Clin. Invest. 35:1286, 1956.

Comroe, J. H., Jr., Forster, R. E., II, Dubois, A. B., Briscoe, W. A. and Carlsen, E.: The Lung. Chicago, Year Book Publishers, 1955.

Davenport, H. W.: The ABC of Acid-Base Chemistry. Chicago, University of Chicago Press, 1958.

Donald, K. W., Renzetti, A., Riley, R. L. and Cournand, A.: Analysis of factors affecting concentrations of oxygen and carbon dioxide in gas and blood of lungs: results. J. Appl. Physiol. 4:497, 1952.

Filley, G. F., Bower, G. C. and Mitchell, R. S.: Report on the Second Aspen Conference on Research in Emphysema. The morphologic basis of pulmonary mechanics. Am. Rev. Resp. Dis. 81:734, 1960.

Fishman, A. P., Turino, G. M. and Bergofsky, E. H.: The syndrome of alveolar hypoventilation. Am. J. Med. 23:33, 1957.

Forster, R. E., II: Exchange of gases between the alveolar air and pulmonary capillary blood: pulmonary diffusing capacity. Physiol. Rev. 37:391, 1957.

Fowler, W. S.: Intrapulmonary distribution of inspired gas. Physiol. Rev. 32:1, 1952.

Gray, J. S.: Pulmonary Ventilation and its Physiological Regulation. Springfield, Ill., Charles C Thomas, 1950.

Gray, J. S.: The multiple factor theory of the control of respiratory ventilation. Science 103:739, 1946.

Hackney, J. D., Sears, C. H. and Collier, C. R.: Estimation of arterial CO_2 tension by rebreathing technique. J. Appl. Physiol. 12:425, 1958.

Hickam, J. B. and Ross, J. C.: Respiratory acidosis in chronic pulmonary heart disease: pathogenesis, clinical features and management. Progr. Cardiovasc. Dis. 1:309, 1959.

Lindskog, G. E.: Collateral respiration in the normal and diseased lung. Yale J. Biol. & Med. 23:311, 1951.

Lilienthal, J. L., Jr. and Riley, R. L.: Circulation through the lung and diffusion of gases. Ann. Rev. Med. 5:237, 1954.

Mead, J.: Mechanical properties of lungs. Physiol. Rev. 41:281, 1961.
Mead, J. and Whittenberger, J. L.: Physical properties of human lungs measured during spontaneous respiration. J. Appl. Physiol. 5:779, 1953.
Naimark, A. and Cherniack, R. M.: The compliance of the respiratory system and its components in health and obesity. J. Appl. Physiol. 15:377, 1960.
Otis, A. B.: The work of breathing. Physiol. Rev. 34:449, 1954.
Riley, R. L.: The work of breathing and its relation to respiratory acidosis. Ann. Int. Med. 41:172, 1954.
Roughton, F. J. W.: Respiratory functions of blood. In Handbook of Respiratory Physiology. Randolph Air Force Base, Texas, U. S. School of Aviation Medicine, 1954.
Woolmer, R.: Symposium on pH and Blood Gas Measurement. London, J. & A. Churchill, 1959.

SECTION 2.   The Manifestations of Respiratory Disease.

Cherniack, L.: Chest movements in respiratory diseases. Canad. M.A.J. 62:266, 1950.
Cherniack, R. M., Cuddy, T. E. and Armstrong, J. B.: The significance of pulmonary elastic and viscous resistance in orthopnea. Circulation 15:859, 1957.
Christie, R. V.: Dyspnea: a review. Quart. J. Med. 7:421, 1938.
Comroe, J. H., Jr.: Dyspnea. Mod. Concepts Cardiovas. Dis. 25:347, 1956.
Coope, R.: Diseases of the Chest. 2nd ed. Edinburgh, E. S. Livingston, 1951.
Fritts, H. W.: Clinical implications of cyanosis. Bull. N.Y. Acad. Med. 37:291, 1961.
Hurtado, A., Velasquez, T., Reynafarje, C., Lozano, R., Chavez, R., Salazar, H. A., Reynafarje, B., Sanchez, C. and Muñoz, J.: Mechanisms of natural acclimatization; studies on the native resident of Morococha, Peru, at an altitude of 14,900 feet. Randolph Air Force Base, Texas, School of Aviation Medicine, Report No. 56-1, 1956, pp. 1–62.
Husson, G. S. and Otis, A. B.: Physiological Adaptation to Chronic Hypoxia. Randolph Air Force Base, Texas, School of Aviation Medicine, 1956.
Jackson, C. and Jackson, C. L.: Diseases of the Nose, Throat and Ear. Philadelphia, W. B. Saunders Co., 1958.
Leopold, S. S.: The Principles and Methods of Physical Diagnosis. Philadelphia, W. B. Saunders Co., 1957.
MacBryde, C. M.: Signs and Symptoms. Philadelphia, J. B. Lippincott Co., 1957.
McIlroy, M. B.: Dyspnea and the work of breathing in diseases of the heart and lung. Progr. Cardiovas. Dis. 1:284, 1959.
Major, R. H. and Delp, M. H.: Physical Diagnosis. Philadelphia, W. B. Saunders Co., 1956.
Prior, J. A. and Silberstein, J. S.: Physical Diagnosis. St. Louis, C. V. Mosby Co., 1959.
Selzer, A.: Chronic cyanosis. Am. J. Med. 10:334, 1951.

SECTION 3.   The Patterns of Respiratory Disease.

Adams, W. and Veith, I.: Pulmonary Circulation. New York, Grune & Stratton, 1959.
Baldwin, E. deF., Cournand, A. and Richards, D. W., Jr.: Pulmonary insufficiency. II. A study of 39 cases of pulmonary fibrosis. Medicine 28:1, 1949.
Baldwin, E. deF., Cournand, A. and Richards, D. W., Jr.: Pulmonary insufficiency.

III. A study of 122 cases of chronic pulmonary emphysema. Medicine 28:201, 1949.

Barach, A. L. and Bickerman, H. A.: Pulmonary Emphysema. Baltimore, Williams & Wilkins, 1956.

Bates, D. V., Knott, J. M. S. and Christie, R. V.: Respiratory function in emphysema in relation to prognosis. Quart. J. Med. 25:137, 1956.

Burwell, C. S., Robin, E. D., Whaley, R. D. and Bickelmann, A. G.: Extreme obesity associated with alveolar hypoventilation—a Pickwickian syndrome. Am. J. Med. 21:811, 1956.

Cherniack, R. M.: Respiratory effects of obesity. Canad. M.A.J. 80:613, 1959.

Cherniack, R. M.: The oxygen consumption and efficiency of the respiratory muscles in health and emphysema. J. Clin. Invest. 38:494, 1959.

Cherniack, R. M.: The physical properties of the lung in chronic obstructive pulmonary emphysema. J. Clin. Invest. 35:394, 1956.

Cherniack, R. M., Cuddy, T. E. and Armstrong, J. B.: The significance of pulmonary elastic and viscous resistance in orthopnea. Circulation 15:859, 1957.

Cooke, F. N. and Blades, B.: Cystic disease of the lungs. J. Thoracic Surg. 23:546, 1952.

Dale, W. A. and Rahn, H.: Rate of gas absorption during atelectasis. Am. J. Physiol. 170:606, 1952.

Ebert, R. V.: Pulmonary emphysema. Ann. Rev. Med. 7:123, 1956.

Fishman, A. P., Turino, G. M. and Bergofsky, E. H.: The syndrome of alveolar hypoventilation. Am. J. Med. 23:33, 1957.

Fleischner, F. G.: The pathogenesis of bronchiectasis. Radiology 53:818, 1949.

Fraser, R. G. and Bates, D. V.: Body section roentgenography in the evaluation and differentiation of chronic hypertrophic emphysema and asthma. Am. J. Roentgenol. 82:39, 1959.

Gould, D. M. and Torrance, D. J.: Pulmonary edema. Am. J. Roentgenol. 73:366, 1955.

Harley, H. R. S.: Subphrenic abscess. Thorax 4:1, 1949.

Heppleston, A. G.: Chronic diffuse interstitial fibrosis of the lungs. Thorax 6:426, 1951.

Heppleston, A. G.: Pathology of honeycomb lung. Thorax 11:77, 1956.

Hickam, J. B. and Ross, J. C.: Respiratory acidosis in chronic pulmonary heart disease: pathogenesis, clinical features and management. Progr. Cardiovasc. Dis. 1:309, 1959.

Hinshaw, H. C. and Garland, L. M.: Diseases of the Chest. Philadelphia, W. B. Saunders Co., 1956.

Hugh-Jones, P.: The functional pathology of emphysema. Brit. J. Anaesth. 30:107, 1958.

Kaufman, B. J., Ferguson, M. H. and Cherniack, R. M.: Hypoventilation in obesity. J. Clin. Invest. 38:500, 1959.

Liebow, A. A., Hales, M. R., Harrison, W., Bloomer, W. and Lindskog, G. E.: The genesis and functional implications of collateral circulation of lungs. Yale J. Biol. & Med. 22:637, 1950.

Leigh, T. F. and Weens, H. S.: The Mediastinum. Springfield, Ill., Charles C Thomas, 1959.

Lilienthal, J. L., Jr. and Riley, R. L.: Circulation through the lung and diffusion of gases. Ann. Rev. Med. 5:237, 1954.

Marshall, R.: The physiology and pharmacology of the pulmonary circulation. Progr. Cardiovasc. Dis. 1:341, 1959.

McLean, K. H.: The pathogenesis of pulmonary emphysema. Am. J. Med. 25:62, 1958.

Mitchell, R. S.: A summary of the Third Conference on Research in Emphysema. Air pollution and chronic pulmonary insufficiency. Am. Rev. Resp. Dis. 83:402, 1961.

Mitchell, R. S. and Filley, G.: Symposium on Emphysema and the "Chronic Bronchitis" Syndrome. Am. Rev. Resp. Dis. 80:(Suppl.), 1959.

Naimark, A. and Cherniack, R. M.: The compliance of the respiratory system in health and obesity. J. Appl. Physiol. 15:377, 1960.

Oswald, N. C.: Recent Trends in Chronic Bronchitis. London, Lloyd-Luke, 1959.

Parker, B. M. and Smith, J. R.: Pulmonary embolism and infarction. A review of the physiologic consequences of pulmonary arterial obstruction. Am. J. Med. 24:402, 1958.

Race, G. A., Scheifly, C. H. and Edwards, J. E.: Hydrothorax in congestive heart failure. Am. J. Med. 22:83, 1957.

Reid, L. and Simon, G.: Pathological findings and radiological changes in chronic bronchitis and emphysema. Brit. J. Radiol. 32:291, 1959.

Riley, R. L.: The work of breathing and its relation to respiratory acidosis. Ann. Int. Med. 41:172, 1954.

Rottenberg, L. A. and Golden, R.: Spontaneous pneumothorax. A study of 105 cases. Radiology 53:157, 1949.

Rushmer, R. F.: Cardiovascular Dynamics. Philadelphia, W. B. Saunders Co., 1961.

Spain, D. M.: Patterns of pulmonary fibrosis as related to pulmonary function. Ann. Int. Med. 33:1150, 1950.

Stringer, C. J., Stanley, A. L., Bates, R. C. and Summers, J. E.: Pulmonary arteriovenous fistula. Am. J. Surg. 89:1054, 1955.

Tysinger, D. S., Jr. and Meneely, G. R.: Spontaneous pneumothorax; clinical diagnosis and management. Am. J. Surg. 89:360, 1955.

Wood, P.: Pulmonary hypertension. Brit. M. Bull. 8:348, 1952.

Xalabarder, C.: What is atelectasis? Tubercle 30:266, 1949.

SECTION 4.   The Assessment of Respiratory Disease.

Baldwin, E. deF., Cournand, A. and Richards, D. W., Jr.: Pulmonary insufficiency. II. A study of 39 cases of pulmonary fibrosis. Medicine 28:1, 1949.

Cherniack, L.: Chest movements in respiratory diseases. Canad. M.A.J. 62:266, 1950.

Comroe, J. H., Jr., Forster, R. E., II, Dubois, A. B., Briscoe, W. A. and Carlson, E.: The Lung. Chicago, Year Book Publishers, 1955.

Coope, R.: Diseases of the Chest. Edinburgh, E. S. Livingston, 1951.

Donohoe, R. F., Katz, S. and Matthews, M. J.: Aspiration biopsy of the parietal pleura: results in 45 cases. Am. J. Med. 22:883, 1957.

Dubos, R. J.: Bacterial and Mycotic Infections of Man. Philadelphia, J. B. Lippincott Co., 1958.

Felson, B.; Fundamentals of Chest Roentgenology. Philadelphia, W. B. Saunders Co., 1960.

Ferris, B. G., Jr.: Studies of pulmonary function. New England J. Med. 262:557, 609, 1960.

Fraser, R. G. and Bates, D. V.: Body section roentgenography in the evaluation and differentiation of chronic hypertrophic emphysema and asthma. Am. J. Roentgenol. 82:39, 1959.

Gaensler, E. A.: Clinical pulmonary physiology. New England J. Med. 252:177, 221, 264, 1955.

Gaensler, E. A.: Evaluation of pulmonary function: methods. Ann. Rev. Med. 12:385, 1961.

Hackney, J. D., Sears, C. H. and Collier, C. R.: Estimation of arterial CO_2 tension by rebreathing technique. J. Appl. Physiol. 12:425, 1958.

Leopold, S. S.: The Principles and Methods of Physical Diagnosis. Philadelphia, W. B. Saunders Co., 1957.

MacBryde, C. M.: Signs and Symptoms. Philadelphia, J. B. Lippincott Co., 1957.

Major, R. H. and Delp, M. H.: Physical Diagnosis. Philadelphia, W. B. Saunders Co., 1956.

Naimark, A. and Cherniack, R. M.: The compliance of the respiratory system and its components in health and obesity. J. Appl. Physiol. 15:377, 1960.

Page, L. R. and Culver, P. J.: A Syllabus of Laboratory Examinations in Clinical Diagnosis. Cambridge, Harvard University Press, 1960.

Prior, J. A. and Silberstein, J. S.: Physical Diagnosis. St. Louis, C. V. Mosby Co., 1959.

Wells, B. B.: Clinical Pathology. Application and Interpretation. Philadelphia, W. B. Saunders, Co., 1956.

Woolmer, R.: Symposium on pH and Blood Gas Measurement. London, J. & A. Churchill, 1959.

INDEX

ABDOMEN
  examination of, 326
  pain in, in embolism, pulmonary, 219
  viscera, as source of chest pain, 109
    herniation of, 268–272
Abscess
  pulmonary, 194–199
    absorption of, 197
    aspiration type, development of, 96
    clinical manifestations, 197
    formation and character of, 196
    functional manifestations, 199
    pathogenesis of, 194
    radiological manifestations, 198
    tension cavity in, 196
  subdiaphragmatic, 274
Acclimatization to hypoxia at high altitude
    and sea level, 125, 126
Acetylcholine, effect on pulmonary circu-
    lation, 211
Acid solution, definition of, 63
Acid-base balance, 63
  disturbances in, metabolic causes, 65
    respiratory causes, 64
  laboratory estimation of, 66
Acidosis, 64
  metabolic, 66
  respiratory, 65
Actinomyces bovis infections, diagnosis of,
    352
Adventitious sounds, 137–141
  assessment of, 323–325
Air. See also Gas(es).
  distribution of, impaired, in emphy-
    sema, chronic obstructive, 172
  in mediastinum, 263–265
  in pleural space, 141, 241. See also
    Pneumothorax.
  in tissues in thoracic injuries, 287

Airway resistance, 22
Alkaline solution, definition of, 63
Alkalosis, 64
  respiratory, 65
Allergy and bronchial asthma, 179, 180
Allergic skin tests, 358
Altitude, and acclimatization to hypoxia,
    125, 126
Alveolocapillary membrane, 49
Alveolus(i) or Alveolar
  anatomy, 4
  and capillaries, gaseous exchange be-
    tween, 57
  ducts, 4
  gas tensions in, 38
  hypoventilation, assessment of, 371,
    372
  pores, 92
  sacs, 4
  ventilation, 41–44
  ventilation-perfusion ratios, 44–47
Amphoric breath sounds, 198
Amyloidosis, diagnosis, 360
Anastomoses, bronchopulmonary, 211
Anatomy
  bronchopulmonary, 147–151
  chest surface, 310–315
  diaphragmatic, 266–268
  lung
    left, 149
    peripheral portion, 4
    right, 147
    segments, surface, 313
  mediastinal, 248–252
  pleural, 231, 232
Anemia
  diagnosis by inspection, 327
  diagnostic significance, 359
  dyspnea in, 101

383

Aneurysm
  aortic, chest pain in, 107
  arteriovenous, pulmonary, 222–225
    clinical manifestations, 224
    functional manifestations, 225
    pathogenesis, 223
    radiological manifestations, 224
Angina of effort, 107
Angiography, 336
  in pulmonary arteriovenous aneurysm, 225
Angle
  kidney, 310
  of Louis, 310
  sternal, 310
Anorexia in respiratory disease, 111
Anteromediastinal lymph nodes, 255
Antibody, 179
Antigen, 179
Aorta, as source of chest pain, 107
Apex beat
  in determining position of mediastinum, 316
  position of, 316
Apneusis, 69
Area postrema, 74
Arrhythmias in pulmonary infarction, 220
Arterial gas tension, 38
Arteriovenous aneurysm, pulmonary, 222–225. See also under *Aneurysm.*
Asbestos bodies in sputum, 343
Ascaris lumbricoides in sputum, 344
Aspiration
  abscess formation, 194, 195
  fibrosis of lung due to, 204
  pneumonia, pulmonary consolidation in, 190
Assessment of respiratory disease, 295–376
  clinical, 297–328
  clinical-pathological, 340–361
  functional, 362–376
  radiological, 329–339
Asthma, bronchial, 179–182
  allergic reaction in, 180
  chronic obstructive emphysema and relationship, 165
  clinical manifestations, 181
  functional manifestations, 182
  heredity in, 180
  pathogenesis, 179–181
  psychic factors in, 180
  radiological manifestations, 182

Asthma, bronchial, vagus nerves and, 181
Atelectasis, 183–188
  clinical manifestations, 186
  compressive, 184
  development of, 184
  functional manifestations, 188
  in bronchial obstruction, signs of, 156
  mediastinal shift in, 129
  obstructive, 184
  pathogenesis of, 183–186
  physiologic, 183
  radiological manifestations, 187
Atrial pressure, left, elevation of, 213
Auditory fremitus, 134, 321
Auscultation of chest, 323–325
Azygos venous system, 251, 253

BACTERIAL pneumonias, 351
  pulmonary consolidation in, 189
Bacteriological diagnosis, 346–354
Barrel-chest in chronic obstructive emphysema, 168
Base angle in digital clubbing, 307, 308
Bicarbonate, formation of, in blood, 61
Biopsy
  lung, needle, 356
    open, 356
  pleural, 356
  scalene node, 355
Biot's respiration, 86, 305
Blastomyces dermatitidis infection, diagnosis of, 353
Blastomycin skin test, 353
Blebs
  pulmonary, 201
  subpleural, 243
Bleeding in pulmonary arteriovenous aneurysm, 224
Blood
  arterial, oxygen saturation of, 57
  buffering action of, 63
    direct effect on respiratory centers, 75
  carbon dioxide in, transport of, 59–63
  chemistry of, in diagnosis, 360
  circulation of, impaired, in emphysema, chronic obstructive, 172
  flow
    capillary, of lungs, distribution of, 44–47
    direct effects of, on respiratory centers, 74

Blood (*cont.*)
  flow, pulmonary, increased, 213
    obstruction of, 214
  gas tensions in, 39
  in sputum, 97, 342
  oxygen in, transport of, 55–59
  pH of, 63–66
  respiratory function of, 55–67
  tests, for fungus infection, 354
    special, 359
  true venous admixture, 47, 373
Blood vessels, pulmonary
  obliteration of, 214
  obstruction of, 214
  vasoconstriction of, 214
Bochdalek's foramen, herniation through, congenital, 270
Bohr's formula, for measurement of physiologic dead space, 42
Bony thorax
  diseases affecting, 283–288
  radiological appearance, 333
Boyle's law, 37
Bradypnea, 305
Breast, pigeon, 116, 315
Breath sounds, 135–137, 323. See also *Sounds, breath.*
Breathing. See also *Respiration.*
  capacity, maximal, determining, 366
  difficult. See *Dyspnea.*
  forces and resistances involved, 10–27
  Kussmaul, 305
  mechanics of, 3–32
    chronic obstructive emphysema and, 170
  oxygen cost of, 30
  periodic, 83
  work of, 27–32
    and control of respiration, 80–82
    mechanical, 27
      relation to alveolar ventilation, 30
      total, 27
Broadbent's sign, 263
Bronchial asthma, 179–182. See also *Asthma, bronchial.*
Bronchial breath sounds, 137, 323
Bronchial circulation, 211
Bronchiectasis, 173–179
  clinical manifestations, 175–178
  cystic, 200
  "dry," 175

Bronchiectasis (*cont.*)
  functional manifestations, 178
  pathogenesis, 174
  plexuses of collateral arterial vessels in, 212
  radiological manifestations, 178
  reversible, 174
  suppurative, 175
Bronchiolar fibrosis, 204
Bronchioles, 4
Bronchitis, 157–163
  acute, 158
    clinical manifestations, 158
  chronic, 159–163
    clinical manifestations, 161
    environmental causes, 160
    functional manifestations, 163
    incidence of, 159
    occupation and, 160
    pathogenesis of, 160
    radiological manifestations, 162
    smoking and, 161
  recurrent, 159
Bronchogram, assessment of, 336
Broncholiths in sputum, 342
Bronchopleural fistula, 241
Bronchopulmonary
  anastomoses, 211
  anatomy, 147–151
  infections, bacteriological diagnosis in, 346–354
  segments, 147–151
  surface anatomy, 313
Bronchoscopy, diagnostic, 355
Bronchospirometry, 45
Bronchovesicular breath sounds, 137
Bronchus(i)
  anatomy of, 4, 147–151
  diseases, patterns of, 147–182
  obstruction of, 151–157
    abscess formation in, 195
    clinical manifestations, 154–156
    complete, 154
    effect on distribution of air, 34
    partial, 152
      by-pass, 152, 153
      check-valve, 153, 154
        expiratory x-ray in, 157
        in emphysema, chronic obstructive, 165
    pathogenesis, 152

Bronchus(i) (*cont.*)
    obstruction of (*cont.*)
        pneumonia in, pulmonary consolida-
            tion due to, 191
        pressure-flow relationship in, 26
        radiological manifestations, 156
        ventilatory changes in, 31
    segmental, 147
    size of, change during respiration, 3
Buccal mucosa, examination of, 306
Buffer system, 63
Buffering action of blood, 63
    direct effect on respiratory centers, 75
Bullae, pulmonary, 201, 243

Candida albicans infections, diagnosis of,
    352
Capillaries
    and alveoli, gaseous exchange between,
        57
    permeability of, increased, as cause of
        pulmonary edema, 227
    systemic, and tissues, gaseous exchange
        between, 56
Carbamino-carbon dioxide, transport of
    carbon dioxide as, 62
Carbon dioxide
    concentration of, in expired gas, ven-
        tilation-perfusion ratio and, 45
    diffusing capacity for, measurement of,
        374
        breath-holding method, 374
        steady-state method, 374
    dissociation curve, 60
    elimination, formula for, 291
        insufficiency of, with insufficiency of
            oxygen exchange, 291
    pressure, partial, 38
    retention of. See *Hypercapnia.*
    tension, 38
        alterations in, assessment of, 370, 371
            effects on respiratory centers, 71,
                77
        alveolar and arterial, 38
    transport of, 59–63
        as bicarbonate, 60
        as carbamino-carbon dioxide, 62
        as dissolved carbon dioxide, 60
    ventilatory response to, 71
Carbon monoxide, mean gradient for,
    measuring, 53
Carbonic acid, formation of, in blood, 60
Cardiac. See also *Heart.*

Cardiac impulse, assessment of, 325
Cardiac insufficiency
    respiratory insufficiency secondary to,
        294
    secondary to respiratory insufficiency,
        292–294
Cardiac pain, 107
Cardiorespiratory insufficiency, 289–294
Cardiovascular manifestations of hyper-
    capnia, 128
Cardiovascular system, review of, in his-
    tory taking, 300
Carotid sheath, 260
Cartilages, rib, as source of chest pain,
    104
Casoni skin test, 358
Cavitation of lung, 194–196
Center(s)
    cough, 93
    higher, influence on respiration, 80
    pneumotaxic, 69
    respiratory, 68–70
        factors acting directly on, 70–75
        factors acting indirectly on, 75–80
Cerebral function, hypoxia and, 125
Chemistry of blood in diagnosis, 360
Chest
    auscultation of, 323–325
    barrel, in emphysema, chronic obstruc-
        tive, 168
    bony structures
        diseases affecting, 283–288
        radiological appearance, 333
    cage
        density of, altered, 131–142
        diseases of, 279–288
        distensibility of, altered, 131
        movement of, examination for, 317–
            321
        resting level of, 8
    deformities, 113–117
        congenital, of anterior wall, 115
        due to abnormalities of thoracic verte-
            brae, 113
        examination for, 315
    examination of, 309–326
        auscultation, 323–325
        fluoroscopic, 337–339
        for signs of pulmonary heart disease,
            325
        inspection, 315
        palpation, 316–321
        percussion, 321–323

Chest (*cont.*)
  examination of (*cont.*)
    radiological, 329–339
    surface anatomy, 310–315
  flail, 285, 286
  funnel, 115, 315
  indrawing movement, 315
  injuries to, 284–288. See also *Injuries to chest.*
  inspection of, 315
  movement, examination for, 315
  normal, radiological appearance of, 329–333
  pain, 102–109, 303. See also *Pain, chest.*
  palpation of, 316–321
  percussion of, 131–133, 321–323
  physical properties, altered, signs of, 128–143
  skin and subcutaneous tissues of, diseases affecting, 279
  veins, collateral, significance of, 316
  wall
    anterior, congenital deformities of, 115
    compliance of, 21
    diseases of, 279–288
    distribution of dermatomes over, 103
Cheyne-Stokes respiration, 84, 305
Chloride shift, 61
Chlorides, sweat, test for, 358
Chyle, 236
Chylothorax, 235
  in tumors of mediastinum, 258
Ciliary activity, protective function of, 91
Circulation
  bronchial, 211
  collateral, in diseased lung, pathology of, 212
  pulmonary, 209–212
    in emphysema, chronic obstructive, 173
Click
  coin, 141, 245, 325
  early systolic ejection, in pulmonary hypertension, 142
Clinical-pathological assessment of respiratory disease, 340–361
Clubbing of digits, 117
  acquired, 118
  examination for, 307–309
  hereditary, 118
  in abscess, pulmonary, 198

Clubbing of digits (*cont.*)
  in aneurysm, pulmonary arteriovenous, 224
  in bronchiectasis, 178
  in fibrosis of lung, 206
  pathogenesis of, 118–120
  unilateral, 118
Coccidioides immitis infection, 353
Coccidioidin skin test, 353
Coin click, 141
  eliciting, 325
  in pneumothorax, 245
Complaints, entrance, eliciting in history, 297
Compliance, 17
  functional, 20
  of chest wall, 21
  of lung, 18
    in chronic obstructive emphysema, 170
  respiratory, assessment of, 363, 364
  total, 17
Congenital
  cysts of lung, 199
  deformities of anterior chest wall, 115
  herniation of diaphragm, 268–271
Consolidation, pulmonary, 188–193
  clinical manifestations, 191
  due to specific pneumonias, 189
  functional manifestations, 193
  mediastinal shift in, 130
  pathogenesis, 189–191
  radiological manifestations, 192
Constitutional symptoms
  history of, taking, 303
  of respiratory disease, 109–112
Control of respiration, 68–86
Cor pulmonale, 143, 173, 207, 212
Coronary occlusion, pain of, 107
Cough
  as symptom of disease, 95
  center, 93
  diaphragm in, 268
  history of, taking, 303
  in bronchial asthma, 181
  in bronchial obstruction, 155
  in bronchiectasis, 175
  in bronchitis, acute, 158
    chronic, 161
  in cysts of lung, 202
  in diaphragmatic disease, 276
  in edema, pulmonary, 228

Cough (*cont.*)
  in embolism, pulmonary, 219
  in emphysema, chronic obstructive, 167
  in mediastinal tumors, 257, 258
  in mediastinitis, acute, 261
  in pleural effusion, 237
  in pneumothorax, 245
  phases of, 93
  reflex, 93–96
    impaired, dangers in, 95
      in thoracic injuries, 287
Coxiella burnetii infections, 354
Crush injuries of chest, 285
Culture of sputum
  in nontuberculous infection, 349
  in tuberculous infection, 347
Cyanosis
  and hypoxia, 121–124
  assessment of, 370
  in aneurysm, pulmonary arteriovenous, 224
  in cysts of lung, 202
  in edema, pulmonary, 229
  in pulmonary consolidation, 191
Cystic bronchiectasis, 200
Cysts of lung, 199–203
  acquired, 201
  clinical manifestations, 202
  congenital, 199
    ballooning, 200
  diffuse multiple, 201, 203
  functional manifestations, 203
  pathogenesis of, 199
  radiological manifestations, 202

DEAD space
  anatomic, 41
  physiologic, 41
    measurement of, 42
Dead-space-like ventilation, 46, 290
Decubitus films, lateral, of chest, 335
Defenses of respiratory tract, 91–96
Deficiency diseases, chest pain in, 105
Deformities of chest, 113–117
  congenital, of anterior wall, 115
  due to abnormalities of thoracic verte-
    brae, 113
  examination for, 315
Dermatomes, distribution of, over chest
  wall, 103

Diagnosis
  bacteriological, 346–354
  clinical, 297–328
  clinical-pathological, 340–361
  functional, 362–376
  histological, 354–357
  radiological, 329–339
Diaphragm
  action of, in respiration, 7
    on costal margins, examination for,
      320
  altered function of, in pleural effusion,
    238
  anatomy of, 266–268
  as source of chest pain, 106
  diseases of, 266–278
    manifestations, 275–278
      clinical, 275
      functional, 278
      radiological, 277
  diseases affecting position of, 272, 273
  displacement of, in bronchiectasis, 177
    in chronic obstructive emphysema,
      168
  eventration of, 273
  fluoroscopy of, 338
  herniation of
    congenital, 268–271
      sites of, 269, 270
    traumatic, 271
  in cough reflex, 268
  inflammation of, primary, 275
  inflammatory diseases of, 274, 275
  involvement of, in fibrothorax, 273
    in intra-abdominal conditions, 273
  normal, radiological appearance, 333
  paralysis of, 272
  role in coughing, 94
  rupture of, in thoracic injuries, 287
  spasmodic conditions affecting, 275
Diaphragmatic flutter, 275
Diffusion
  capacity of lungs, altered, assessment of,
    373–376
  defect, effect on gas exchange, 49
  gradient, 37, 49
  of gas, 37, 48–54
Digits, clubbing of, 117, 307–309. See also
  Clubbing of digits.
Dissociation curve
  carbon dioxide, 60
  oxyhemoglobin, 58

Dittrich's plugs, 176, 342
Dysphagia
  in mediastinitis, acute, 261
  in tumors of mediastinum, 258
Dyspnea, 98–102
  and hypoxia, 124
  clinical assessment of, 102
  history of, taking, 302
  in aneurysm, pulmonary arteriovenous, 224
  in asthma, bronchial, 181
  in atelectasis, 186
  in bronchial obstruction, 155
  in bronchiectasis, 176
  in bronchitis, chronic, 162
  in cysts of lung, 202
  in diaphragmatic disease, 276
  in edema, pulmonary, 228
  in embolism, pulmonary, 218, 219
  in emphysema, chronic obstructive, 166
  in fibrosis of lung, 205
  in mediastinal tumors, 258
  in mediastinitis, acute, 261
  in organic disease, 100
  in pleural effusion, 237
  in psychogenic diseases, 101
  in pulmonary consolidation, 191
  in pulmonary hypertension, primary, 215
  mechanism of, 99
  nocturnal, in chronic bronchitis, 162
    in pulmonary edema, 229
  paroxysmal, nocturnal, 229

Echinococcus granulosus in sputum, 344
Edema, pulmonary, 225–230
  clinical manifestations, 228
  functional manifestations, 230
  in thoracic injuries, 287
  pathogenesis, 225–228
  radiological manifestations, 229
Egophony, 134, 177, 192
Elasticity of lungs and chest wall, 13, 14, 15
  assessment of, 363
  loss of, in chronic obstructive emphysema, 165
Electrocardiography, 361
Embolism, pulmonary, 216–222
  chest pain in, 108
  clinical manifestations, 218

Embolism, pulmonary (*cont.*)
  functional manifestations, 222
  low diffusing capacity of lung in, 375
  pathogenesis, 216
  radiological manifestations, 221
  vasoconstriction in, 214, 215
Emphysema, obstructive, chronic, 163–173
  bronchial asthma and, relationship, 165
  centrilobular and generalized forms, 166
  clinical manifestations, 166–169
  functional manifestations, 170–173
  in chronic bronchitis, 162, 163
  lung volumes and, 172
  mechanics of breathing and, 170
  nitrogen washout during oxygen inhalation, 35, 36
  pathogenesis, 164–166
  pulmonary circulation and, 173
  radiological manifestations, 169
  regulation of respiration and, 173
  ventilatory function in, 367, 368
  ventilatory response to carbon dioxide in, 72
Empyema, 233
  causes of, 234
  clinical manifestations, 237
  clinical picture, 234
Endamoeba histolytica in sputum, 344
Environment, history of, 298
Enzymes, serum, determination of, diagnostic value, 359
Epinephrine, effect on pulmonary circulation, 211
Epistaxis in pulmonary arteriovenous aneurysm, 224
Erythrocyte sedimentation rate, diagnostic significance, 360
Esophageal hiatus, hernia of
  chest pain in, 105
  congenital, 270
Esophagogram, assessment of, 336
Esophagus as source of chest pain, 108
Eventration of diaphragm, 273
Examination
  fluoroscopic, of chest, 337–339
  of pleural fluid, 344, 345
  of sputum, 341–344
  of urine, 360
  of x-ray films of chest, 333, 334
  radiological, of chest, 329–339
  physical, 303–328
    abdomen, 326

Examination (*cont.*)
  physical (*cont.*)
    chest, 309–326
      auscultation, 323–325
      inspection, 315
      palpation, 316–321
      percussion, 321–323
      signs of pulmonary heart disease,
        325, 326
    extremities, 327
    eyes, 305
    genitalia, external, 327
    hands and feet, for clubbing, 307–
      309
    head, 304
    inspection, general, 304
    neck, 306
    skin, 327
    upper respiratory tract, 305
Expectoration
  history of, taking, 302
  of blood, 97, 98
  of sputum, 96, 97
Expiratory center, 69
Expiratory obstruction, test for, 365
Extremities, examination of, 327
Eyes, examination of, 305

FAMILY history, taking of, 299
Fascial layers of mediastinum, 259
Fatigue in respiratory disease, 111
Feet, examination of, for clubbing, 307–
  309
Ferritin, reduced, clubbing and, 119
Fever
  in empyema, 237
  in respiratory disease, 109
  unexplained, in pulmonary embolism,
    218, 219, 220
Fibrosis
  bronchiolar, 204
  parenchymal, 205
  pleural, 205, 206
  pulmonary, 203–205
    clinical manifestations, 205
    functional manifestations, 208
    low diffusing capacity of lung in, 375
    pathogenesis of, 204
    radiological manifestations, 207
    rales in, 141
    vascular, 205
    ventilatory function in, 367, 368

Fibrothorax, 206, 236
  clinical signs of, 238, 239
  diaphragmatic involvement in, 273
  functional manifestations, 240
Fingers, clubbing of, 117, 307–309. See
  also *Clubbing of digits.*
Fissures of lung, surface anatomy, 312,
  313
Fistula, bronchopleural, 241
Flail chest, 285, 286
Flow rate, mid-expiratory, maximal, 365
Fluid, pleural, 232
  signs associated with, 141
Fluoroscopic examination of chest, 337–
  339
  contour of heart, 338
  diaphragm, 338
  general survey, 337
  lung fields, 338
  mediastinum, 338
Fluoroscopy, findings
  in aneurysm, pulmonary arteriovenous,
    225
  in bronchial obstruction, 156
  in bronchitis, chronic, 162
  in emphysema, chronic obstructive,
    170
  in pneumothorax, 246
Flutter, diaphragmatic, 275
Foramina of Bochdalek and Morgagni,
  herniation through, congenital, 270
Fremitus
  auditory, 134, 321
  tactile, 134, 320
  vocal, 134
    assessment of, 320
    in atelectasis, 187
    in bronchiectasis, 177
    in emphysema, chronic obstructive,
      168
    in pneumothorax, 245
Friedländer's bacillus infections, diagnosis
  of, 350
Functional assessment of respiratory disease, 362–376
  gaseous exchange, 370–376
  ventilation, 362–370
Fungus infections, diagnosis of, laboratory, 352–354
Fungus skin tests, 353
Funnel-chest, 315
  depression deformity, 115

Gas(es)
  acid, increased capillary permeability
    in lungs due to, 227
  diffusion of, 48–54
  distribution in lungs, 33–36
  exchange in lungs, 37–41
    between pulmonary alveoli and capil-
      laries, 57
    between systemic capillaries and tis-
      sues, 57
    effects of alterations in ventilation-
      perfusion ratios on, 44–47
    of true venous admixture on, 47–48
    impaired
      assessment of, 370–376
      in chronic obstructive emphysema,
        172
      signs of, 120–128
  in pleural space, 241. See also *Pneumo-
    thorax.*
  inspired, distribution of, assessment,
    366
  partial pressures, in alveolar air and
    mixed venous blood, 185
  pressure of, factors influencing, 37
    partial, 38
  properties of, 37
  tension of, 37
    alveolar and arterial, 38
Gastrointestinal system, review of, in history taking, 300
Gay-Lussac's law, 37
Genitalia, external, examination of, 327
Genitourinary system, review of, in history
  taking, 301
Giddiness in vena caval obstruction, 256
Gradient diffusion, 49
  mean, between alveolus and capillary,
    52
Granules, sulphur, 352
Grooves, Harrison's, 116
Guinea pig inoculation in diagnosis of
  tuberculous infection, 347

Habits, personal, history of, 298
Hands, examination of, for clubbing, 307–
  309
Harrison's grooves, 116

Head, examination of, 304
Headache
  in hypercapnia, 127
  in vena caval obstruction, 256
Heart
  apex beat. See *Apex beat.*
  as source of chest pain, 107
  contour of, fluoroscopic study, 339
  disease, pulmonary, signs of, 325, 326
  failure
    mechanism of development, in re-
      spiratory disease, 293
    respiratory failure secondary to, 294
    right-sided, chronic, in emphysema,
      chronic obstructive, 169
    secondary to respiratory insufficiency,
      292–294
  normal, radiological appearance of, 332
  sounds
    assessment of, 326
    in emphysema, chronic obstructive,
      168
    second pulmonic in pulmonary hyper-
      tension, 142
  surface anatomy, 314
Heartburn, 109
Hematology, test findings, significance,
  359
Hemiazygos veins, 251, 253
Hemoglobin
  combination of oxygen with, 56
  reduced, 57
Hemophilus influenzae infections, diagnosis of, 350
Hemoptysis, 97, 98
  clinical assessment of, 98
  history of, taking, 302
  in aneurysm, pulmonary arteriovenous,
    224
  in bronchiectasis, cystic, 202
  in embolism, pulmonary, 219
  in pulmonary hypertension, primary,
    215
  in tumors of mediastinum, 258
Hemorrhage, intrapulmonary or intrapleural, in thoracic injuries, 287
Hemothorax, 235
  in thoracic injuries, 287
Henderson-Hasselbach equation, 63, 292
Heredity, and bronchial asthma, 180
Hering-Breuer reflexes, 78

Herniation
 hiatus, chest pain in, 109
 of abdominal viscera, 268–272
 of diaphragm
  congenital, 268–271
   sites of, 269, 270
  traumatic, 271
 of mediastinum, 265
 of stomach, mediastinal shift in, 130, 131
Herpes zoster, chest pain in, 105
Hiatus hernia
 chest pain in, 109
 congenital, 270
Hiccup, 275
Histological diagnosis, 354–357
Histoplasma capsulatum infection, 353
Histoplasmin skin test, 353
History taking, 297–303
 entrance complaints, 297
 family, 299
 past illnesses, 299
 personal, 297–299
 present illness, 301–303
 review of nonrespiratory systems, 300, 301
H₂O shift, 61
Honeycombing, 201, 203
Horner's syndrome in tumors of mediastinum, 258
Hydatid disease, Casoni skin test for, 358
Hydrogen ion concentration. See pH.
Hydrostatic pressure, increased, as cause of pulmonary edema, 226
Hydrothorax, 234
Hypercapnia, 126–128
 assessment of, 370, 371
 clinical manifestations, 127
  cardiovascular, 128
  neurological, 127
 in emphysema, chronic obstructive, 169, 172, 173
 in flail chest, 286
 in kyphoscoliosis, 284
 in pneumothorax, 246
 in respiratory insufficiency, mechanism of, 290, 291
 pulmonary circulation and, 210
Hypertension
 and hypoxia, 125
 pulmonary, 212–216
  chest pain in, 108

Hypertension (cont.)
 pulmonary (cont.)
  in bronchitis, chronic, 163
  in embolism, pulmonary, 222
  in fibrosis of lung, 206, 208
  in infarction, pulmonary, 221
  primary, manifestations of, 215
  second pulmonic heart sound in, 142
  signs of, 142
Hyperventilation syndrome, 102
Hypocapnia
 in aneurysm, pulmonary arteriovenous, 225
 in edema, pulmonary, 230
 in embolism, pulmonary, 222
 in respiratory insufficiency, 289, 290
Hypotension, and hypercapnia, 128
Hypoventilation, alveolar, assessment of, 371, 372
Hypoxemia, 120
Hypoxia, 120
 acclimatization to, at high altitude, 125
 and cerebral function, 125
 and cyanosis, 121–124
 and dyspnea, 124
 and hypertension, 125
 and tachycardia, 124
 anemic, 121
 arterial, in chronic obstructive emphysema, 172, 173
 assessment of, 370, 371
 circulatory, 121
 clinical manifestations, 121–125
 effects on respiratory centers, 75
 histotoxic, 121
 hypoxic, 120
 in aneurysm, pulmonary arteriovenous, 225
 in asthma, bronchial, 182
 in bronchiectasis, 179
 in cysts of lung, 203
 in diaphragmatic disease, 278
 in edema, pulmonary, 230
 in embolism, pulmonary, 222
 in emphysema, chronic obstructive, 169
 in fibrosis of lung, 208
 in flail chest, 288
 in kyphoscoliosis, 284
 in pleural effusion, 240
 in pneumothorax, 246
 in pulmonary consolidation, 193
 in respiratory insufficiency, mechanism of, 289, 290

Hypoxia (*cont.*)
increased capillary permeability in lungs due to, 227
pulmonary circulation and, 210
tissue, as cause of clubbing, 119
ventilatory response to, 75

ICTERUS in infarction, pulmonary, 220
Illness(es)
past history of, 299
present, taking history of, 301
Impulse, cardiac, assessment of, 325
Index of intrapulmonary mixing, 35
Indrawing movement of chest, 315
Infarction, pulmonary, 216–222
abscess formation in, 196
clinical manifestations, 218
functional manifestations, 222
pathogenesis, 218
radiological manifestations, 221
Infections, bronchopulmonary, bacteriological diagnosis in, 346–354
Inflammation of mediastinum, 259–263
Inflammatory diseases of diaphragm, 274, 275
Influenza, diagnosis of, laboratory, 351
Injuries to chest, 284–288
clinical and radiological manifestations, 288
complications, 287
crush, 285
nonpenetrating, 285
penetrating, 286
pneumothorax due to, 243
pulmonary consolidation due to, 191
Inspection
of chest, 315
of hands and feet, 307
of neck, 306
of patient, general, 304
Inspiration-expiration films of chest, 334
Inspiratory
capacity, 10
center, 69
obstruction, assessment of, 365
reserve volume, 10
Insufficiency
cardiac, respiratory insufficiency secondary to, 294
secondary to respiratory insufficiency, 292–294

Insufficiency (*cont.*)
cardiorespiratory, 289–294
of oxygen exchange, 289
and of carbon dioxide elimination, 291
respiratory, 289–294
cardiac insufficiency secondary to, 292–294
secondary to cardiac insufficiency, 294
Intensity of sound, 133
Intercostal muscles, action in respiration, 6, 8
Intra-abdominal conditions, diaphragmatic involvement in, 273
Intrapulmonary pressure, 11
Intrathoracic pressure, 11
Irradiation of thorax, pulmonary consolidation due to, 191
Ischemia, myocardial, pain of, 107

JOINTS, receptors in, influence on respiration, 79

KIDNEY angle, 310
Kussmaul breathing, 305
Kyphoscoliosis, 115
as cause of cardiorespiratory disability, 283
examination for, 315
mediastinal shift in, 114, 129
ventilatory function in, 369
Kyphosis, 114
as cause of cardiorespiratory disability, 283
examination for, 315

LAMINAR resistance, 22
Larynx
inspection of, 306
protective function of, 91
L.E. cells, demonstration of, 359
Leukocytosis
eosinophilic, diagnostic significance, 360
neutrophilic, diagnostic significance, 359

Lingula, 150
  movement of, palpation for, 319
Liver, displacement of, in pneumothorax, 245
Locomotor system, review of, in history taking, 301
Lordotic films of chest, 335
Louis, angle of, 310
Lung
  abscess of, 194–199. See also *Abscess, pulmonary.*
  air distribution in, uneven, tests for, 366
  biopsy of, needle, 356
    open, 356
  blebs of, 201
  bullae of, 201, 243
  cavitation of, 194–196
  collapse of, 183–188. See also *Atelectasis.*
  compliance of, 18
    assessment of, 363
    in chronic obstructive emphysema, 170
  consolidation of, 188–193. See also *Consolidation, pulmonary.*
  cysts of, 199–203. See also *Cysts of lung.*
  density of, altered, 131–142
  diffusing properties of, 48–54
    altered, assessment of, 373–376
  distensibility of, altered, 131
  distribution of gas in, 33–36
  edema of, 225–230. See also *Edema, pulmonary.*
  elastic properties of, 13, 14, 15
    assessment of, 363
  expiratory reserve volume of, 10
  fibrosis of, 203–205. See also *Fibrosis, pulmonary.*
  fissures of, surface anatomy, 312, 313
  fluoroscopy of, 338
  functional residual capacity of, 10
  gaseous exchange in, 37–41, 370–376.
    See also *Gas(es), exchange in lungs.*
  honeycomb, 201, 203
  inspiratory capacity of, 10
  inspiratory reserve volume of, 10
  left, anatomy of, 149
  lobes, movement of, palpation for, 318–320
  mechanical work on, during breathing, 28
  minute ventilation of, 10

Lung (*cont.*)
  nitrogen elimination from, study of, 35
    test for, 367
  nonelastic resistance, assessment of, 364
  normal, radiological appearance of, 330–332
  parenchyma of, as source of chest pain, 106
  parenchymal disease, patterns of, 183–208
  peripheral portion of, anatomy, 4
  right, anatomy of, 147
  segments of, surface anatomy, 313
  size of, alterations in, 128
  surface markings, 310–314
  tidal volume of, 9
  total capacity of, 9
  tumor of, abscess development in, 195
  vascular disease of, 209–230. See also *Vascular disease, pulmonary.*
  ventilation-perfusion ratios, 44–47
  ventilatory function, assessment of, 362
  vital capacity of, 9
    determination of, 363
    timed, 365
  volumes of, 8–10
    alterations in, in chronic obstructive emphysema, 172
    assessment of, 362
    residual, 10
      measurement of, 362, 363
    three-dimensional increase in, 4
Lymph flow, interference with, as cause of pulmonary edema, 228
Lymph nodes
  anteromediastinal, 255
  mediastinal, 250
    anterior, 251
    posterior, 252
    tracheobronchial, 250
  tracheobronchial, 250, 255
Lymphocytosis, relative, diagnostic significance, 360

Mammary venous system, collateral, of mediastinum, 254
Manifestations of respiratory disease, 87–143
Mean gradient between alveolus and capillary, 52
Mean oxygen tension, 52
Mechanics of breathing, 3–32

Mediastinal air, 263–265
  clinical manifestations, 264
  in thoracic injuries, 287
  pathogenesis, 263
  radiological manifestations, 265
Mediastinitis, 259–263
  acute, 260–262
    clinical manifestations, 261
    radiological manifestations, 262
  chronic fibrous, 262, 263
    manifestations of, 263
Mediastinum
  anatomy of, 248–252
  anterior, 249
  disease of, 248–265
  fascial layers of, 259
  fluoroscopy of, 338
  herniation of, 265
  inflammation of, 259–263
  lymph nodes of, 250
    anterior, 251
    posterior, 251
    tracheobronchial, 250
  middle, 249
  position of, palpation for, 316
  posterior, 249
  shift of, 128–130
    diagnosis of, 316
    in abscess, pulmonary, 198
    in pleural effusion, 237, 238, 239
    in pneumothorax, 241, 242, 245
  superior, 249
  tumors of, 257–259
    clinical manifestations, 257
    radiological manifestations, 259
  venous systems of, collateral, 253
Membrane, alveolocapillary, 49
Membrane component of alveolar oxygen
  tension, 40
Metabolic system, review of, in history
  taking, 301
Mid-axillary line, 310
Mid-clavicular line, 310
Mid-scapular line, 310
Mixing, intrapulmonary, index of, 35
Morgagni's foramen, herniation through,
  congenital, 270
Mouth, examination of, 306
Mucosa, buccal, examination of, 306
Mucus, bronchial
  hypersecretion of, in bronchitis, 158
  production of, normal, 158

Muscles
  air in, in thoracic injuries, 287
  disturbances of, in hypercapnia, 127
  intercostal, action in respiration, 6, 8
  receptors in, influence on respiration,
    79
  respiratory
    accessory, 8
    action of, 4–8
    diseases affecting, 282
    efficiency of, 32
    oxygen consumption of, 30
  scalene, action in respiration, 6, 8
  thoracic, as source of chest pain, 105
Muscoviscidosis, sweat chlorides in, 358
Mycotic infections, diagnosis of, laboratory, 352–354
Mycotic pneumonias, pulmonary consolidation in, 190
Myocardial ischemia, pain of, 107

NASAL passages, examination of, 306
Nasopharynx, protective function of, 90
Neck, examination of, 306
Nerves as source of chest pain, 104
Nervous system
  review of, in history taking, 300
  sympathetic, bronchial asthma and, 181
Neurological manifestations
  of hypercapnia, 127
  of pulmonary arteriovenous aneurysm,
    224
Neuromuscular disease, dyspnea in, 101
Neutropenia, diagnostic significance, 360
Nickerson-Kveim skin test, 357
Night sweats, 111
Nitrogen
  elimination from lung
    study of, 35
    test for, 367
  pressure, partial, 38
  tension, alveolar and arterial, 38
Nocardia asteroides infection, diagnosis
  of, 352
Norepinephrine, effect on pulmonary circulation, 211
Nose, examination of, 306
  protective function of, 90

OBESITY
  respiratory disturbances due to, 280–282
  ventilatory function in, 369
Oblique fissure of lung, surface anatomy, 312
Observation, general, of patient, 304
Occupation
  and chronic bronchitis, 160
  history of, 298
Oil droplets in sputum, 343
Organic disease, dyspnea in, 100
Orthopnea, 99
  in tumors of mediastinum, 258
Osmotic pressure, diminished, as cause of pulmonary edema, 227
Osteo-arthropathy, pulmonary, hypertrophic, 118
  in pulmonary arteriovenous aneurysm, 224
Oxygen
  combination with hemoglobin, 56
  consumption, alterations in, in emphysema, chronic obstructive, 171
    by respiratory muscles, 30
  deficiency of. See *Hypoxia.*
  diffusing capacity of lung for, 54
    measurement of, 373
  exchange, insufficiency of, 289
    and insufficiency of carbon dioxide elimination, 291
  in physical solution, 55
  mean gradient for, measuring, 52
  pressure, partial, 38
  saturation of arterial blood, 57
    assessment of, 370
  tension
    alveolar and arterial, 38
    assessment of, 371
    mean, 52
  transport of, 55–59
Oxyhemoglobin, 56
  dissociation curve, 58

PAIN
  abdominal, in pulmonary embolism, 219
  brachial, in tumors of mediastinum, 258
  cardiac, 107
  chest, 102–109
    distribution of dermatomes and, 103
    history of, taking, 303

Pain (*cont.*)
  chest (*cont.*)
    in atelectasis, 186
    in embolism, pulmonary, 218, 219
    in emphysema, chronic obstructive, 167
    in mediastinal tumors, 258
    in mediastinitis, acute, 261
    in pleurisy, 237
    in pneumothorax, spontaneous, 245
    in pulmonary hypertension, primary, 215
    sources of, 104–109
    pleural, 105
      in embolism, pulmonary, 218, 219
      in pleural effusion, 237
    referred, in diaphragmatic disease, 275
    root, in chest, 105
    substernal, in mediastinal air accumulation, 264
Palpation
  for movement of chest cage, 317–321
  for position of trachea, 315, 316
  of chest, 316–321
  of mediastinum, 316
Palpitation in primary pulmonary hypertension, 215
Paradoxical movement in flail chest, 285, 286, 288
Paralysis of diaphragm, 272
Parenchyma of lung as source of chest pain, 106
Parenchymal disease, pulmonary, patterns of, 183–208
Parenchymal fibrosis, 205
Patterns of respiratory disease, 145–294
Pectoriloquy, whispering, 177, 192, 238, 259, 321
Pendaluft
  in flail chest, 285, 286
  in penetrating injuries of chest, 286
  in pneumothorax, open, 242
Peptic ulcer in chronic obstructive emphysema, 167
Percussion
  in abscess, pulmonary, 198
  in asthma, bronchial, 182
  in atelectasis, 187
  in bronchiectasis, 177
  in bronchitis, chronic, 162
  in fibrosis of lung, 206
  in mediastinal air accumulation, 265

Percussion (*cont.*)
in mediastinal tumors, 258
in pleural effusion, 238
in pneumothorax, 245
in pulmonary consolidation, 192
in thoracic injuries, 288
of chest, 131–133, 321, 323
Perfusion
pulmonary, in relation to ventilation, 44–47
venous-admixture-like, 45
Pericardium as source of chest pain, 108
Periodic breathing, 83
Personal history, taking of, 297–299
Perspiration, insensible, 111
pH
arterial, action of, on respiratory centers, 70, 77
of blood, 63–66
Pharmacologic agents
effect of, on pulmonary circulation, 211
on respiratory centers, 75, 77
Phlebothrombosis as source of pulmonary emboli, 217
Physical examination, 303–328. See also *Examination physical.*
Pigeon-breast protrusion deformity, 116, 315
Pitch of sound, 133
Pleura
anatomy of, 231
as source of chest pain, 105
biopsy of, 356
disease of, 231–247
fibrosis of, 205, 206
surface markings, 311
Pleural cavity
air or fluid in, signs associated with, 141
pressure within, 231
Pleural effusion, 232–240
absorption of, 240
chyliform, 236
chylous, 235
clinical manifestations, 131, 236
functional manifestations, 240
hemorrhagic, 235
inflammatory, 233
mediastinal shift in, 130
noninflammatory, 234
radiological manifestations, 238

Pleural effusion (*cont.*)
serosanguineous, 235
serous or serofibrinous, 233
Pleural fluid
coagulability of, 345
examination of, 344, 345
chemical, 345
macroscopic, 344
microscopic, 345
odor of, 345
protein content, 345
specific gravity, 345
Pleural pain
in embolism, pulmonary, 218, 219
in pleural effusion, 237
Pleural rubs, 141
assessment of, 325
Pleurisy, "dry" or fibrinous, 233
Plugs, Dittrich's, 176, 342
Pneumatoceles, 201, 203
Pneumococcus infection, diagnosis of, 350
Pneumoconiosis, 204
Pneumonia(s)
abscess formation in, 195
atypical, diagnosis of, laboratory, 351
influenzal, diagnosis of, laboratory, 351
physicochemical, pulmonary consolidation in, 190
psittacosis-ornithosis, diagnosis of, laboratory, 351
specific, pulmonary consolidation in, 189
Pneumonitis, 189
Pneumotaxic center, 69
Pneumothorax, 241–247
absorption of, 247
clinical manifestations, 141, 244
closed, 242–244
in penetrating injuries of chest, 286
diagnostic, 244
functional manifestations, 246
open, 241
in penetrating injuries of chest, 286
radiological manifestations, 246
signs associated with, 141
spontaneous, 242
tension, 244
in penetrating injuries of chest, 286
therapeutic, 243
traumatic, 243
valvular, 244
vocal fremitus in, 134, 135

Poliomyelitis, ventilatory function in, 368
Pores, alveolar, 92
Postesophageal fascia, 260
Posture, effect on distribution of inspired air, 35
Pressoreceptors, influence on respiration, 79
Pressure(s)
  intrapulmonary, 11
  intrathoracic, 11
    and intrapulmonary, relationship during breathing, 12
  of gas, factors influencing, 37
    partial, 37, 38
  relaxation, 16
  respiratory, 11
Pressure-flow relationship, 26
Pressure-volume loop, 24, 365
Pretracheal fascia, 260
Prevertebral fascia, 260
Pseudochyle, 236
Psittacosis- ornithosis, diagnosis of, laboratory, 351
Psychic factors in bronchial asthma, 180
Psychogenic disease
  chest pain in, 109
  dyspnea in, 101
Pulmonary. See also *Lung.*
  abscess, 194–199. See also *Abscess, pulmonary.*
  arteriovenous aneurysm, 222–225
  blebs, 201
  blood flow, increased, 213
    obstruction of, 214
  circulation, 209–212
    anastomoses with bronchial, 211
    in emphysema, chronic obstructive, 173
  consolidation, 188–193. See also *Consolidation, pulmonary.*
  edema, 225–230. See also *Edema, pulmonary.*
  embolism, 216–222. See also *Embolism, pulmonary.*
  fibrosis, 203–205. See also *Fibrosis, pulmonary.*
  heart disease, signs of, 325, 326
  hypertension, 212–216. See also *Hypertension, pulmonary.*
  infarction, 216–222. See also *Infarction, pulmonary.*
  osteoarthropathy, hypertrophic, 118, 224

Pulmonary (*cont.*)
  receptors, influence on respiration, 78
  vascular disease, 209–230. See also *Vascular disease, pulmonary.*
  vascular resistance
    alterations in, signs of, 142
    formula for determining, 213
  vasculature
    obliteration of, 214
    obstruction of, 214
    vasoconstriction of, 214
  vessels, as source of chest pain, 108
Pyrexin, 110

Q FEVER, diagnosis, 354

RADIOLOGICAL appearance of normal chest, 329
  bony structures, 333
  diaphragm, 333
  heart, 332, 333
  lungs, 330–332
Radiological assessment of chest disease, 329–339
Radiological examination of chest
  assessment of films, 333, 334
  special techniques, 334–337
  standard technique, 333
Radiological manifestations
  of abscess, pulmonary, 198
  of aneurysm, pulmonary arteriovenous, 224
  of asthma, bronchial, 182
  of atelectasis, 187
  of bronchial obstruction, 156
  of bronchiectasis, 178
  of bronchitis, chronic, 162
  of cysts of lung, 202
  of diaphragmatic disease, 277
  of edema, pulmonary, 229
  of embolism, pulmonary, 221
  of emphysema, chronic obstructive, 169
  of fibrosis of lung, 207
  of injuries of chest, 288
  of mediastinal air accumulation, 265
  of mediastinal tumors, 259
  of mediastinitis, acute, 262
    chronic fibrous, 263
  of pleural effusions, 238
  of pneumothorax, 246

Radiological manifestations (*cont.*)
  of pulmonary consolidation, 192
  of pulmonary hypertension, 215
  of vena caval obstruction, 256
Rales, 138–141
  assessment of, 324
  in abscess, pulmonary, 198
  in atelectasis, 187
  in bronchiectasis, 177
  in edema, pulmonary, 229
  in pulmonary consolidation, 192
  in pulmonary fibrosis, 141
  origin of, in relation to their temporal
    position, 139, 140
  pitch of, significance, 139, 324
  post-tussic, 140, 324
Reaction of solution, expressing, 63
Receptors, pulmonary, presso-, muscle and
  joint, and thermo-, influence on respiration, 79, 80
Reflex(es)
  cough, 93–96
  Hering-Brewer, 78
  pathological, and clubbing, 120
  sneeze, 90
Regulation of respiration, 68–86
Relaxation pressures, 16
  curve, 16, 17
Reserve volume, expiratory, 10
Residence, history of, 298
Residual capacity, functional, 10
Residual volume of lungs, 10
  measurement of, 362, 363
Resistance
  airway, 22
  elastic, 13
    assessment of, 363
  laminar, 22
  nonelastic, 21
    assessment of, 364
  turbulent, 23
  viscous, tissue, 23
Respiration. See also *Breathing.*
  Biot's, 86, 305
  Cheyne-Stokes, 84, 305
  factors influencing, 70–80
  regulation of, 68–86
    impaired, in emphysema, chronic ob-
      structive, 172
    in respiratory diseases, 82–86
Respiratory centers, 68–70
  factors acting directly on, 70–75

Respiratory centers, factors acting indirectly on, 75–80
Respiratory disease
  assessment of, 295–376
    clinical, 297–328
    clinical-pathological, 340–361
    functional, 362–376
    radiological, 329–339
  patterns of, 145–294
  regulation of ventilation in, 82
  signs of, 113–143
  symptoms of, 89–112
    constitutional, 109
Respiratory function of blood, 55–67
Respiratory insufficiency, 289–294
  cardiac insufficiency secondary to, 292–
    294
  secondary to cardiac insufficiency, 294
Respiratory muscles, diseases affecting,
  282
Respiratory pressures, 11
Respiratory tract
  defenses of, 91–96
  upper
    chronic infections of, and bronchi-
      ectasis, 176
    examination of, 305
    infections of, pneumonia and, 191
    protective function of, 89
    symptoms, taking history of, 303
Resting level, 8
Rhonchi, 137
  assessment of, 323, 324
  in bronchial obstruction, 155
  in bronchiectasis, 177
  in bronchitis, chronic, 162
  in emphysema, chronic obstructive, 168
  in fibrosis of lung, 206
  in pulmonary consolidation, 192
  medium-pitched, 138
  sibilant, 138
  sonorous, 138
Ribs
  as source of chest pain, 104
  motions of, during respiration, 5, 6
Rickettsial infection, diagnosis, 354
Rickettsial pneumonias, pulmonary consolidation in, 190
Roentgenological. See *Radiological.*
Root pain in chest, 105
Rub, pleural, 141
  assessment of, 325

SARCOIDOSIS, Nickerson-Kveim skin test
for, 357
Scalene muscles, action in respiration, 6, 8
Scalene node biopsy, 355
Scleroderma, chest symptoms in, due to
fibrosed skin, 280
Scoliosis, 113
as cause of cardiorespiratory disability,
283
examination for, 315
Secretions, abnormal, assessment of, 340–
345
Segments, bronchopulmonary, 147–151
Septum transversum, 269
Serological tests
in mycotic infections, 354
special, 359
Serotonin, effect on pulmonary circulation,
211
Shock in pulmonary embolism, 219
Signs of respiratory disease, 113–143
Skin
as source of chest pain, 104
examination of, 327
of chest, diseases affecting, 279
tests, 357–359
allergic, 358
Casoni, 358
fungus, 353
Nickerson-Kveim, 357
tuberculin, 348
Smear, stained, in diagnosis of tuberculous
infection, 347
Smoking, and chronic bronchitis, 161
Sneeze reflex, 90
Sniffing test for diaphragmatic paralysis,
278
Solution, reaction of, expressing, 63
Sounds, 131–143
adventitious, 137–141
assessment of, 323–325
breath, 135–137
amphoric, 198
assessment of, 323
bronchial, 137, 323
bronchovesicular, 137
in abscess, pulmonary, 198
in atelectasis, 187
in bronchiectasis, 177
in emphysema, chronic obstructive,
168
in fibrosis of lung, 206
in pleural effusion, 238

Sounds (cont.)
breath (cont.)
in pneumothorax, 245
in pulmonary consolidation, 192
vesicular, 136
heart, assessment of, 326
in chronic obstructive emphysema,
168
second pulmonic, in pulmonary hypertension, 142
intensity of, 133
percussion, in respiratory disease, 132
pitch of, 133
timbre of, 133
transmission of, alterations in, 133
vocal, 133
Spasmodic conditions affecting diaphragm, 275
Spine, thoracic, deformities of, 113
cardiorespiratory disability in, 283
Spinous processes of thoracic vertebrae,
examination of, 310
Splash, succussion, 141, 325
Sputum, 340
abnormal substances in, 342, 343
amount and character, significance of,
97
asbestos bodies in, 343
Ascaris lumbricoides in, 344
bloody, 97, 342
broncholiths in, 342
collection of, 340
by bronchoscopic aspiration, 341
by gastric aspiration, 341
color and consistency, 342
culture of, in nontuberculous infection,
349
in tuberculous infection, 349
Dittrich's plugs in, 342
Echinococcus granulosus in, 344
Endamoeba histolytica in, 344
examination of
bacteriological, 344
macroscopic, 341–343
microscopic, 343
expectoration of, 96, 97
in abscess, pulmonary, 197
in bronchiectasis, 175
in bronchitis, chronic, 161
in edema, pulmonary, 229
in embolism, pulmonary, 219
in emphysema, chronic obstructive, 167
in tumors of mediastinum, 258

Sputum (*cont.*)
  odor of, 342
  oil droplets in, 343
  tuberculous, bacteriological examination, 346
  volume of, 341
Staphylococcus infections, diagnosis of, 350
Status asthmaticus, 181
Stereoscopic films of chest, 335
Sternal angle, 310
Stomach
  dilatation of, in thoracic injuries, 287
  herniation of, mediastinal shift, 130, 131
Streptococcus, hemolytic, infections, diagnosis of, 350
Subcutaneous tissues
  air in, in thoracic injuries, 287
  of chest, diseases affecting, 279
Subdiaphragmatic abscess, 274
Subpleural blebs, 243
Succussion splash, 141, 325
  in pneumothorax, 245
Sulphur granules, 352
Surface anatomy of chest, 310–315
Sweat chlorides, test for, 358
Sweating in respiratory disease, 110
Sweats, night, 111
Symptoms of respiratory disease, 89–112
  constitutional, 109–112
Syncope
  in pulmonary embolism, 218
  in pulmonary hypertension, primary, 215
Syphilis, test for, 359

TACHYCARDIA
  and hypercapnia, 128
  and hypoxia, 124
  in pulmonary edema, 229
  in pulmonary infarction, 220
Tachypnea, 305
Tactile fremitus, 134, 320
Telangiectasis, cutaneous, pulmonary arteriovenous aneurysm and, 223
Tenderness at site of chest pain in pulmonary infarction, 220
Tension of gas, 37
Tension pneumothorax, 244, 286

Tests
  nonspecific, 359
  serological, for fungus infection, 354
  special, 359
  skin, 348, 353, 357–359. See also *Skin tests.*
  special, in blood, 359
Thermoreceptors, influence on respiration, 79
Thoracic duct, 251, 252
Thoracic vertebrae
  deformities of, 113
    cardiorespiratory disability in, 283
  spinous processes, examination of, 310
Thoraco-epigastric venous system, collateral, of mediastinum, 254
Thorax. See *Chest.*
Thrombophlebitis as source of pulmonary emboli, 216
Thrombosis, venous
  pulmonary embolism and, 216
  signs of, 220
Tidal volume, 9
Timbre of sound, 133
Tissue viscous resistance, 23
Tissues and systemic capillaries, gaseous exchange between, 56
Toes, clubbing of, 117, 307–309. See also *Clubbing of digits.*
Tomogram
  in abscess, pulmonary, 198
  in aneurysm, pulmonary arteriovenous, 225
  in asthma, bronchial, 182
  in emphysema, chronic obstructive, 170
Tomography, 335
  full chest, 335
Toxemia, clubbing and, 119
Trachea
  anatomy of, 147
  palpation of, for position of mediastinum, 316, 317
Tracheobronchial lymph nodes, 249, 255
Tracheobronchial tree
  as source of chest pain, 107
  change in size of, during respiration, 3
Transport
  of carbon dioxide, 59–63
  of oxygen, 55–59
Transverse fissure of lung, surface anatomy, 313
Trauma. See *Injuries.*

Tuberculin skin test, 348
Tuberculous infection, bacteriological diagnosis in, 346–349
Tumors of mediastinum, 257–259
  clinical manifestations, 257
  radiological manifestations, 259
Turbulent resistance, 23

URINE, examination of, 360

VAGUS nerves, role of, in bronchial asthma, 180
Vascular disease, pulmonary, 209–230
Vascular fibrosis, pulmonary, 205
Vascular resistance, pulmonary, alterations in, signs of, 142
  formula for determining, 213
Vasculature. See Blood vessels.
Vasoconstriction, pulmonary, 214
Veins
  collateral, in chest, significance of, 316
  dilatation of, in vena cava obstruction, 256
Vena azygos system, 251, 253
Vena cava, superior, obstruction of, 252–256
  clinical manifestations, 255
  in tumors of mediastinum, 257
  pathogenesis, 254
  radiological manifestations, 256
Venous admixture, true, 47
  assessment of, 373
  effects on gas exchange in lungs, 47–48
  in pneumothorax, 246
  in pulmonary arteriovenous aneurysm, 225
Venous admixture component of alveolar oxygen tension, 40
Venous-admixture-like perfusion, 45
  in pleural effusion, 240
  in pulmonary edema, 230
Venous systems, collateral, of mediastinum, 253
  azygos, 253
  internal mammary, 254
  thoraco-epigastric, 254
  vertebral, 254

Venous thrombosis
  pulmonary embolism and, 216
  signs of, 220
Ventilation
  alveolar, 41–44
    relation to mechanical work of breathing, 30
  collateral, 92
  dead-space-like, 46, 290
  minute, 10
  regulation of, 68–86
    in respiratory disease, 82–86
  uneven, tests for, 366
  voluntary, maximal, determination of, 366
Ventilation-perfusion ratios, 44–47
  altered, assessment of, 372
Ventilatory function, assessment of, 362–370
Ventricular failure secondary to respiratory failure, 292–294
Vertebrae, thoracic
  abnormalities of, 113
    chest deformities due to, 113
  spinous processes, examination of, 310
Vertebral venous system, collateral, of mediastinum, 254
Viral infections, diagnosis of, laboratory, 350
Viral pneumonias, pulmonary consolidation in, 189
Viscera, abdominal
  as source of chest pain, 109
  herniation of, 268–272
Vital capacity, 9
  determination of, 363
  timed, 365
Vocal fremitus, 133
  assessment of, 320
Vocal sounds, 133
Volumes, lung, 8–10
  alterations in, in chronic obstructive emphysema, 172
  assessment of, 362

WEAKNESS
  in pulmonary hypertension, primary, 215
  in respiratory disease, 111

Weight loss
  in emphysema, chronic obstructive, 167
  in respiratory disease, 111
  in tumors of mediastinum, 258
Wheezing
  in bronchial asthma, 181
  in bronchiectasis, 176
  in bronchitis, acute, 159
    chronic, 162
  in diaphragmatic disease, 276
  in edema, pulmonary, 228, 229
  in emphysema, chronic obstructive, 166
  in fibrosis of lung, 205

Whispering pectoriloquy, 177, 192, 238, 259, 321
Work of breathing, 27–32
  and control of respiration, 80–82
  mechanical, 27
    relation to alveolar ventilation, 30
    total, 27

X-RAY. See *Radiological.*

YEAST infections, diagnosis of, 352